CARDIOVASCULAR DISEASE IN THE ELDERLY

CONTEMPORARY CARDIOLOGY

CHRISTOPHER P. CANNON, MD
SERIES EDITOR

Cardiovascular Disease in the Elderly,
edited by *Gary Gerstenblith, MD,*
2005

Platelet Function: Assessment,
Diagnosis, and Treatment, edited
by *Martin Quinn, MB BCh BAO,*
PhD, and Desmond Fitzgerald,
MD, FRCPI, 2005

Diabetes and Cardiovascular Disease,
Second Edition, edited by
Michael T. Johnstone, MD, CM,
FRCP(C), and Aristidis Veves, MD,
DSC, 2005

Angiogenesis and Direct Myocardial
Revascularization,
edited by *Roger J. Laham, MD,*
and *Donald S. Baim, MD,* 2005

Interventional Cardiology:
Percutaneous Noncoronary
Intervention, edited by *Howard*
C. Herrmann, MD, 2005

Principles of Molecular Cardiology,
edited by *Marschall S. Runge,*
MD, and Cam Patterson, MD, 2005

Heart Disease Diagnosis and Therapy:
A Practical Approach, Second
Edition, M. Gabriel Khan, MD,
FRCP(LONDON), FRCP(C), FACC,
2005

Cardiovascular Genomics:
Gene Mining for Pharmaco-
genomics and Gene Therapy,
edited by *Mohan K. Raizada,*
PhD, Julian F. R. Paton, PhD,
Michael J. Katovich, PhD, and
Sergey Kasparov, MD, PhD, 2005

Surgical Management of Congestive
Heart Failure, edited by *James*
C. Fang, MD and Gregory S.
Couper, MD, 2005

Cardiopulmonary Resuscitation,
edited by *Joseph P. Ornato, MD,*
FAP, FACC and Mary Ann Peberdy,
MD, FACC, 2005

CT of the Heart: Principles
and Applications, edited by *U.*
Joseph Schoepf, MD, 2005

Heart Disease and Erectile
Dysfunction, edited by
Robert A. Kloner, MD, PhD, 2004

Cardiac Transplantation:
The Columbia University
Medical Center/New York-Pres-
byterian Hospital Manual, edited
by *Niloo M. Edwards, MD,*
Jonathan M. Chen, MD,
and *Pamela A. Mazzeo,* 2004

Coronary Disease in Women:
Evidence-Based Diagnosis
and Treatment, edited by *Leslee J.*
Shaw, PhD and Rita F. Redberg,
MD, FACC, 2004

Complementary and Alternative
Cardiovascular Medicine,
edited by *Richard A. Stein, MD*
and *Mehmet C. Oz, MD,* 2004

Nuclear Cardiology, The Basics:
How to Set Up and Maintain a
Laboratory, by *Frans J. Th.*
Wackers, MD, PhD, Wendy Bruni,
BS, CNMT, and Barry L. Zaret, MD,
2004

Minimally Invasive Cardiac Surgery,
Second Edition, edited by *Daniel*
J. Goldstein, MD, and Mehmet C.
Oz, MD 2004

Cardiovascular Health Care
Economics, edited by
William S. Weintraub, MD, 2003

Platelet Glycoprotein IIb/IIIa
Inhibitors in Cardiovascular
Disease, Second Edition, edited
by *A. Michael Lincoff, MD,* 2003

Heart Failure: A Clinician's Guide
to Ambulatory Diagnosis and
Treatment, edited by
Mariell L. Jessup, MD
and *Evan Loh, MD,* 2003

CARDIOVASCULAR DISEASE IN THE ELDERLY

Edited by

GARY GERSTENBLITH, MD

Johns Hopkins University School of Medicine
Baltimore, MD

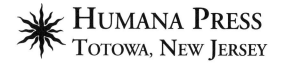

HUMANA PRESS
TOTOWA, NEW JERSEY

Production Editor: Robin B. Weisberg
Cover design by Patricia F. Cleary

This publication is printed on acid-free paper. ∞
ANSI Z39.48-1984 (American National Standards Institute) Permanence of Paper for Printed Library Materials.

Printed in the United States of America.   10 9 8 7 6 5 4 3 2 1

e-ISBN: 1-59259-941-9

Library of Congress Cataloging-in-Publication Data

Cardiovascular disease in the elderly / edited by Gary Gerstenblith.
       p. ; cm.
 Includes bibliographical references and index.
 ISBN 1-58829-282-7 (alk. paper)
 1. Geriatric cardiology.
 [DNLM: 1. Cardiovascular Diseases--physiopathology--Aged. 2.
Aging--physiology. 3. Cardiovascular Diseases--therapy--Aged. WG 120
C26733 2005] I. Gerstenblith, Gary.
  RC669.C2782 2005
  618.97'612--dc22   2005007405

PREFACE

The number of older individuals, and the proportion that they represent of the total population, are rapidly increasing. Even more striking is the high proportion the elderly represent of the patient population with cardiovascular disease (CVD). This is due in part to demographic trends, but also to more successful identification, prevention, and management strategies employed in the middle-aged population. As the number of older individuals and the multitude of new treatments for them continue to grow, health care providers are increasingly called on to make decisions as to whether or not to recommend these therapies. It is unclear, however, whether or not diagnostic and therapeutic interventions employed in the younger age groups can be extrapolated to the elderly because of differences in physiology, expected life span, complication rates, and increased co-morbidities.

Cardiovascular Disease in the Elderly is intended for physicians and other health care providers who care for older patients with or at risk for CVD. It reviews physiological changes associated with the normal aging process that increase the likelihood for the development of disease and for adverse consequences once disease develops, and which alter the benefit–risk equation for medical and other interventions designed to diagnose, assess, and treat CVD. This text discusses primary and secondary prevention strategies as well as the treatment of acute and chronic ischemic disease and complications. It focuses on presentations that are particularly common in the elderly as well, including cardiac failure with normal ejection fraction, isolated systolic hypertension, and atrial fibrillation, and has endeavored to take an evidenced-based approach to recommendations that rely heavily on prospective clinical trials. This text emphasizes new risk factors associated with age, including insulin resistance, and the value of lifestyle changes in the aging population. The chapters are written by leading experts in their fields who have studied extensively, and in many cases conducted, the studies on which current recommendations are based.

Gary Gerstenblith, MD

CONTENTS

CONTRIBUTORS

PHILIP A. ADES, MD, *Division of Cardiology, University of Vermont College of Medicine, Burlington VT*

JOSEPH S. ALPERT, MD, *Department of Medicine, University of Arizona College of Medicine, Tucson, AZ*

LOFTY L. BASTA, MD, FRCP, FACC, *Project GRACE, Clearwater, FL; Department of Medicine, University of South Florida College of Medicine, Tampa, FL*

WILLIAM A. BAUMGARTNER, MD, *Division of Cardiac Surgery, Johns Hopkins University School of Medicine, Baltimore, MD*

HUGH CALKINS, MD, *Division of Cardiology, Johns Hopkins University School of Medicine, Baltimore, MD*

CHRISTOPHER P. CANNON, MD, *Cardiovascular Division, Brigham and Women's Hospital and Harvard Medical School, Boston, MA*

MILIND Y. DESAI, MD, *Division of Cardiology, Johns Hopkins University School of Medicine, Baltimore, MD*

W. DANIEL DOTY, MD, FACC, FAHA, *Project GRACE, Clearwater, FL; Sacred Heart Regional Heart and Vascular Institute, Pensacola, FL*

MICHAEL D. D. GELDART, ESQ, *Project GRACE, Clearwater, FL*

GARY GERSTENBLITH, MD, *Division of Cardiology, Johns Hopkins University School of Medicine, Baltimore, MD*

WILLIAM RUSSELL HAZZARD, MD, *Division of Gerontology and Geriatric Medicine, University of Washington School of Medicine, VA Puget Sound Health Care System, Seattle, WA*

WILLIAM R. HIATT, MD, *Section of Vascular Medicine, University of Colorado Health Sciences Center and the Colorado Prevention Center, Divisions of Geriatrics and Cardiology, Denver, CO*

EDWARD G. LAKATTA, MD, *Gerontology Research Center, Intramural Research Program, National Institute on Aging, National Institutes of Health, Baltimore, MD*

BETH R. MALASKY, MD, *The Native American Cardiology Program, Sarver Heart Center, University of Arizona College of Medicine, Tucson, AZ*

MICHAEL J. MCWILLIAMS, MD, *Department of Cardiovascular Medicine, The Cleveland Clinic Foundation, Cleveland, OH*

EMILE R. MOHLER III, MD, *Cardiovascular Division, Department of Medicine, University of Pennsylvania School of Medicine, Philadelphia, PA*

SAMER S. NAJJAR, MD, *Gerontology Research Center, Intramural Research Program, National Institute on Aging, National Institutes of Health, Baltimore, MD*

JONATHAN P. PICCINI, MD, *Division of Cardiology, Johns Hopkins University School of Medicine, Baltimore, MD*

MICHAEL W. RICH, MD, *Cardiovascular Division, Washington University School of Medicine, St. Louis, MO*

STEVEN P. SCHULMAN, MD, *Division of Cardiology, Johns Hopkins University School of Medicine, Baltimore, MD*

JANICE B. SCHWARTZ, MD, *Department of Research, Jewish Home, San Francisco; Departments of Medicine, Cardiology, and Clinical Pharmacology, University of California, San Francisco School of Medicine, San Francisco, CA*

ERIC J. TOPOL, MD, *Department of Cardiovascular Medicine, The Cleveland Clinic Foundation, Cleveland, OH*

STEPHEN D. WIVIOTT, MD, *Cardiovascular Division, Brigham and Women's Hospital and Harvard Medical School, Boston, MA*

DAVID D. YUH, MD, *Division of Cardiac Surgery, Johns Hopkins University School of Medicine, Baltimore, MD*

SUSAN J. ZIEMAN, MD, *Division of Cardiology, Johns Hopkins University School of Medicine, Baltimore, MD*

1

Aging of the Heart and Arteries
Relevance to Cardiovascular Disease

Samer S. Najjar, MD
and Edward G. Lakatta, MD

INTRODUCTION

The world population in both industrialized and developing countries is aging. For example, in the United States, 35 million people are over the age of 65 years, and the number of older Americans is expected to double by the year 2030. The clinical and economic implications of this demographic shift are staggering because age is the most powerful risk factor for cardiovascular diseases (CVDs). The incidence and prevalence of hypertension, coronary artery disease (CAD), congestive heart failure, and

From: *Contemporary Cardiology: Cardiovascular Disease in the Elderly*
Edited by: G. Gerstenblith © Humana Press Inc., Totowa, NJ

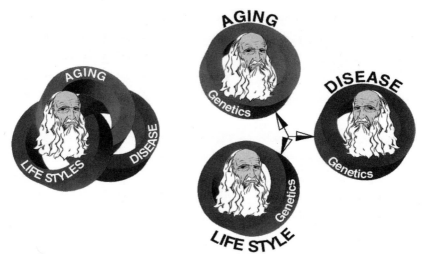

Fig. 1. The interaction of age, disease, lifestyle and genetics determines cardiovascular structure and function. The Baltimore Longitudinal Study of Aging continues to make a sustained effort to study these components and their interactions.

stroke, the quintessential diseases of Western society, increase exponentially with age. Although epidemiological studies have discovered that some aspects of lifestyle and genetics are risk factors for these diseases, age, *per se*, confers the major risk. Thus, it is reasonable to hypothesize that specific pathophysiological mechanisms that underlie these diseases become superimposed on cardiac and vascular substrates that have been modified by an "aging process," and that the latter modulates disease occurrence and severity. In other words, age-associated changes in cardiovascular structure and function become "partners" with pathophysiological disease mechanisms, lifestyle, and genetics in determining the threshold, severity, and prognosis of CVD occurrence in older persons (Fig. 1).

The nature of age–disease interactions is complex and involves mechanisms of aging, multiple defined disease risk factors, and as yet undefined risk factors (e.g., those that may have a genetic basis). The role of specific age-associated changes in cardiovascular structure and function in such age–disease interactions has formerly been, and largely continues to be, unrecognized by those who shape medical policy. Thus, specific aspects of cardiovascular aging have remained largely outside the bailiwick of clinical cardiology, and until recently, have not been considered in most epidemiological studies of CVD.

Quantitative information on age-associated alterations in cardiovascular structure and function in health is essential to unravel age–disease interactions and to target the specific characteristics of cardiovascular aging that render it such a major risk factor for CVDs. Such information is also of practical value because it is required to differentiate between the limitations of an older person that relate to disease, and those that might be expected, within limits, to accompany advancing age or a sedentary lifestyle.

SUCCESSFUL VS UNSUCCESSFUL CARDIOVASCULAR AGING

To define why age (or an aging process × exposure-time interaction) is so risky, the specific components of the risk associated with age must be identified. Two complimentary approaches have evolved. On the one hand, epidemiologists are searching for novel measures of "subclinical disease" (in addition to the more established risk factors that have already been well characterized) in large, unselected study cohorts composed of persons both with and without CVD. In contrast, gerontologists are attempting to develop quantitative information on cardiovascular structure and function in apparently healthy individuals to define and target the specific characteristics of aging that render it such a major risk factor for CVD, even in the absence of clinically apparent co-morbidity. The latter approach consists of identifying and selecting community-dwelling individuals who have not yet experienced clinical disease and who do not have occult disease that can be detected by noninvasive methods. These individuals are then grouped by age and stratified according to the level of a given variable, which may include some of the novel measures of subclinical disease identified by the epidemiologists. If the variable is perceived as beneficial or deleterious with respect to cardiovascular structure or function, those with extreme measures are considered to be aging "successfully" or "unsuccessfully," respectively. "Unsuccessful" aging in this context is not synonymous with having clinical disease, as individuals with defined overt or occult clinical disease have been excluded from consideration *a priori*. Instead, unsuccessful aging, that is, falling within the poorest category with respect to the measure viewed as deleterious, may be viewed as a risk factor for future clinical CVD. In this regard, unsuccessful aging is a manifestation of the interaction of the cardiovascular aging process and specific aspects of vascular disease pathophysiology. Thus, gerontologists and epidemiologists have become part of a joint effort in the quest to define why aging confers such an enormous risk for CVD.

AGE-ASSOCIATED CHANGES
IN HEART STRUCTURE AND FUNCTION
IN APPARENT HEALTH AT REST AND IN RESPONSE
TO INCREASED DEMAND FOR BLOOD FLOW

During the past two decades, a sustained effort has been ongoing to characterize the effects of aging on multiple aspects of cardiovascular structure and function in a single study population in the Baltimore Longitudinal Study of Aging (BLSA) (1). These community-dwelling volunteers are rigorously screened to detect both clinical and occult CVD and are characterized with respect to lifestyle (e.g., diet and exercise habits) in an attempt to identify and clarify the interactions among these factors and those changes that result from aging (1).

The most notable impact of aging on the cardiovascular system is on cardiovascular reserve utilized in response to demands that go beyond those of the resting state, i.e., in response to acute physical stress, or in response to the chronic stress of pathophysiological mechanisms that underlie CVDs.

In the basal state, only a fraction of the maximum cardiovascular function is utilized. During stress (e.g., dynamic exercise), cardiovascular reserve functions become engaged: a substantial volume of blood is shifted from the venous system, where most blood resides at rest, to the arterial system, increasing the rate of blood flow returning to the heart; and the rate at which blood is pumped by the heart acutely increases owing to both faster and stronger beating, mediated, in a large measure, by signaling via the autonomic nervous system. Released neurotransmitters, norepinephrine (NE) and epinephrine, bind to β-adrenergic receptors (β-AR) on pacemaker cells comprising the sinoatrial node, and to β-ARs on myocytes to modulate cellular mechanisms that govern the frequency and amplitude, respectively, of the duty cycles of these cells. The net result is an increase in heart rate (HR), stroke volume (SV), and ejection fraction (EF).

The acute reserve capacity of specific cardiac functions that determine overall cardiac performance can be conveniently illustrated by depicting these over a wide range of demand for blood flow and pressure regulation, e.g., assumption of the sitting posture and during submaximal and exhaustive (maximal) upright exercise (Fig. 2).

Fig. 2. Least-squares linear regression on age of left ventricular volumes, heart rate (HR), and cardiac index (CI), at rest and during graded cycle exercise in 149 healthy males from the Baltimore Longitudinal Study of Aging (BLSA), who (a) had a resting brachial blood pressure of less than160/90 mmHg; (b) had no evidence of silent ischemia by electrocardiogram or thallium scan during a prior maximal stress test; and (c) exercised to at least a 100-W workload. The asterisk (*)

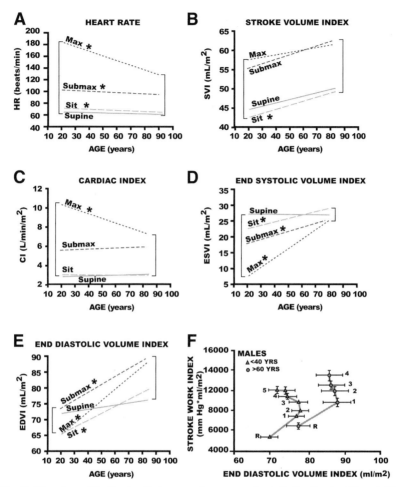

Fig. 2. *(Continued)* indicates that regression on age is statistically significant. The overall magnitude of the acute, dynamic range of reserve of a given function in younger compared with older subjects can quickly be gleaned from the length of the brackets depicted at the extremes of the regression lines *(1)*. (**A**) The maximum acute dynamic reserve range of HR is reduced by about one-third between 20 and 85 years of age. (**B**) The stroke volume index (SVI)is preserved in older persons over a wide range of performance. (**C**) The loss of acute cardiac output reserve from seated rest to exhaustive, seated cycle exercise averages about 30% in healthy, community-dwelling BLSA volunteer men. This reduction is entirely due to a reduction in HR reserve, as SVI at maximum exercise is preserved. (**D**) There is a remarkable age-associated reduction in the range of reserve in the end-systolic volume index (ESVI). (**E**) For end-diastolic volume index (EDVI), the average, acute, dynamic EDV reserve range during the postural change and during graded upright exercise is moderately greater at 85 than at 20 years. (**F**) Stroke work index (SVI × brachial blood pressure) as a function of EDVI at rest and throughout graded exercise.

Heart Rate, Cardiac Volumes, and Cardiac Index
at Rest and During Graded Exercise to Exhaustion

In the supine position at rest, the HR in healthy BLSA men is not age-related (Fig. 2A). In other populations, a reduction in the spontaneous and respiratory variations in resting HR is observed and reflects altered autonomic modulation with aging (*see* section on impaired responses to β-adrenergic receptor stimulation). With assumption of the seated resting position, HR increases slightly less in older than in younger men. The magnitude of this age-associated reduction increases progressively during exercise. The net result is that maximum acute dynamic reserve range of HR is reduced by about one-third between 20 and 85 years of age.

The maximum SV indexed (SVI) to body surface area does not decline with age in carefully screened individuals (Fig 2B). It is the reduction in the HR response to exercise, then, that underlies the maximum acute cardiac output reserve in healthy BLSA volunteers, which decreases, on average, by about 30% between ages 20 and 85 years (Fig 2C). Thus, healthy individuals at the older end of the age range can augment their cardiac index (CI) about 2.5-fold over that at seated rest, whereas those at the younger end of the age spectrum can increase their CI about 3.5-fold. As the age-associated decline in peak oxygen consumption during these studies averages about 50%, deficits in O_2 extraction from the blood associated with aging occur in this population, and average about 20% (1).

If our queries of age-associated changes in heart reserve function were to have ended here, a most remarkable pattern of adaptation utilized to maintain the SV in older persons during stress would have gone undetected. Actually, the older heart fails to empty as well as the younger heart. Figure 2D illustrates a remarkable age-associated reduction in the range of reserve of the end-systolic volume index (ESVI): in younger men, the ESVI becomes progressively reduced with increasing demands for cardiovascular perfusion from supine rest to maximum upright exercise, but the range of acute ESVI reserve at age 85 is only about one-fifth of that at age 20.

In addition to impaired ejection, the left ventricle (LV) also exhibits filling impairments with aging. The early diastolic filling rate progressively slows after the age of 20 years, so that, by 80 years, the rate is reduced up to 50% (Fig. 3A). This reduction in filling rate is likely attributable either to structural (fibrous) changes within the LV myocardium or to residual myofilament Ca^{2+} activation from the preceding systole. More filling occurs in late diastole, owing, in part, to a more vigorous atrial contraction. Hence, the ratio of early to late LV filling decreases with age (Fig. 3B). The augmented atrial contraction is accompanied by

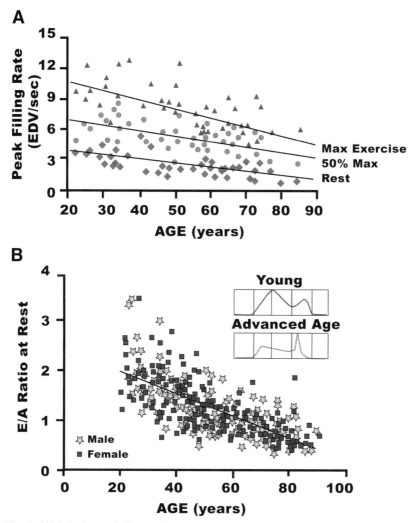

Fig. 3. (**A**) Maximum left ventricular (LV) filling rate at rest and during vigorous cycle exercise, assessed via equilibrium gated blood-pool scans in healthy volunteers from the Baltimore Longitudinal Study of Aging (BLSA) prescreened for study as in Fig. 2. EDV, end-diastolic volume. (**B**) The ratio of early LV diastolic filling rate (E) to the atrial filling component (A) declines with aging in healthy BLSA volunteers prescreened for study as in Fig. 2. (A and B from ref. *160*.)

atrial enlargement and can be manifested on auscultation as a fourth heart sound (atrial gallop).

Despite the altered LV filling pattern, in the supine position end-diastolic volume index (EDVI) is greater in older vs younger men (Fig. 2E).

Assumption of the sitting from the supine position reduces EDVI to a greater extent in younger, than in older individuals (Fig. 2E). During submaximal cycle-seated exercise EDVI increases equivalently at all ages, owing to the acute increase in venous return to the heart (Fig. 2E,F). But during increasingly vigorous exercise, EDVI progressively drops to the seated rest level in young men but remains elevated in older men (Fig. 2E, F). Thus, for EDVI, the average, acute, EDV utilization range from supine to the sitting state through graded upright exercise is moderately greater at 85 than at 20 years. Regardless of age, the normal response to an acute increase in venous return to the heart during submaximal exercise is an increase in LV EDV, but in younger persons as the exercise time or workload intensify, the HR increase and ESV reduction permit the EDVI to return to about the resting level (Fig. 2E,F). The persistent increase in LV EDVI in older vs younger persons during vigorous exercise is due both to a failure of the LV to empty as completely, and to an increase in the filling time that accompanies a slower HR. In other words, persistent LV dilation at end diastole during vigorous exertion in older persons is linked to mechanisms that underlie the deficits in the regulation of both maximum HR, LV contractility, and afterload (*see* section on LV afterload).

The net result of the age-associated changes in EDVI and ESVI regulation depicted in Fig. 2, preserves the SVI (Fig. 2B) and stroke work (Fig. 2F) in older persons at that level achieved by younger persons over a wide range of performance. In fact, the Frank-Starling mechanism is utilized in older men in an upright, seated posture at rest (Fig. 2E) to produce a modest age-associated increase in SVI (Fig. 2B). During progressive exhaustive exercise, however, the failure of older men to reduce ESVI (Fig. 2D) prevents their SVI and stroke work index (Fig. 2F) from remaining higher than younger men, as would be anticipated on the basis of their augmented EDVI. In other words, although healthy older persons utilize the Frank-Starling mechanism throughout upright, graded exercise, this mechanism is impaired during vigorous exercise because of factors that impair LV ejection.

AGE–GENDER INTERACTIONS

The patterns of hemodynamic reserve function measured across the range of demands as illustrated in Fig. 2 for males are nearly identical in females *(1)*. Exceptions are that, at seated rest, females do not exhibit a modest age-associated increase in EDVI because, unlike males, assumption of the upright posture does not produce a greater reduction in EDVI in younger than in older women. Owing to the absence of an age-associated increase in EDVI in women in the seated position, the SVI does not increase with age at seated rest, and, in contrast to males, the calculated

CI at seated rest decreases modestly with age in women. At maximum exercise, the age-associated increase of EDVI is of borderline statistical significance in women. However, the change in EDVI from rest to exercise varies with the intensity of exercise, and within given individuals significantly increases with age, in both men and women (1). The age-associated changes in diastolic function do not exhibit prominent gender differences (Fig 3).

In summary, Fig. 2 illustrates that when basal and reserve cardiovascular function in adult volunteer community-dwelling subjects ranging in age from 20 to 85 years are compared, impaired cardio-acceleration and LV ejection reserve capacity are the most dramatic changes in cardiac function with aging in health. Impaired ejection reserve during graded upright exercise, indicated by the failure of older persons to regulate ESV (Fig. 2D) as effectively as younger ones do, is accompanied by LV dilation at end diastole (Fig. 2E,F) and an altered diastolic filling pattern (Fig. 3A).

AGE–DISEASE INTERACTIONS FURTHER IMPAIR LV EJECTION RESERVE CAPACITY IN OLDER PERSONS

In older BLSA persons with asymptomatic coronary disease, but with both electrocardiographic and thallium scintigraphic evidence of ischemia during vigorous exercise (2), the LV EDVI increase at maximum exercise is greater than that in healthy age-matched subjects, as is the increase in LV ESVI (3) (Fig. 4). The SVI during vigorous exercise in these persons with asymptomatic coronary disease is preserved at the expense of EF (cf. Fig. 9). Note that these differences among the age groups or between these older persons with silent coronary disease and those without disease are not evident at rest.

Cardiac Function During Prolonged Submaximal Exercise

Traditional laboratory assessment of cardiovascular exercise performance as depicted in Figs. 2, 3A, and 4 involves maximal graded exercise protocols of 8 to 12 minutes in total duration. Although such protocols provide useful insight into the maximum capacity of an individual to augment cardiac function and the mechanisms involved in this process, their relevance is not directly applicable to the usual aerobic activities of everyday living, which are typically submaximal, but sustained for longer time periods. Classical exercise recommended cardiovascular conditioning regimens, for example, consist of no less than 20 minutes of exercise at a work level between 50% and 70% of maximal oxygen consumption (VO_2max).

Prolonged submaximal cycle exercise at 70% of peak-cycle exercise VO_2 for up to 2 hours in a thermoneutral environment elicits a progres-

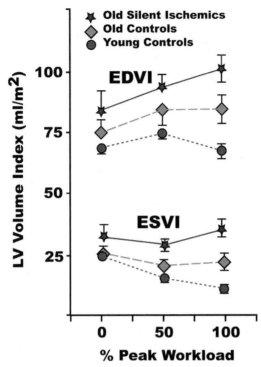

Fig. 4. Left ventricular (LV) volumes as function of relative workload in young and older, healthy subjects prescreened for study as in Fig. 2 and in older subjects with silent ischemia. Values are mean ± SE. Both end-diastolic volume index (EDVI) and end-systolic volume index (ESVI) were similar at rest among groups and diverged progressively with exercise, indicating differing rates of volume change with increasing relative work loads *(3)*.

sive increase in cardiac performance throughout exercise *(4)*. Older, healthy BLSA volunteers demonstrate a lesser augmentation of HR and systolic LV ejection between 10 minutes and exercise termination than younger ones (Fig. 5), analogous to findings during the traditional graded maximal exercise protocol in Fig. 2.

Heterogeneity of Cardiac Performance Measures Among Older Persons

Although the format of characterizing average age-associated changes in various facets of cardiac function across a graded range of demands as in Figs. 2, 3A, 4, and 5 is instructive, it does not portray variations among individuals. For many functions, the variation about the mean increases

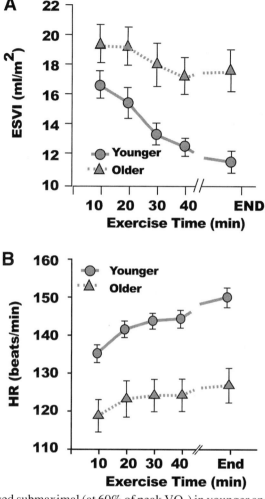

Fig. 5. Prolonged submaximal (at 60% of peak VO_2) in younger and older Baltimore Longitudinal Study of Aging subjects. (A) End-systolic volume index (ESVI) declines between 10 and 40 minutes in both groups, though to a greater extent in younger subjects (3). (B) An increase in heart rate occurs with time in each age group but this increase is less in older vs younger subjects.

with aging. Increased heterogeneity among older persons in the ability of the heart to beat faster and stronger during vigorous exercise is illustrated in Fig. 6. Note that some older individuals have a maximum HR and ESV at maximum exhaustive exercise that are equivalent to their younger counterparts, whereas other older individuals exhibit marked

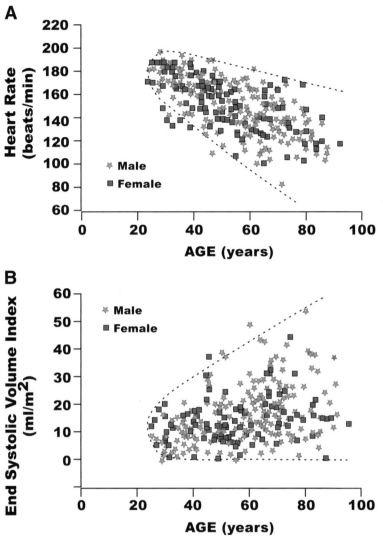

Fig. 6. Scatter plots of (**A**) heart rate and (**B**) end-systolic volume index in healthy sedentary men from the Baltimore Longitudinal Study of Aging (BLSA) depicted in Fig. 2 and for 113 BLSA women who exercised to a 75-W workload, prescreened for study as in Fig. 2. Note the increased heterogeneity among individuals at older age *(1)*.

compromises. The former individuals might be described as having aged "successfully" with respect to these functions, whereas the latter might be described as having aged "unsuccessfully." Those who age "unsuccessfully" with respect to cardiac structure and reserve function and vascular structure and function are at increased risk for clinical manifestations of the occurrence of CVD and for the severity and adverse prognosis of these diseases (*see* section on age-associated changes in vascular structure and function).

Impaired Responses to β-Adrenergic Receptor Stimulation

The essence of sympathetic modulation of the cardiovascular system is to ensure that the heart beats faster; to ensure that it retains a small size, by reducing the diastolic filling period, reducing LV afterload, and augmenting myocardial contractility and relaxation; and to redistribute blood to working muscles, and to skin so as to dissipate heat. Each of the deficient components of cardiovascular regulation with aging, i.e., HR (and thus filling time), afterload (both cardiac and vascular), myocardial contractility, and redistribution of blood flow exhibits a deficient sympathetic modulation.

Multiple lines of evidence support the idea that the efficiency of postsynaptic β-adrenergic signaling declines with aging (*see* ref. 5 for review). One line of evidence stems from the observations that cardiovascular responses at rest to β-adrenergic agonist infusions decrease with age (*see* ref. 5 for review). A second type of evidence for a diminished efficacy of synaptic β-AR signaling is that acute β-AR blockade changes the exercise hemodynamic profile of younger persons to resemble that of older individuals. Significant β-blockade-induced LV dilatation occurs only in younger subjects (Fig. 7A); the HR reduction during exercise in the presence of acute β-adrenergic blockade is greater in younger vs older subjects (Fig. 7B) as are the age-associated deficits in LV early diastolic filling rate, both at rest and during exercise (Fig. 7C). It has also been observed in older dogs, that the age-associated increase in impedance during exercise is also abolished by acute β-adrenergic blockade (6).

Apparent deficits in sympathetic modulation of cardiac and arterial functions with aging occur in the presence of exaggerated neurotransmitter levels. Plasma levels of norepinephrine (NE) and epinephrine, during any perturbation from the supine basal state, increase to a greater extent in older compared with younger healthy humans (*see* ref. 7 for review). The age-associated increase in plasma levels of NE results from an increased spillover into the circulation and, to a lesser extent, to reduced plasma clearance. The degree of NE spillover into the circulation differs among body organs; increased spillover occurs within the heart (8). Deficient NE re-uptake at nerve endings is a primary mechanism for increased spillover during acute graded exercise as in Fig. 2. During prolonged exercise, as in Fig. 5, however, diminished neurotransmitter re-uptake might also be associated with depletion and reduced release and spillover (9).

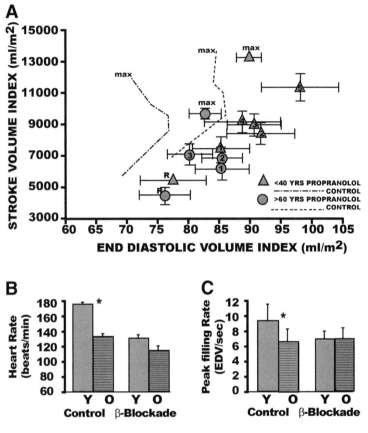

Fig. 7. **(A)** Stroke volume index (SVI) as a function of end-diastolic volume index (EDVI) at rest (R) and during graded cycle workloads in the upright seated position in healthy Baltimore Longitudinal Study of Aging (BLSA) men in the presence and absence (dashed lines) of β-adrenergic blockade. R, seated rest; 1–4 or 5, graded submaximal workloads on cycle ergometer; max, maximum effort. Stroke volume vs end-diastolic functions with symbols are those measured in the presence of propranolol; dashed line functions without symbols are the stroke volume vs end-diastolic functions measured in the absence of propranolol. Note that in the absence of propranolol the SVI vs EDVI relation in older persons (dashed lines) is shifted rightward from that in younger ones (dashed lines with points). This indicates that the left ventricle (LV) of older persons in the sitting position compared to that of younger ones operates from a greater preload both at rest and during submaximal and max exercise. Propranolol markedly shifts the SV–EDV relationship in younger persons (▲ without points) rightward, but does not markedly offset the curve in older persons (●). Thus, with respect to this assessment of ventricular function curve, β-adrenergic blockade with propranolol makes younger men appear like older ones. The abolition of the age associated differences in the LV function curve after propranolol are accompanied by a reduction or abolition of the age-associated reduction in heart rate, which, at max, is shown in B. Note, however, that

The well-documented age-associated reduction in the postsynaptic response of myocardial cells to β-AR stimulation appears to be the result of multiple changes in the molecular and biochemical steps that couple the receptor to postreceptor effectors. However, the major limiting modification of this signaling pathway with advancing age in rodents appears to be at the coupling of the β-AR to adenylyl cyclase via the G_s protein, and to changes in adenylyl cyclase protein, leading to a reduction in the ability to sufficiently augment cell cyclic adenosine monophosphate and to activate protein kinase A to drive the phosphorlyation of key proteins that are required to augment cardiac contractility. In contrast, the apparent desensitization of β-AR signaling with aging does not appear to be mediated via increased β-adrenergic receptor kinase (β-ARK) or increased G_i activity.

Left-Ventricular Afterload, Arterial-Ventricular Load Matching, and Ejection Fraction

AFTERLOAD

Cardiac afterload results from factors that inhibit myocardial displacement and the ejection of blood during systole and has two major components, one generated by the heart itself, and the other by the vasculature. The cardiac component of afterload during exercise can be expected to increase slightly with age because heart size increases in older persons throughout the cardiac cycle *(1)* (Fig. 2). The vascular load on the heart has four components: conduit artery compliance characteristics, reflected pulse waves, inertance, and resistance (Fig. 8). Studies in large populations of broad age range demonstrate that arterial pressure, a major factor of vascular loading, is a major determinant of LV mass. Thus, the relative impact of age on LV wall thickness varies with the manner in which study subjects are screened with respect to hypertension *(10)*. There is

---

Fig. 7. *(Continued)* β-adrenergic blockade in younger individuals in (A) causes SVI to increase to a greater extent than during β-blockade in older ones, suggesting that mechanisms other than deficient β-adrenergic regulation compromises LV ejection. One potential mechanism is an age-associated decrease in maximum intrinsic myocardial contractility. Another likely mechanism is enhanced vascular afterload, owing to the structural changes in compliance arteries noted above, and possibly also to impaired vasorelaxation during exercise. (From ref. *161.)* (B) Peak exercise heart rate in the same subjects as in A in the presence and absence of acute β-adrenergic blockade by propranolol. (C) The age associated reduction in peak LV diastolic filling rate at max exercise in healthy BLSA subjects is abolished during exercise in the presence of β-adrenergic blockade with propranolol. Y, <40 years; O, >60 years *(14)*. (From ref. *160.*)

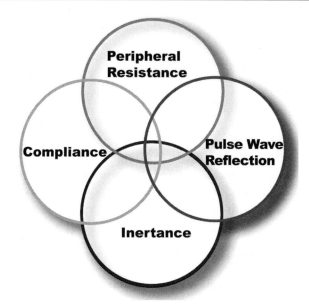

Fig. 8. Components of arterial afterload on the left ventricle.

considerable evidence to indicate that during aging the vascular load on the LV increases with age, and that this is a likely cause of an increase in LV wall thickness that occurs with aging in both men and women (Fig. 9). The increase in LV wall thickness with aging likely reduces the expected increase in cardiac afterload owing to increased LV volume in older persons during exercise stress *(1)*.

ARTERIAL-VENTRICULAR LOAD MATCHING

Optimal and efficient ejection of blood from the heart occurs when ventricular and vascular energies or loads are matched. Effective arterial elastance (EaI) is a steady-state arterial measure that characterizes the functional properties of the arterial system on the basis of SVI and central end-systolic pressure. Characterization of the functional properties of LV elastance ($E_{LV}I$) incorporates the end-systolic pressure and EDVI. EaI and $E_{LV}I$ share common units, and their ratio (EaI/$E_{LV}I$), an index of atrioventricular (A-V) coupling *(11)*, is mathematically related to EF *(12)*: $Ea/E_{LV} = (1/EF-1)$. Thus, although EF is often considered an important clinical index of LV systolic function, it is not exclusively governed by LV properties. Rather, EF is determined by the coupling of arterial and ventricular loads *(11,13,14)*.

At rest, the noninvasively determined resting ventricular–vascular coupling index, EaI/$E_{LV}I$ averages 0.5 to 0.6 and does not vary with age

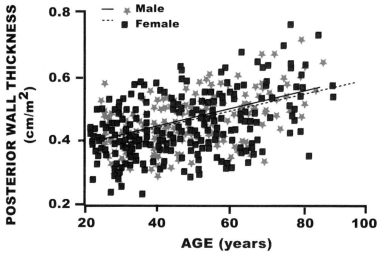

Fig. 9. Left ventricular (LV) posterior wall thickness, measured by M-mode echocardiography, increases with age in healthy Baltimore Longitudinal Study of Aging (BLSA) men and women and who had a brachial blood pressure of <160/90 mmHg. Note that the marked age-associated increase in LV wall thickness in these healthy BLSA participants is within what is considered to be the clinically "normal" range (16).

in young and old men and women of the BLSA, in whom basal brachial blood pressure (BP) is less than 140/90 mmHg (Fig. 10A), and is similar to that measured invasively in other studies. This value of Ea/E$_{LV}$ is that at which the work efficiency of the heart is maximal (5,15) and its similarity in older and younger persons suggests that LV work efficiency at rest does not vary appreciably with aging. As expected, the normal EF at rest averages about 65%, and does not differ with age (Fig. 10B). Thus, a resting EF of 50% in patients with heart failure, particularly "diastolic heart failure" should not be accepted as normal regardless of age.

Important age differences in EaI/E$_{LV}$I are observed during graded cycle exercise (Fig. 10A). In both men and women, younger subjects had greater declines in EaI/E$_{LV}$I, i.e., had better coupling, from rest to maximal workload compared to older subjects (69% and 62% vs 38% and 35% for young men and women, respectively). Thus, although in the resting state, A-V coupling is maintained in a range that maximizes the efficiency of the heart, during stress energetic efficiency is sacrificed in favor of cardiac efficacy, manifest by a decrease in the coupling index (i.e., a greater relative increase in ventricular contractility than arterial load); and aging is associated with the inability to attain maximal efficacy, manifest by a lesser reduction in the coupling index. As expected from the

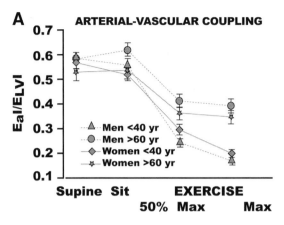

A ARTERIAL-VASCULAR COUPLING

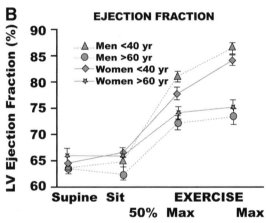

B EJECTION FRACTION

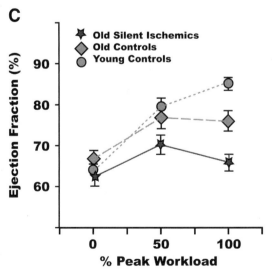

C

age-associated reduction in EaI/E_{LV}I during exercise, the increase in EF during exercise is reduced in older persons *(1,5)* (Fig. 10B).

Interestingly, men and women display mechanistic differences in their predisposition for the age associated suboptimal A-V coupling efficiency during exercise. Indeed, in the healthy BLSA cohort, exercise E_{LV}I is higher in younger compared to older men, but in women this age difference is less impressive. In contrast, exercise EaI is higher in older compared to younger women, but no age differences are observed in men. In other words, gender differences in younger persons in E_{LV}I and EaI during exercise become blunted with aging.

Because the LVEF encompasses a dynamic range, characterization of EF in the context of heart failure should employ stress to determine the EF reserve, and thus, the A-V coupling reserve, with respect to diagnosis and treatment. Moreover, because EF is not solely determined by the heart, but by both Ea and $E_{LV,}$ both of these parameters need to be assessed in order to interpret the meaning of an EF value, particularly in a nondilated heart, with respect to the presence or severity of heart failure. In other words, an apparently normal EF could result from normal, enhanced or reduced ventricular elastance, coupled to normal, increased or reduced arterial elastance. Figure 10C shows that the age-associated EF impairment during exercise, and therefore the impairment in A-V coupling reserve, is more pronounced in older persons with silent ischemia.

AGE-ASSOCIATED CHANGES IN VASCULAR STRUCTURE AND FUNCTION

As noted earlier, advancing age is the most powerful predictor of cardiovascular morbidity, mortality, and disability. Age has traditionally been ignored as a risk factor for CVD because it is considered a nonmodifiable risk. However, close examination of the age-associated changes in vascular structure and function may help explain why aging is such a strong predictor of adverse events. Findings from recent clinical studies have

---

Fig. 10. *(Opposite page)* Rest and exercise of EaI/E_{LV}I (**A**) and ejection fraction (EF) (**B**) in men ($\triangle$) and women ($\Diamond$) <40 years of age, and in men (O) and women ($\star$) >60 years of age who had a resting brachial blood pressure <140/90 mmHg. EF increases with exercise in both age groups and genders. In both men and women, there is a greater increase in EF at maximal exercise in younger compared to older subjects. EaI/E_{LV}I decreases with exercise in both age groups and genders. In both men and women, there is a greater decrease in EaI/E_{LV}I at maximal exercise in younger men and women compared to older ones. (From ref. *162*.) (**C**) EF is similar among younger and older healthy subjects and older subjects with silent ischemia at rest but diverges progressively with increasing effort *(3)*.

Table 1
Age-Associated Changes
in Human Arterial Structure and Function

Increases with age
    Lumen size
    Intimal-medial thickness
    Collagen content and cross-linking
    Vessel wall stiffness
    Systolic blood pressure
    Pulse pressure
    Elastin fragmentation
Decreases with age
    Elastin content
    Endothelial function

show that the age-associated changes in vascular structure and function, previously not defined as clinical or subclinical diseases, are themselves risk factors for CVDs. These novel risk factors, including intimal-medial thickness (IMT), vascular stiffness, and endothelial dysfunction, alter the substrate on which the CVDs are superimposed; therefore, they affect the development, manifestation, severity, and prognosis of these diseases.

Many age-associated changes are seen in the large arteries of humans (Table 1). Cross-sectional studies show that central elastic arteries dilate with age, leading to an increase in lumen size *(16)*, which results in an increased inertance (Fig. 8). In addition, postmortem studies have indicated an age-associated increase in arterial wall thickening, which is caused mainly by an increase in intimal thickening *(17)*. In cross-sectional studies, carotid IMT increases nearly threefold between the ages of 20 and 90 years *(18)* (Fig. 11A). The range of values for IMT in Fig. 11A is much greater in older individuals than in younger ones. The increase in arterial wall thickening is accompanied by an increase in vascular stiffening

Fig. 11. *(Opposite page)* Age-associated changes in vascular structure and function in humans. (**A**) The common carotid intimal-medial thickness (IMT) in healthy Baltimore Longitudinal Study of Aging (BLSA) volunteer subjects, as a function of age and gender. Note that the values for IMT are much greater in older individuals than in younger ones. (**B**) Aortic pulse wave velocity (PWV) in healthy BLSA volunteer subjects, as a function of age and gender. PWV is an index of arterial stiffness. (**C**) Endothelial flow-mediated and nonendothelial (glyceryl trinitrate)-induced arterial dilatation in apparently healthy individuals. Note that the marked age-associated accelerated decline in endothelial-mediated dilatation occurs about a decade later in women than in men. (Reprinted with permission from ref. *21*.)

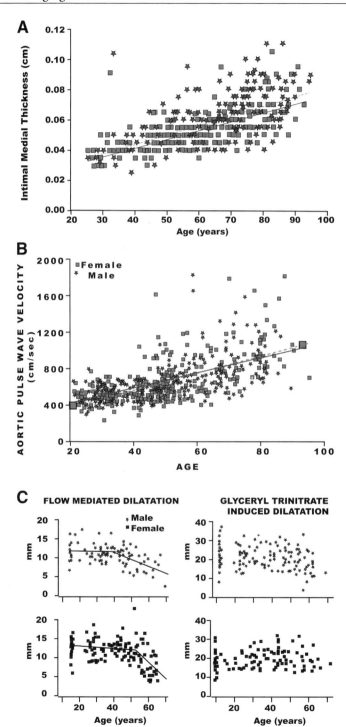

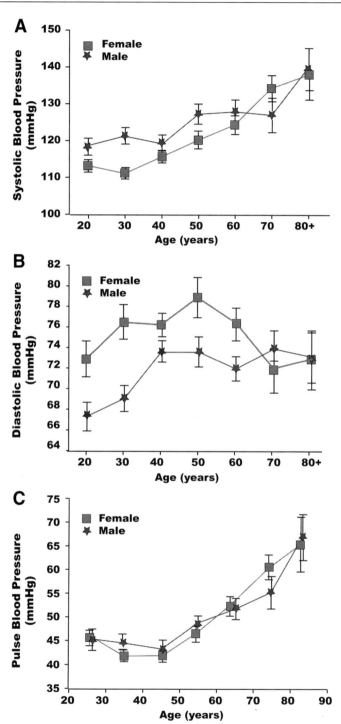

(reduction in vascular compliance) *(19)* (Fig. 11B), which is the result of several structural changes in the arterial wall *(5)*. These changes include an increase in collagen content, cross-linking of adjacent collagen molecules to form advanced glycosylation end products *(20)*, fraying of elastin, and a decrease in the amount of elastin. In addition to structural changes, functional alterations include an age-associated decline in vascular endothelial vasoreactivity *(21,22)* (Fig. 11C).

Blood Pressure

Both systolic and pulse pressures increase with age in all adults, whereas diastolic blood pressure (DBP) increases until the fifth decade and then levels off before decreasing after 60 years of age *(23,24)* (Fig. 12A–C). These age-dependent changes in systolic, diastolic, and pulse pressures are consistent with the idea that in younger people, BP is determined largely by peripheral vascular resistance, whereas in older people BP is determined mainly by the stiffness of central conduit vessels *(23)*.

HYPERTENSION

As clinical studies have shown the deleterious effects of hypertension, recommendations for the treatment of elevated BPs have been adjusted accordingly. The emphasis was initially on treating increases in DBP. However, the finding that systolic hypertension is a predictor of adverse events prompted the use of increased systolic blood pressure (SBP) as an indication for treatment. Although the initial cut-off value for normal SBP was 160 mmHg, the value was adjusted downward when studies showed that pressures between 140 and 160 mmHg conferred added risk. The systolic value was recently further lowered to 130 mmHg for patients with diabetes mellitus (DM) *(25)*.

In older individuals, isolated systolic hypertension (ISH) is the most common form of hypertension. ISH is defined as a SBP greater than 140 mmHg and a DBP less than 90 mmHg (i.e., a widened pulse pressure), and it could be described as a disease related, in part, to arterial stiffening *(26)*. Even mild ISH (stage 1) is associated with an appreciable increase in CVD risk *(27,28)*.

Intimal-Medial Thickness

Studies of morphological, cellular, enzymatic, and biochemical changes in animal models have increased our understanding of age-associated arterial remodeling in humans. For example, the age-associated intimal-

---

Fig. 12. *(Opposite page)* (A–C) Average systolic **(A)**, diastolic **(B)**, and pulse **(C)** pressures and age, in Baltimore Longitudinal Study of Aging participants stratified by gender. Values are mean ± SEM.

medial thickening seen in humans is often ascribed to "subclinical" atherosclerosis *(29–32)*. This idea has become so well accepted that IMT is used as a surrogate measure of atherosclerosis *(33,34)*. However, IMT, which is usually measured in areas devoid of atherosclerotic plaque, is only weakly associated with the extent and severity of CAD *(35)*. Furthermore, findings in rodent *(36)* and nonhuman primate *(37)* models of aging clearly indicate that IMT is an age-related process that is separate from atherosclerosis because atherosclerosis is absent in both of these animal models. Thus, excessive IMT is not necessarily synonymous with early or subclinical atherosclerosis *(38)*.

Nonetheless, an association between IMT and carotid *(39–41)*, aortic *(42)*, and coronary *(34)* atherosclerosis is documented in humans. In individuals rigorously screened for the absence of CVD, excessive IMT at a given age predicts silent CAD *(18)* (Fig. 13A), which, in turn, progresses to clinical ischemic heart disease. In the Atherosclerosis Risk In Communities (ARIC) study, which comprised middle-aged adults, IMT was associated with a greater prevalence of CVDs *(43)* and was an independent predictor of stroke *(44)*. In the Cardiovascular Health Study (CHS), which comprised individuals over the age of 65, IMT was an independent predictor of future myocardial infarction and stroke *(45)* (Fig. 13B). In the CHS study, subjects were grouped according to quintiles of IMT, and the results indicated a nonlinear gradation in risk, with higher quintiles conferring a greater risk for CVDs *(31)* (Fig. 13B). Compared to the lowest quintile, the fifth quintile had a 3.15 relative risk for cardiovascular events, even after adjusting for traditional risk factors. In fact, the strength of IMT as a risk factor for CVDs equals or exceeds that of most other traditional risk factors (Fig. 13C).

Thus, IMT is not a manifestation of atherosclerosis but is associated with it. IMT is an aging-related process that is separate from the pathophysiological process of atherosclerosis, yet IMT is a risk factor for atherosclerosis. IMT has been previously classified in the same disease category as atherosclerosis, but should be correctly reclassified as a marker of arterial aging. When the extent of thickening exceeds the value in age and

---

Fig. 13. *(Opposite page)* Carotid intimal-medial thickness (IMT) and cardiovascular diseases. **(A)** Common carotid intimal-medial thickness (CCA IMT) as a function of age, stratified by coronary artery disease (CAD) classification, in Baltimore Longitudinal Study of Aging subjects. CAD-1 denotes a subset with positive exercise electrocardiogram (ECG) but negative thallium scans; CAD-2 represents a subset with concordant positive exercise ECG and thallium scans. **(B)** CCA IMT as a predictor of future cardiovascular events in the Cardiovascular Health Study (CHS). Note the nonlinear increase in the risk for cardiovascular event rates with

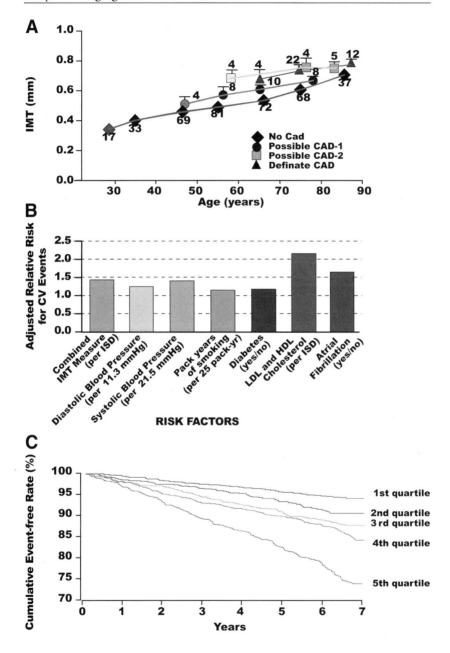

Fig. 13 *(Continued)* increasing quintiles. (From ref. *45*, with permission.) **(C)** Comparisons of the associations of age- and gender-adjusted cardiovascular risk factors with the combined events of stroke or myocardial infarction in the CHS study, using Cox proportional hazards models. Note that IMT is a potent risk factor for future cardiovascular events. (Adapted with permission from ref. *45*.)

gender-matched controls, it is a risk factor associated with adverse cardiovascular outcomes. The threshold or cut-off values above which the risk from IMT becomes clinically significant have not been defined, but some investigators are beginning to address these issues *(46)*.

Studying the relationship between primary age-associated vascular wall remodeling and CVDs has led researchers to search for new phenotypic manifestations of arterial remodeling to explore their clinical and prognostic significance. For example, the various carotid geometric patterns that are derived by combining the measurements of vascular mass with wall-to-lumen ratio were recently associated with unique functional and hemodynamic profiles that are largely independent of age and hypertension *(47)*. These patterns were recently found to have differing prognostic implications *(48)*.

Vascular Stiffness

In addition to IMT, increased vascular stiffness has been observed with advancing age in humans *(19,23,49,50)* and in animal models of aging *(51,52)*. Studies in animals have shown several structural changes in the vascular wall, including increased collagen content, reduced elastin content, and calcification and fragmentation of elastin, as well as alterations in smooth muscle tone and endothelial function, which underlie the observed phenotypic compliance changes *(5)*. Strictly speaking, stiffness and its inverse, distensibility, depend on intrinsic structural properties of the blood vessel wall that relate a change in pressure with a corresponding change in volume. However, in this chapter, the terms stiffness and compliance are used in a broader sense, to denote the overall lumped stiffness and compliance, which include the additional effects of vascular tone, BP, and other modulating factors, all of which impact LV afterload (Fig. 8).

Pulse Wave Velocity

With each systolic contraction of the ventricle, a propagation wave is generated in the arterial wall and travels centrifugally down the arterial tree. This propagation wave accompanies (and slightly precedes) the luminal flow wave generated during systole. The velocity of propagation of this wave is directly proportional to the stiffness of the arterial wall. This situation is analogous to the flow of a wave on a string; as the string is stretched, it becomes less compliant, and the velocity of the flow wave increases. The velocity of the pulse wave in vivo is determined not only by the intrinsic stress–strain relationship (stiffness) of the vascular wall, but also by smooth muscle tone, which is reflected by the mean arterial pressure (MAP) *(53)*.

The availability of noninvasive measures of the velocity of this pulse wave allows for large-scale epidemiological studies. Pulse wave velocity (PWV) was assessed in BLSA participants who were rigorously screened for the absence of overt or silent CVD *(19)* and in other populations with varying degrees of prevalence of CVD *(23,49,54–57)*. In all these studies, a significant age-associated increase in PWV was observed in both men and women.

Elegant experiments in canines have shown several detrimental hemodynamic effects when the heart is switched from ejecting into a compliant vessel to ejecting into a stiff conduit, especially in the setting of myocardial ischemia *(58)*. In support of these animal studies, several clinical studies demonstrate the adverse cardiovascular effects of accelerated vascular stiffening. In the ARIC study, several vascular compliance indices were predictors of hypertension *(59)* (Fig. 14A). In hypertensive patients, PWV was a marker of cardiovascular risk *(60)* and coronary events *(61)* (Fig. 14B) and an independent predictor of mortality *(62)*. In addition, pulse wave velocity was an independent predictor of mortality in subjects over 70 years of age (63) and in patients with end-stage renal disease (ESRD) *(64)*. Other noninvasive indices of vascular compliance, including SV divided by pulse pressure *(65)* (Fig. 14C) and the incremental modulus of elasticity *(66)*, were independent predictors of adverse outcomes. Thus, vascular stiffening, like IMT, should be viewed as another marker of aging, which, when accelerated, also becomes a risk factor for CVDs.

The interaction between vascular wall stiffening and CVDs may set in motion a vicious cycle. PWV is determined, in part, by smooth muscle cell (SMC) tone, which, in turn, is partially regulated by endothelial cells. Moreover, endothelial dysfunction is seen early in several cardiovascular disorders including atherosclerosis *(67)*, diabetes *(68)*, and hypertension *(69)*. Thus, in this cycle, alterations in the mechanical properties of the vessel wall contribute to endothelial cell dysfunction and, ultimately, vascular stiffening.

REFLECTED WAVES

In addition to the forward pulse wave, each cardiac cycle generates a reflected wave, which travels back up the arterial tree toward the central aorta. This reflected wave, which probably originates in the smaller arteries and arterioles, alters the arterial pressure waveform *(70)* and is modulated, in part, by nitric oxide (NO) *(71)*. The velocity of the reflected flow wave is directly proportional to the stiffness of the arterial wall *(53)*. Thus, in young individuals whose vascular wall is compliant, the reflected wave does not reach the large elastic arteries until diastole. With advancing age

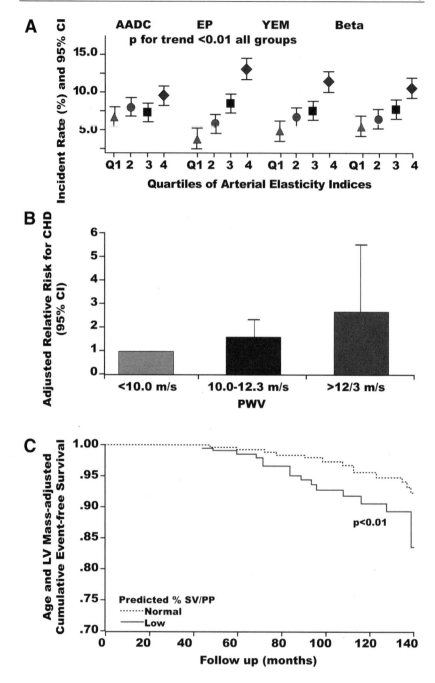

Fig. 14. Vascular stiffness and cardiovascular outcomes. (A) Reduced arterial elasticity and incidence of hypertension in the Atherosclerosis Research In Communities (ARIC) study. Values 1–4 denote the highest to lowest quartiles. Note that for all

and increasing vascular stiffening, the velocity of the reflected wave increases, and the wave reaches the central circulation earlier in the cardiac cycle, during the systolic phase. This reflected wave can be noninvasively assessed from recordings of the carotid *(72,73)* or radial *(72, 74,75)* arterial pulse waveforms by arterial applanation tonometry and high-fidelity micromanometer probes. Inspection of the recorded arterial pulse wave contour shows an inflection point, which heralds the arrival of the reflected wave *(76)* (Fig. 15A). The amplitude distance from the inflection point to the peak of the arterial waveform is the pressure pulse augmentation that results from the early arrival of the reflected wave. Dividing this augmentation by the distance from the peak to the trough of the arterial waveform (corresponding to the pulse pressure) yields the augmentation index *(76)*. The augmentation index, like the PWV, increases with age *(19,70,72,75,77)* (Fig. 15B).

Because reflected waves originate in small arteries and arterioles, the age-associated changes in this index are probably determined, in part, by the age-associated changes in the structure and function of distal vessels, as well as by age-associated alterations in the structure and function of large elastic arteries. Although attention has focused on the transmission velocity of reflected waves as an index of arterial stiffness, evaluation of the pulse wave contour may provide valuable insight into the characteristics and the pathology of more distal vessels, where reflected waves originate *(78)*.

The pressure pulse augmentation provided by the early return of the reflected wave is an added load against which the ventricle must contract *(79)*. Furthermore, the loss of the diastolic augmentation seen in compliant vessels, owing to the early return of the reflected waves, decreases DBP and thus has the potential to reduce coronary blood flow because most coronary flow occurs during diastole *(79)*. These considerations suggest that excessively early return of the reflected waves, which can be assessed with the augmentation index, may be detrimental to the cardio-

Fig. 14. *(Continued)* indices, decreased elasticity is associated with an increased incidence of hypertension ($p < 0.01$). CI, confidence interval; AADC, adjusted arterial diameter change; EP, Peterson's elastic modulus; YEM, Young's elastic modulus; BETA, β-stiffness index. (Reprinted with permission from ref. *58*.) **(B)** Relative risk for coronary heart disease (CHD) events, adjusted for age, gender, blood pressure, heart rate, diabetes mellitus, smoking, and previous antihypertensive treatment, by tertiles of pulse wave velocity (PWV). CI, confidence interval. (Adapted with permission from ref. *60*.) **(C)** Cumulative event-free survival, adjusted for age and left ventricular mass, relative to total arterial compliance indexed as stroke volume (SV)/pulse pressure (PP). Note that reduced arterial compliance is a predictor of cardiovascular events. (Reprinted with permission from ref. *64*.)

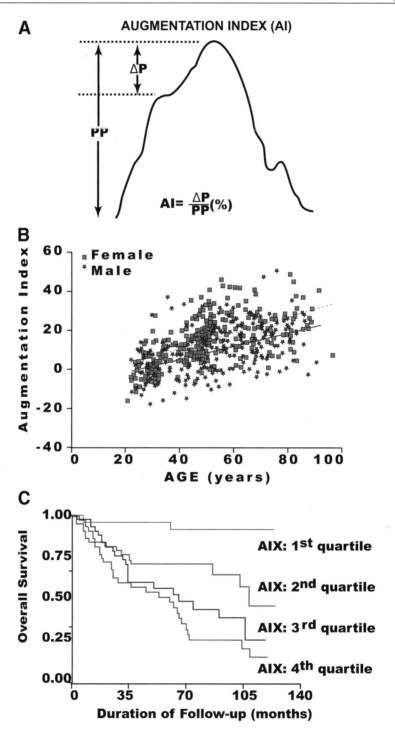

vascular system. In fact, the augmentation index is a predictor of adverse events in ESRD patients *(80)* (Fig. 15C). Thus, this index is another marker of vascular aging that is a risk factor for CVDs.

PULSE PRESSURE

As blood vessels stiffen, their diameter increases, which decreases wall strain. Moreover, the combination of arterial wall stiffening and early return of the reflected waves (*see* below) widens the pulse pressure *(81)*. Indeed, a high SBP generates a similar distention of hardened capacitance vessels, wheras a lower DBP results, in part, from the loss of diastolic augmentation. Thus, pulse pressure is a useful hemodynamic marker of the vascular stiffness of conduit arteries. Clinical and epidemiological studies in several different populations with varying prevalences of CVDs have confirmed the prognostic importance of pulse pressure *(82–96)*. Furthermore, in several studies, pulse pressure was a stronger predictor of outcome than SBP or DBP. This suggests the need for studies to evaluate whether pulse pressure should be added to SBP or DBP as a screening criterion or as a therapeutic endpoint in the treatment of hypertension.

VASCULAR STIFFNESS AND HYPERTENSION

Recent studies showing that increased vascular stiffness may precede the development of hypertension underscore the relationship between hypertension and arterial wall stiffening *(59)*. This concept has been overshadowed by the notion that an increase in MAP (or peripheral resistance) is the predominant cause of increased stiffness of large arteries. The increase in mean BP that occurs with hypertension can lead to a secondary increase in large-artery stiffness; however, the primary age-associated increase in large-artery stiffness can lead to an increase in arterial pressures. Thus, hypertension can be defined as a disease that is, in part, determined or modulated by properties of the arterial wall. An even broader view recognizes hypertension as a syndrome *(97)*, with BP increases representing only one (albeit late) manifestation.

Recognizing the independence of arterial wall stiffening from hypertension has important clinical implications. In a study of patients with ESRD who required dialysis, Guerin et al. *(98)* reported that treatment of hyper-

---

Fig. 15. *(Opposite page)* (**A**) Graphic representation of the augmentation index, which is defined as the ratio of the distance from the inflection point to the peak of the arterial waveform ($\triangle$P), over the pulse pressure (PP). (**B**) The augmentation index in healthy Baltimore Longitudinal Study of Aging volunteer subjects, as a function of age and gender. (**C**) Probability of overall survival in patients with end-stage renal failure, stratified by quartiles of augmentation index (AIX). (Reprinted with permission from ref. *79*.)

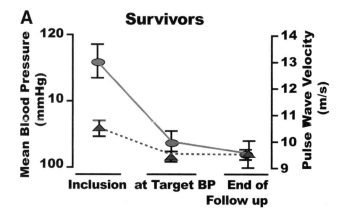

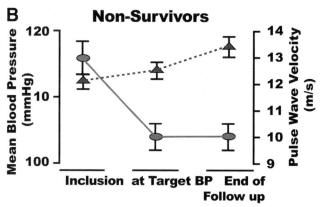

Fig. 16. Changes in mean blood pressure (solid circles) and aortic pulse wave velocity (open circles) in survivor and nonsurvivor patients with end-stage renal failure.
Follow-up occurred at a mean of 51 ± 38 months. Values are means $\pm$ standard
error. (Reprinted with permission from ref. *98*.)

tension had differing effects on PWV, despite having similar BP-lowering effects *(98)* (Fig. 16). Mortality was higher in the group in whom
PWV increased in spite of therapy, and progression of vascular stiffening was an independent predictor of mortality. These observations suggest
that treating BP is necessary but not sufficient therapy for the syndrome
of hypertension.

Vascular Stiffness and Metabolic Diseases

The incidence and prevalence of DM and the metabolic syndrome
increase with advancing age. Several studies document a robust association between DM and increased vascular stiffening *(99–102)*. Increased
levels of hemoglobin A1c *(54)* and fasting glucose *(99)* are associated

with greater arterial stiffness, even in non-diabetic subjects. This association may be due to the increased glycosylation of long-lived matrix proteins (such as collagen) in the vascular wall during hyperglycemia, and the subsequent irreversible covalent cross-linking of these proteins to form advanced glycation end products *(20)*.

The metabolic syndrome, which includes insulin resistance, obesity (particularly abdominal adiposity), hypertension, and dyslipidemia (increased triglycerides and low high-density lipoprotein), is associated with a markedly increased incidence of CVDs. Greater waist circumference *(54)* and levels of insulin *(54,56,99)*, triglycerides *(54,99)*, and visceral adiposity *(56)* are all associated with arterial stiffening. A recent analysis showed that even after taking into account each individual component of the metabolic syndrome, the clustering of at least three of these components is independently associated with increased IMT and stiffness *(103)*. This suggests that the components of the metabolic syndrome interact to synergistically impact vascular thickness and stiffness, and that the deleterious effects of the metabolic syndrome may be mediated, in part, via acceleration of vascular stiffening and thickening.

Endothelial Function

Endothelial cells are extremely important and powerful regulators of the vasculature. Several cardiovascular conditions and risk factors are associated with endothelial dysfunction, including hypercholesterolemia, insulin resistance, cigarette smoking, and heart failure *(104)*. Endothelial cell dysfunction contributes to the pathogenesis of hypertension *(69)* and atherosclerosis *(67,105)*. In addition, endothelial cells play a pivotal role in regulating vascular tone, vascular permeability, and the response to inflammation *(105–107)*. Several features of these arterial properties undergo age-associated alterations in function.

VASOREACTIVITY

With advancing age, NO-dependent mechanical and agonist-mediated endothelial vasodilatation is reduced in humans *(21,22,108,109)* (Fig. 11C) and animals *(37,110)*. This vasoreactivity depends on NO generated by endothelial nitric oxide synthase (eNOS). In aging rats *(111)* and rabbits *(112)*, activity of the eNOS isoform is markedly reduced. In addition, the bioavailability of NO may be reduced to age-associated increases in the amounts of superoxide and nitrated tyrosine residues of proteins *(113)*.

INFLAMMATION

Aging is associated with increased expression of adhesion molecules in rats *(36)* and increased adherence of monocytes to the endothelial surface in rabbits *(112)*. Adhesion molecules on the luminal surface of endothelial cells mediate leukocyte binding to endothelial cells and subendothelial migration *(114)*. This process is probably facilitated by the actions of matrix metalloproteinases (MMPs) *(115–117)*. Serum levels of adhesion molecules show age-associated alterations in humans *(118,119)*. In patients with hypercholesterolemia and ischemic heart disease, serum levels of soluble vascular cell adhesion molecule-1, but not soluble intercellular adhesion molecule (ICAM)-1, are positively associated with aging *(119)*.

PERMEABILITY

In rat aortae, aging is associated with increased permeability to albumin *(120)*. Moreover, glycosaminoglycans *(112)*, which help regulate several arterial properties including vascular permeability *(121)*, accumulate in greater number in the intima of older rabbits. Within hours of an acute arterial balloon injury to the rabbit carotid artery, the pericellular distribution of glycosaminoglycans is significantly reduced in the arterial wall, and this loss is associated with a significant expansion of the extracellular space. The glycosaminoglycans were rapidly replaced in the media but not in the developing neointima by SMCs *(122)*.

VASCULAR-WALL SHEAR STRESS

Vascular-wall shear stress is important in modulating endothelial morphology and function *(105,107,123)*. The identities of the mechanoreceptors that transduce the frictional forces of blood, the various effector systems and component molecules that are activated, and the disparate second-messenger signaling systems involved are not well defined. Nonetheless, changes in vascular-wall shear stress result in acute and chronic alterations in the synthetic and metabolic activities of endothelial cells *(107,123)*. Arterial regions with low shear stress are particularly vulnerable to the development of atherosclerosis *(123)*.

ENDOTHELIAL DYSFUNCTION AND CELLULAR SENESCENCE

Telomeres, which are DNA–protein complexes that form the ends of chromosomes, and telomerase, a unique enzyme that regulates telomere length, may be important in cellular senescence *(124)*. Because telomeres shorten with each replicative cell division *(125)*, they may be good indicators of biological aging. Telomere length is a marker of cellular turnover in human vascular tissue *(126)*, where it is inversely associated with age *(127)* and with atherosclerotic grade *(128)*. In a study of Danish twins, telomere length of chromosomes in white blood cells was negatively associated with pulse pressure *(129)*. In a normotensive French cohort, telomere length of chromosomes in white blood cells was longer in women than in men but contributed significantly to variations in pulse pressure and PWV only in men *(130)*. Loss of telomere function induces endothelial dysfunction in vascular endothelial cells, whereas inhibition of telomere shortening suppresses age-associated dysfunction in these cells *(131)*.

ENDOTHELIAL DYSFUNCTION AND ANGIOGENESIS

Endothelial cells play a pivotal role in angiogenesis in which new vessels grow from the existing microvasculature. Studies in animal models of aging indicate that angiogenesis is impaired with advancing age *(132)*, which could be, in part, related to an age-associated decrease in endothelial progenitor cells from the bone marrow *(133)*. Angiogenesis requires the migration and proliferation of endothelial cells in response to cytokines. Migration of endothelial cells, in turn, requires an optimal level of adhesion to matrix proteins, which is regulated by matrix-degrading metalloproteases such as MMP-1. In microvascular endothelial cells from aged mice, expression of MMP-1 is decreased, whereas expression of its inhibitor tissue inhibitor of metalloproteinase (TIMP)1 is increased *(134)*. Furthermore, in these aged animals, expression of the growth factor transforming growth factor (TGF)-β1 and the matrix protein type-1 collagen is decreased *(135)*. Recent evidence suggests that the expression of growth factors is modulated by advanced glycosylation end products *(136)*. Thus, the age-associated impairment in angiogenesis is, in part, owing to changes in the levels of extracellular enzymes, matrix proteins, and growth factors, which affect endothelial cell migration.

An Integrated View of Vascular Aging

An integrated and comprehensive conceptualization of arterial aging requires improved methods for studying endothelial function and an understanding of as yet unrecognized genetic and polymorphic components of arterial structure and function. Furthermore, interactions among traditional vascular variables need to be defined. These vascular variables have been studied separately, and the emphasis has been placed on their relationship to CVDs, not on their relationship with each other. In addition to being intimately involved with CVDs, these traditional vascular factors are interrelated to and interdependent on each other. For example, in a longitudinal study of a large population of relatively aged subjects, increased baseline levels of pulse pressure were associated with progression of IMT, and baseline IMT, in turn, was associated with greater widening of the pulse pressure *(137)*. After all the components of arterial aging are identified, a comprehensive vascular aging profile may be developed for each individual that represents the integrated sum of all the vascular processes.

CARDIOVASCULAR AGING
AND CLINICAL MEDICINE

Despite the interest in the physiology of the age-associated changes in cardiovascular structure and function, cardiovascular aging has remained, for the most part, outside of mainstream clinical medicine. This is because their pathophysiological implications are largely underappreciated and are not well disseminated in the medical community. In fact, age has traditionally been considered a nonmodifiable risk factor. However, as noted in the preceding sections, many of the age-associated alterations in cardiovascular structure and function, at both the cellular and molecular levels, ought not to be simply considered as part of a "normal or physiological aging" process, but rather, should be construed as specific risk factors for CV diseases. This highlights the urgency to incorporate cardiovascular aging into clinical medicine, which as a requisite, will require that the following steps be implemented.

First, clinicians should be educated regarding those aspects of cardiovascular aging that are "risky." This educational process should be geared toward all physicians taking care of middle-aged or older individuals, not just geriatricians, because many of the "risky" components—often referred to as "subclinical disease"—begin to appear in middle age, which is when they start exacting their toll, and which is when preventive strategies (once they are developed, *see* below) should be implemented in order to obtain the most benefit. Beyond presenting the epidemiological data implicating the markers of cardiovascular aging as risk factors for disease, the educational curriculum should also include several important concepts discussed in this chapter, which would enable a fuller appreciation of the impact of these risk factors, including the differentiation among successful, usual, and unsuccessful cardiovascular aging, which are in many ways the products of age–disease interactions.

This educational process needs to be complemented by aggressive efforts to set up normative values for each risk marker within a specific population, and adjusted for age groups and gender. This, in turn, is dependent on standardizing the methodologies, techniques, and protocols utilized for acquiring and interpreting these measurements. Findings from the epidemiological studies can then be incorporated to determine the specific thresholds, or cut-off values, that would distinguish successful (or desired) values, from normal values, from preclinical values, and from disease values.

Concomitantly, aggressive efforts should be undertaken to develop effective therapies to prevent, delay, or attenuate the cardiovascular changes that accompany aging. This is a critical step because if such interventions are not developed in a timely manner, then the recognition of cardiovascular aging as a risk marker for disease would remain an epidemiological finding of historical interest only. Thus, investigating these preventive measures should be a top research priority, and future efforts will require the close collaboration of a consortium of researchers, including molecular cardiologists, cardiovascular physiologists, and translational clinical trialists. In the next section, we discuss a number of lifestyle and pharmacological interventions to retard the rate of progression of subclinical disease, which have already been explored.

LIFESTYLE INTERVENTIONS
Physical Activity

With respect to lifestyle, the risk factor of lack of vigorous exercise increases dramatically with age in otherwise healthy persons *(138)*, including the community-dwelling BLSA volunteer participants (Fig. 17A). Thus, a reduction in physical conditioning status might be implicated as a factor in the reduced cardiovascular reserve of older, healthy sedentary individuals, as discussed. But, the issue arises as to whether physical conditioning via aerobic training of sedentary older persons can affect deficits in cardiovascular reserve capacity owing to an aging process, *per se*.

It has been amply documented that physical conditioning of older persons can substantially increase their maximum aerobic work capacity and peak oxygen consumption. The extent to which this conditioning effect results from enhanced central cardiac performance or from augmented peripheral circulatory and O_2 utilization mechanisms, including changes in skeletal muscle mass, varies with the characteristics of the population studied, genetic factors, the type and degree of conditioning achieved, gender, and body position during study (*see* ref. 5 for review). A longitudinal study of older males in the upright position indicates that an enhanced physical conditioning status increases O_2 consumption and work capacity, in part by increases in the maximum cardiac output, by increasing the maximum SV, and in part by increasing the estimated total body oxygen utilization *(139)*. The augmentation of maximum SVI is the result of an augmented reduction of LV ESV (Fig. 17B), thus, a concomitant increase in LV EF occurs. The vascular exercise afterload is also reduced by physical conditioning. Thus, the exercise EF is also enhanced *(139)*. Pulse pressure, PWV, and carotid augmentation index are lower (Fig. 17C) *(19,140)* and baroreceptor reflex function is improved *(141)*

A

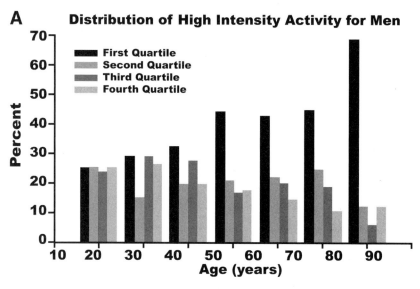

Distribution of High Intensity Activity for Men

B

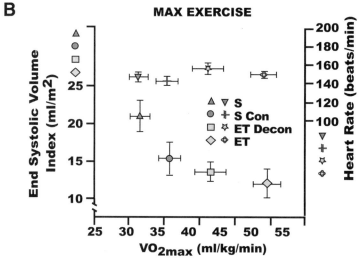

MAX EXERCISE

C

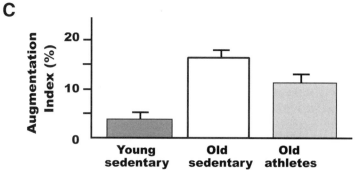

in older persons who are physically conditioned than in sedentary persons. Exercise conditioning also improves endothelial function in older persons *(142)*.

In contrast to the improved LV ejection, the maximal HR of older persons does not vary with physical conditioning status (Fig. 17A). There is no strong evidence at hand that physical conditioning of older persons can offset the deficiency in sympathetic modulation.

Diet

There is some evidence to indicate that diets low in sodium are associated with reduced arterial stiffening with aging in humans *(143)*. In rodents, consumption of diets high in ω-3 polyunsaturated fatty acids (PUFAs) lead to increases in ω-3 PUFAs in mitochrondrial membranes, increased efficacy of adenosine triphosphate production and reduction of Ca^{2+} and arrhythmias following ischemic–reperfusion stress. Diets high in coenzyme Q (COQ) reduce post-ischemic systolic and diastolic dysfunction and Ca^{2+} overload. Treatment of isolated ventricular myocytes with COQ increases the threshold required for reactive oxygen species (ROS) to induce the mitochondrial permeability transition.

Pharmacotherapy

Therapies that improve the coupling of ventricular and vascular elastances are likely to improve exercise tolerance and cardiac function, not only in patients with heart failure, but even in healthy subjects. This concept is supported by two studies. In healthy, older BLSA subjects treated with the direct vasodilator, sodium nitroprusside showed marked reductions in reflected pulse waves at rest indexed by carotid tonometry (Fig. 18A), as well as reductions in arterial pressure, EDVs and ESVs and improved cardiac function (Fig. 18B), including a higher EF at rest and during maximal exercise as compared to placebo therapy (Fig. 18C). This

---

Fig. 17. *(Opposite page)* (**A**) High-intensity physical activity becomes reduced with aging. (**B**) Heart rate and end-systolic volume during peak seated, upright exercise on a cycle ergometer across a broad range of aerobic capacity in healthy males who have been exercise conditioned or deconditioned. S, sedentary; ET, exercise trained; Scon, sedentary men after conditioning; ET Decon, men who had been exercise trained but stopped their training for the study to become detrained or deconditioned (DeCon). The figure shows that the extent to which the left ventricle empties, as manifest by the end-systolic volume, varies with the level of aerobic capacity (VO_2 max), which was varied among the four groups by either conditioning or deconditioning protocols. In contrast, the peak heart rate achieved does not vary with aerobic capacity. (**C**) Carotid augmentation index in older athletes is reduced compared to their sedentary counterparts *(139)*.

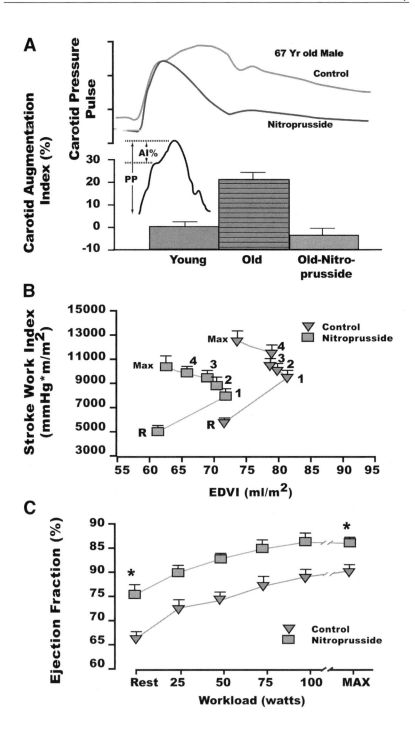

result emphasizes the role of reflected pulse waves in LV function. In another study, an acute intravenous Ca^{2+} channel blocker administered to healthy older subjects reduced noninvasive indices of arterial stiffness and ventricular systolic stiffness and improved exercise tolerance and oxygen consumption before reaching anaerobic threshold *(144)*. A novel breaker of nonenzymatic crosslinks owing to advanced glycation end products reduces EaI in older nonhuman primates and improves the EaI/E_{LV}I ratio and EF *(145)*. This agent also reduced pulse pressure in a human clinical trial in older hypertensive patients *(146)*.

An emerging concept in the treatment of hypertension recognizes that progressive vascular damage can continue to occur even when arterial pressure is controlled. It is conceivable that drugs that retard or reverse age-associated vascular wall remodeling and increased stiffness will be preferable to those that lower pressure without affecting vascular wall properties. The chronic administration of angiotensin-converting enzyme inhibitors to rodents attenuate mitochondrial dysfunction, reduce ROS, enhance NO bioavailability, reduce fibrosis, retard vascular and cardiac aging and prolong life *(51,147–154)*. Retardation or reduction in IMT and arterial stiffness in humans has been achieved by drug–diet intervention *(23,64,91,95,155–159)*. It is thus far not known whether if such treatment can "prevent" unsuccessful aging of the vasculature in individuals of younger-middle age who exhibit excessive subclinical evidence of unsuccessful aging.

In summary, accelerated heart and vascular aging in apparently healthy younger and middle-aged adults, that is those who exhibit measurements of heart or vascular aging that usually occur later in life, may indicate the need for interventions designed to decrease the occurrence and/or manifestations of CVD at later ages. Similarly, exaggerated heart or vascular aging in older persons, that is, those with age-associated vascular measurements in the upper tercile, may merit similar consideration. Specifically, prime targets for intervention are those persons presently perceived as "normal" individuals without a textbook CVD diagnosis whose arteries

---

Fig. 18. *(Opposite page)* Intravenous sodium nitroprusside reduces reflected pulse wave and improves left ventricular function. (**A**) Carotid augmentation index. (**B**) Ventricular function, depicted as stroke work index vs end-diastolic volume index (EDVI) relationship at upright, at seated rest, and during exercise in the presence and absence of sodium nitroprusside (SNP). The relationship is shifted leftward and downward with SNP, indicating a smaller EDVI and lower stroke work index at any exercise load. (**C**) Ejection fraction at seated, at upright rest, at intermediate common submaximal workloads, and at maximum effort in healthy volunteers aged 71 ± 7 prior to and during SNP infusion. At any level of effort, ejection fraction is substantially increased by SNP. (From ref. *163*.)

and hearts are "unsuccessfully" placing them at increased risk for the occurrence of CVD. Such a strategy would thus advocate treating "unsuccessful" aging. Although these preventive lifestyle and pharmacological strategies can be undertaken even now, future genetic characterization of individuals will likely allow person-specific stratification with respect to the risk, efficacy, and cost-effectiveness of measures to retard cardiovascular aging in order to reduce cardiovascular functional disability and disease at older ages. Additional studies of the effectiveness of pharmacological treatment regimens to delay or prevent each change are required for this strategy to be put into practice. Recommendations regarding the impact of lifestyle on cardiovascular aging should be repetitively sounded, loud and clear, so they can be put into practice early in life!

ACKNOWLEDGMENT

The authors would like to thank Christina R. Link for her editorial assistance in preparing this chapter.

REFERENCES

1. Fleg JL, O'Connor FC, Gerstenblith G, et al. Impact of age on the cardiovascular response to dynamic upright exercise in healthy men and women. J Appl Physiol 1995;78:890–900.
2. Fleg JL, Gerstenblith G, Zonderman AB, et al. Prevalence and prognostic significance of exercise-induced silent myocardial ischemia detected by thallium scintigraphy and electrocardiography in asymptomatic volunteers. Circulation 1990;81: 428–436.
3. Fleg JL, Schulman SP, Gerstenblith G, et al. Additive effects of age and silent myocardial ischemia on the left ventricular response to upright cycle exercise. J Appl Physiol 1993;75:499.
4. Correia LCL, Lakatta EG, O'Connor FC, et al. Attenuated cardiovascular reserve during prolonged submaximal cycle exercise in healthy older subjects. J Am Coll Cardiol 2002;40:1290–1297.
5. Lakatta EG. Cardiovascular regulatory mechanisms in advanced age. Physiol Rev 1993;73:413–465.
6. Yin FCP, Weisfeldt ML, Milnor WR. Role of aortic input impedance in the decreased cardiovascular response to exercise with aging in dogs. J Clin Invest 1981; 68:28–38.
7. Lakatta EG. Deficient neuroendocrine regulation of the cardiovascular system with advancing age in healthy humans [Point of view]. Circulation 1993;87:631.
8. Esler MD, Turner AG, Kaye DM, et al. Aging effects on human sympathetic neuronal function. Am J Physiol 1995;268:R278–285.
9. Seals DR, Dempsey JA. Aging, exercise and cardiopulmonary function. In: Lamb DR, Gisolfi CV, Nadel E. (eds.), Perspectives in Exercise Science and Sports Medicine, Vol 8. Loopa Publishing, Carmel, IN, 1995, pp. 237–304.
10. Chen C-H, Ting C-T, Lin S-J, et al. Which arterial and cardiac parameters best predict left ventricular mass? Circulation 1998;98:422.

11. Sunagawa K, Maughan WL, Bukhoff D, Sagawa K. Left ventricular interaction with arterial load studied in isolated canine ventricle. Am J Physiol 1983;245(Heart Circ Physiol 14):H773–H780.

12. Cohen-Solal A, Caviezel B, Laperche T, Gourgon R. Effects of aging on left ventricular-arterial coupling in man: assessment by means of arterial effective and left ventricular elastances. J Human Hypertens 1996;10:111–116.

13. Chen C-H, Nakayama M, Nevo E, et al. Coupled systolic-ventricular and vascular stiffening with age. J Am Coll Cardiol 1998;32:1221–1227.

14. Saba PS, Roman MJ, Ganau A, et al. Relationship of effective arterial elastance to demographic and arterial characteristics in normotensive and hypertensive adults. J Hypertens 1995;13:971–977.

15. Ishihara H, Yokota M, Sobue T, Saito H. Relationship between ventriculoarterial coupling and myocardial energetics in patients with idiopathic dilated cardiomyopathy. J Am Coll Cardiol 1994;23:406–416.

16. Gerstenblith G, Frederiksen J, Yin FC, et al. Echocardiographic assessment of a normal adult aging population. Circulation 1977;56:273–278.

17. Virmani R, Avolio AP, Mergner WJ, et al. Effect of aging on aortic morphology in populations with high and low prevalence of hypertension and atherosclerosis. Comparison between occidental and Chinese communities. Am J Pathol 1991;139: 1119–1129.

18. Nagai Y, Metter EJ, Earley CJ, et al. Increased carotid artery intimal-medial thickness in asymptomatic older subjects with exercise-induced myocardial ischemia. Circulation 1998;98:1504–1509.

19. Vaitkevicius PV, Fleg JL, Engel JH, et al. Effects of age and aerobic capacity on arterial stiffness in healthy adults. Circulation 1993;88:1456–1462.

20. Brownlee M, Cerami A, Vlassara H. Advanced glycosylation end products in tissue and the biochemical basis of diabetic complications. N Engl J Med 1988;318: 1315–1321.

21. Celermajer DS, Sorensen KE, Spiegelhalter DJ, et al. Aging is associated with endothelial dysfunction in healthy men years before the age-related decline in women. J Am Coll Cardiol 1994;24:471–476.

22. Gerhard M, Roddy MA, Creager SJ, Creager MA. Aging progressively impairs endothelium-dependent vasodilation in forearm resistance vessels of humans. Hypertension 1996;27:849–853.

23. Franklin SS, Gustin WT, Wong ND, et al. Hemodynamic patterns of age-related changes in blood pressure. The Framingham Heart Study. Circulation 1997;96:308–315.

24. Burt VL, Whelton P, Roccella EJ, et al. Prevalence of hypertension in the US adult population. Results from the Third National Health and Nutrition Examination Survey, 1988–1991. Hypertension 1995;25:305–313.

25. The sixth report of the Joint National Committee on prevention, detection, evaluation, and treatment of high blood pressure. Arch Intern Med 1997;157:2413–2446.

26. Franklin SS. Is there a preferred antihypertensive therapy for isolated systolic hypertension and reduced arterial compliance? Curr Hypertens Rep 2000;2:253–259.

27. Sagie A, Larson MG, Levy D. The natural history of borderline isolated systolic hypertension. N Engl J Med 1993;329:1912–1917.

28. Kannel WB. Elevated systolic blood pressure as a cardiovascular risk factor. Am J Cardiol 2000;85:251–255.

29. Salonen R, Nyssonen K, Porkkala-Sarataho E, Salonen JT. The Kuopio Atherosclerosis Prevention Study (KAPS): effect of pravastatin treatment on lipids, oxida-

tion resistance of lipoproteins, and atherosclerotic progression. Am J Cardiol 1995; 76:34C–39C.

30. Hodis HN, Mack WJ, LaBree L, et al. Reduction in carotid arterial wall thickness using lovastatin and dietary therapy: a randomized controlled clinical trial. Ann Intern Med 1996;124:548–556.

31. Markus RA, Mack WJ, Azen SP, Hodis HN. Influence of lifestyle modification on atherosclerotic progression determined by ultrasonographic change in the common carotid intima-media thickness. Am J Clin Nutr 1997;65:1000–1004.

32. Woo KS, Chook P, Raitakari OT, et al. Westernization of Chinese adults and increased subclinical atherosclerosis. Arterioscler Thromb Vasc Biol 1999;19:2487–2493.

33. Crouse JR 3rd, Byington RP, Bond MG, et al. Pravastatin, Lipids, and Atherosclerosis in the Carotid Arteries (PLAC-II). Am J Cardiol 1995;75:455–459.

34. Barth JD. An update on carotid ultrasound measurement of intima-media thickness. Am J Cardiol 2002;89:32B–38B.

35. Adams MR, Nakagomi A, Keech A, et al. Carotid intima-media thickness is only weakly correlated with the extent and severity of coronary artery disease. Circulation 1995;92:2127–2134.

36. Li Z, Froehlich J, Galis ZS, Lakatta EG. Increased expression of matrix metalloproteinase-2 in the thickened intima of aged rats. Hypertension 1999;33:116–123.

37. Asai K, Kudej RK, Shen YT, et al. Peripheral vascular endothelial dysfunction and apoptosis in old monkeys. Arterioscler Thromb Vasc Biol 2000;20:1493–1499.

38. Homma S, Hirose N, Ishida H, Ishii T, Araki G. Carotid plaque and intima-media thickness assessed by b-mode ultrasonography in subjects ranging from young adults to centenarians. Stroke 2001;32:830–835.

39. Wendelhag I, Wiklund O, Wikstrand J. On quantifying plaque size and intima-media thickness in carotid and femoral arteries. Comments on results from a prospective ultrasound study in patients with familial hypercholesterolemia. Arterioscler Thromb Vasc Biol 1996;16:843–850.

40. Rosfors S, Hallerstam S, Jensen-Urstad K, Zetterling M, Carlstrom C. Relationship between intima-media thickness in the common carotid artery and atherosclerosis in the carotid bifurcation. Stroke 1998;29:1378–1382.

41. Zureik M, Ducimetiere P, Touboul PJ, et al. Common carotid intima-media thickness predicts occurrence of carotid atherosclerotic plaques: longitudinal results from the Aging Vascular Study (EVA) study. Arterioscler Thromb Vasc Biol 2000;20:1622–1629.

42. Kallikazaros IE, Tsioufis CP, Stefanadis CI, Pitsavos CE, Toutouzas PK. Closed relation between carotid and ascending aortic atherosclerosis in cardiac patients. Circulation 2000;102:III263–III268.

43. Burke GL, Evans GW, Riley WA, et al. Arterial wall thickness is associated with prevalent cardiovascular disease in middle-aged adults. The Atherosclerosis Risk in Communities (ARIC) Study. Stroke 1995;26:386–391.

44. Chambless LE, Folsom AR, Clegg LX, et al. Carotid wall thickness is predictive of incident clinical stroke: the Atherosclerosis Risk in Communities (ARIC) study. Am J Epidemiol 2000;151:478–487.

45. O'Leary DH, Polak JF, Kronmal RA, et al. Carotid-artery intima and media thickness as a risk factor for myocardial infarction and stroke in older adults. Cardiovascular Health Study Collaborative Research Group. N Engl J Med 1999;340: 14–22.

46. Aminbakhsh A, Mancini GB. Carotid intima-media thickness measurements: what defines an abnormality? A systematic review. Clin Invest Med 1999;22:149–157.

47. Scuteri A, Chen CH, Yin FC, et al. Functional correlates of central arterial geometric phenotypes. Hypertension 2001;38:1471–1475.
48. Scuteri A, Manolio TA, Marino EK, Arnold AM, Lakatta EG. Prevalence of specific variant carotid geometric patterns and incidence of cardiovascular events in older persons. The Cardiovascular Health Study (CHS E-131). J Am Coll Cardiol 2004;43:187–193.
49. Avolio AP, Chen SG, Wang RP, et al. Effects of aging on changing arterial compliance and left ventricular load in a northern Chinese urban community. Circulation 1983;68:50–58.
50. Smulyan H, Asmar RG, Rudnicki A, London GM, Safar ME. Comparative effects of aging in men and women on the properties of the arterial tree. J Am Coll Cardiol 2001;37:1374–1380.
51. Michel JB, Heudes D, Michel O, et al. Effect of chronic ANG I-converting enzyme inhibition on aging processes. II. Large arteries. Am J Physiol 1994;267:R124–135.
52. Fornieri C, Quaglino D Jr, Mori G. Role of the extracellular matrix in age-related modifications of the rat aorta. Ultrastructural, morphometric, and enzymatic evaluations. Arterioscler Thromb 1992;12:1008–1016.
53. Nichols WW, O'Rourke MF. Aging. In: Nichols WW, O'Rourke MF. (eds.), McDonald's Blood Flow in Arteries. Edward Arnold, London, 1998, pp. 378–395.
54. Sutton-Tyrrell K, Newman A, Simonsick EM, et al. Aortic stiffness is associated with visceral adiposity in older adults enrolled in the study of health, aging, and body composition. Hypertension 2001;38:429–433.
55. Asmar R, Rudnichi A, Blacher J, London GM, Safar ME. Pulse pressure and aortic pulse wave are markers of cardiovascular risk in hypertensive populations. Am J Hypertens 2001;14:91–97.
56. Mackey RH, Sutton-Tyrrell K, Vaitkevicius PV, et al. Correlates of aortic stiffness in elderly individuals: a subgroup of the Cardiovascular Health Study. Am J Hypertens 2002;15:16–23.
57. Safar ME, Blacher J, Pannier B, et al. Central pulse pressure and mortality in end-stage renal disease. Hypertension 2002;39:735–738.
58. Saeki A, Recchia F, Kass DA. systolic flow augmentation in hearts ejecting into a model of stiff aging vasculature. Influence on myocardial perfusion-demand balance. Circ Res 1995;76:132–141.
59. Liao D, Arnett DK, Tyroler HA, et al. Arterial stiffness and the development of hypertension. The ARIC study. Hypertension 1999;34:201–206.
60. Blacher J, Pannier B, Guerin AP, et al. Carotid arterial stiffness as a predictor of cardiovascular and all-cause mortality in end-stage renal disease. Hypertension 1998; 32:570–574.
61. Boutouyrie P, Tropeano AI, Asmar R, et al. Aortic stiffness is an independent predictor of primary coronary events in hypertensive patients: a longitudinal study. Hypertension 2002;39:10–15.
62. Laurent S, Boutouyrie P, Asmar R, et al. Aortic stiffness is an independent predictor of all-cause and cardiovascular mortality in hypertensive patients. Hypertension 2001;37:1236–1241.
63. Meaume S, Benetos A, Henry OF, Rudnichi A, Safar ME. Aortic pulse wave velocity predicts cardiovascular mortality in subjects >70 years of age. Arterioscler Thromb Vasc Biol 2001;21:2046–2050.
64. Blacher J, Guerin AP, Pannier B, et al. Impact of aortic stiffness on survival in end-stage renal disease. Circulation 1999;99:2434–2439.
65. de Simone G, Roman MJ, Koren MJ, et al. Stroke volume/pulse pressure ratio and cardiovascular risk in arterial hypertension. Hypertension 1999;33:800–805.

66. Blacher J, Asmar R, Djane S, London GM, Safar ME. Aortic pulse wave velocity as a marker of cardiovascular risk in hypertensive patients. Hypertension 1999;33: 1111–1117.
67. Shimokawa H. Primary endothelial dysfunction: atherosclerosis. J Mol Cell Cardiol 1999;31:23–37.
68. Goligorsky MS, Chen J, Brodsky S. Workshop: endothelial cell dysfunction leading to diabetic nephropathy: focus on nitric oxide. Hypertension 2001;37:744–748.
69. Boulanger CM. Secondary endothelial dysfunction: hypertension and heart failure. J Mol Cell Cardiol 1999;31:39–49.
70. McVeigh GE, Bratteli CW, Morgan DJ, et al. Age-related abnormalities in arterial compliance identified by pressure pulse contour analysis: aging and arterial compliance. Hypertension 1999;33:1392–1398.
71. McVeigh GE, Allen PB, Morgan DR, Hanratty CG, Silke B. Nitric oxide modulation of blood vessel tone identified by arterial waveform analysis. Clin Sci (Lond) 2001;100:387–393.
72. Kelly R, Hayward C, Avolio A, O'Rourke M. Noninvasive determination of age-related changes in the human arterial pulse. Circulation 1989;80:1652–1659.
73. Chen CH, Nevo E, Fetics B, et al. Estimation of central aortic pressure waveform by mathematical transformation of radial tonometry pressure. Validation of generalized transfer function. Circulation 1997;95:1827–1836.
74. Chen CH, Ting CT, Nussbacher A, et al. Validation of carotid artery tonometry as a means of estimating augmentation index of ascending aortic pressure. Hypertension 1996;27:168–175.
75. Cameron JD, McGrath BP, Dart AM. Use of radial artery applanation tonometry and a generalized transfer function to determine aortic pressure augmentation in subjects with treated hypertension. J Am Coll Cardiol 1998;32:1214–1220.
76. Murgo JP, Westerhof N, Giolma JP, Altobelli SA. Aortic input impedance in normal man: relationship to pressure wave forms. Circulation 1980;62:105–116.
77. Wilkinson IB, Prasad K, Hall IR, et al. Increased central pulse pressure and augmentation index in subjects with hypercholesterolemia. J Am Coll Cardiol 2002;39: 1005–1011.
78. McVeigh GE, Hamilton PK, Morgan DR. Evaluation of mechanical arterial properties: clinical, experimental and therapeutic aspects. Clin Sci (Lond) 2002;102:51–67.
79. O'Rourke MF. Towards optimization of wave reflection: therapeutic goal for tomorrow? Clin Exp Pharmacol Physiol 1996;23:S11–S15.
80. London GM, Blacher J, Pannier B, et al. Arterial wave reflections and survival in end-stage renal failure. Hypertension 2001;38:434–438.
81. Dart AM, Kingwell BA. Pulse pressure—a review of mechanisms and clinical relevance. J Am Coll Cardiol 2001;37:975–984.
82. Darne B, Girerd X, Safar M, Cambien F, Guize L. Pulsatile versus steady component of blood pressure: a cross-sectional analysis and a prospective analysis on cardiovascular mortality. Hypertension 1989;13:392–400.
83. Madhavan S, Ooi WL, Cohen H, Alderman MH. Relation of pulse pressure and blood pressure reduction to the incidence of myocardial infarction. Hypertension 1994;23:395–401.
84. Mitchell GF, Moye LA, Braunwald E, et al. Sphygmomanometrically determined pulse pressure is a powerful independent predictor of recurrent events after myocardial infarction in patients with impaired left ventricular function. SAVE investigators. Survival and Ventricular Enlargement. Circulation 1997;96:4254–4260.
85. Chae CU, Pfeffer MA, Glynn RJ, et al. Increased pulse pressure and risk of heart failure in the elderly. JAMA 1999;281:634–639.

86. Domanski MJ, Sutton-Tyrrell K, Mitchell GF, et al. Determinants and prognostic information provided by pulse pressure in patients with coronary artery disease undergoing revascularization. The Balloon Angioplasty Revascularization Investigation (BARI). Am J Cardiol 2001;87:675–679.

87. Franklin SS, Khan SA, Wong ND, Larson MG, Levy D. Is pulse pressure useful in predicting risk for coronary heart Disease? The Framingham heart study. Circulation 1999;100:354–360.

88. Millar JA, Lever AF, Burke V. Pulse pressure as a risk factor for cardiovascular events in the MRC Mild Hypertension Trial. J Hypertens 1999;17:1065–1072.

89. Domanski MJ, Davis BR, Pfeffer MA, Kastantin M, Mitchell GF. Isolated systolic hypertension: prognostic information provided by pulse pressure. Hypertension 1999;34:375–380.

90. Benetos A, Gautier S, Lafleche A, et al. Blockade of angiotensin II type 1 receptors: effect on carotid and radial artery structure and function in hypertensive humans. J Vasc Res 2000;37:8–15.

91. Glynn RJ, Chae CU, Guralnik JM, Taylor JO, Hennekens CH. Pulse pressure and mortality in older people. Arch Intern Med 2000;160:2765–2772.

92. Sesso HD, Stampfer MJ, Rosner B, et al. Systolic and diastolic blood pressure, pulse pressure, and mean arterial pressure as predictors of cardiovascular disease risk in men. Hypertension 2000;36:801–807.

93. Fang J, Madhavan S, Alderman MH. Pulse pressure: a predictor of cardiovascular mortality among young normotensive subjects. Blood Press 2000;9:260–266.

94. Domanski M, Norman J, Wolz M, Mitchell G, Pfeffer M. Cardiovascular risk assessment using pulse pressure in the first national health and nutrition examination survey (NHANES I). Hypertension 2001;38:793–797.

95. Fagard RH, Pardaens K, Staessen JA, Thijs L. The pulse pressure-to-stroke index ratio predicts cardiovascular events and death in uncomplicated hypertension. J Am Coll Cardiol 2001;38:227–231.

96. Domanski MJ, Mitchell GF, Norman JE, et al. Independent prognostic information provided by sphygmomanometrically determined pulse pressure and mean arterial pressure in patients with left ventricular dysfunction. J Am Coll Cardiol 1999;33: 951–958.

97. Neutel JM. Beyond the sphygmomanometric numbers: hypertension as a syndrome. Am J Hypertens 2001;14:250S–257S.

98. Guerin AP, Blacher J, Pannier B, et al. Impact of aortic stiffness attenuation on survival of patients in end-stage renal failure. Circulation 2001;103:987–992.

99. Salomaa V, Riley W, Kark JD, Nardo C, Folsom AR. Non-insulin-dependent diabetes mellitus and fasting glucose and insulin concentrations are associated with arterial stiffness indexes. The ARIC Study. Atherosclerosis Risk in Communities Study. Circulation 1995;91:1432–1443.

100. Lambert J, Smulders RA, Aarsen M, Donker AJ, Stehouwer CD. Carotid artery stiffness is increased in microalbuminuric IDDM patients. Diabetes Care 1998;21: 99–103.

101. Aoun S, Blacher J, Safar ME, Mourad JJ. Diabetes mellitus and renal failure: effects on large artery stiffness. J Hum Hypertens 2001;15:693–700.

102. Bella JN, Devereux RB, Roman MJ, et al. Separate and joint effects of systemic hypertension and diabetes mellitus on left ventricular structure and function in American Indians (the Strong Heart Study). Am J Cardiol 2001;87:1260–1265.

103. Scuteri A, Najjar SS, Muller DC, et al. Metabolic syndrome amplifies the age-associated increases in vascular thickness and stiffness. J Am Coll Cardiol; 2004; 63:1388–1395.

104. Anderson TJ. Assessment and treatment of endothelial dysfunction in humans. J Am Coll Cardiol 1999;34:631–638.
105. Toborek M, Kaiser S. Endothelial cell functions. Relationship to atherogenesis. Basic Res Cardiol 1999;94:295–314.
106. Vane JR, Anggard EE, Botting RM. Regulatory functions of the vascular endothelium. N Engl J Med 1990;323:27–36.
107. Gimbrone MA. Vascular endothelium, hemodynamic forces, and atherogenesis. AJP 1999;155:1–5.
108. Chauhan A, More RS, Mullins PA, et al. Aging-associated endothelial dysfunction in humans is reversed by L-arginine. J Am Coll Cardiol 1996;28:1796–1804.
109. Taddei S, Virdis A, Mattei P, et al. Aging and endothelial function in normotensive subjects and patients with essential hypertension. Circulation 1995;91:1981–1987.
110. Hongo K, Nakagomi T, Kassell NF, et al. Effects of aging and hypertension on endothelium-dependent vascular relaxation in rat carotid artery. Stroke 1988;19:892–897.
111. Cernadas MR, Sanchez de Miguel L, Garcia-Duran M, et al. Expression of constitutive and inducible nitric oxide synthases in the vascular wall of young and aging rats. Circ Res 1998;83:279–286.
112. Orlandi A, Marcellini M, Spagnoli LG. Aging influences development and progression of early aortic atherosclerotic lesions in cholesterol-fed rabbits. Arterioscler Thromb Vasc Biol 2000;20:1123–1136.
113. Csiszar A, Ungvari Z, Edwards JG, Kaminski P, Wolin MS, Koller A, Kaley G. Aging-induced phenotypic changes and oxidative stress impair coronary arteriolar function. Circ Res. 2002;90:1159–1166.
114. Ross R. Atherosclerosis—an inflammatory disease. N Engl J Med 1999;340:115–126.
115. Romanic AM, Madri JA. T cell adhesion to endothelial cells and extracellular matrix is modulated upon transendothelial cell migration. Lab Invest 1997;76:11–23.
116. Amorino GP, Hoover RL. Interactions of monocytic cells with human endothelial cells stimulate monocytic metalloproteinase production. Am J Pathol 1998;152:199–207.
117. Rosenberg GA, Estrada EY, Dencoff JE. Matrix metalloproteinases and TIMPs are associated with blood–brain barrier opening after reperfusion in rat brain. Stroke 1998;29:2189–2195.
118. Blann AD, Daly RJ, Amiral J. The influence of age, gender and ABO blood group on soluble endothelial cell markers and adhesion molecules. Br J Haematol 1996; 92:498–500.
119. Morisaki N, Saito I, Tamura K, et al. New indices of ischemic heart disease and aging: studies on the serum levels of soluble intercellular adhesion molecule-1 (ICAM-1) and soluble vascular cell adhesion molecule-1 (VCAM-1) in patients with hypercholes-terolemia and ischemic heart disease. Atherosclerosis 1997;131:43–48.
120. Belmin J, Corman B, Merval R, Tedgui A. Age-related changes in endothelial permeability and distribution volume of albumin in rat aorta. Am J Physiol 1993;264 (3 Pt 2):H679–H685.
121. Wight TN. Cell biology of arterial proteoglycans. Arteriosclerosis 1989;9:1–20.
122. Bingley JA, Hayward IP, Campbell GR, Campbell JH. Relationship of glycosaminoglycan and matrix changes to vascular smooth muscle cell phenotype modulation in rabbit arteries after acute injury. J Vasc Surg 2001;33:155–164.
123. Malek AM, Alper SL, Izumo S. Hemodynamic shear stress and its role in atherosclerosis. JAMA 1999;282:2035–2042.
124. Weng NP, Hodes RJ. The role of telomerase expression and telomere length maintenance in human and mouse. J Clin Immunol 2000;20:257–267.

125. Harley CB, Futcher AB, Greider CW. Telomeres shorten during ageing of human fibroblasts. Nature 1990;345:458–460.
126. Chang E, Harley CB. Telomere length and replicative aging in human vascular tissues. Proc Natl Acad Sci USA 1995;92:11190–11194.
127. Aviv H, Khan MY, Skurnick J, et al. Age dependent aneuploidy and telomere length of the human vascular endothelium. Atherosclerosis 2001;159:281–287.
128. Okuda K, Khan MY, Skurnick J, et al. Telomere attrition of the human abdominal aorta: relationships with age and atherosclerosis. Atherosclerosis 2000;152:391–398.
129. Jeanclos E, Schork NJ, Kyvik KO, et al. Telomere length inversely correlates with pulse pressure and is highly familial. Hypertension 2000;36:195–200.
130. Benetos A, Okuda K, Lajemi M, et al. Telomere length as an indicator of biological aging: the gender effect and relation with pulse pressure and pulse wave velocity. Hypertension 2001;37:381–385.
131. Minamino T, Miyauchi H, Yoshida T, et al. Endothelial cell senescence in human atherosclerosis: role of telomere in endothelial dysfunction. Circulation 2002;105:1541–1544.
132. Rivard A, Fabre JE, Silver M, et al. Age-dependent impairment of angiogenesis. Circulation 1999;99:111–120.
133. Rauscher FM, Goldschmidt-Clermont PJ, Davis BH, et al. Aging, progenitor cell exhaustion, and atherosclerosis. Circulation 2003;108:457–463.
134. Reed MJ, Corsa AC, Kudravi SA, McCormick RS, Arthur WT. A deficit in collagenase activity contributes to impaired migration of aged microvascular endothelial cells. J Cell Biochem 2000;77:116–126.
135. Reed MJ, Corsa A, Pendergrass W, et al. Neovascularization in aged mice: delayed angiogenesis is coincident with decreased levels of transforming growth factor beta1 and type I collagen. Am J Pathol 1998;152:113–123.
136. Treins C, Giorgetti-Peraldi S, Murdaca J, Van Obberghen E. Regulation of vascular endothelial growth factor expression by advanced glycation end products. J Biol Chem 2001;276:43836–43841.
137. Zureik M, Touboul PJ, Bonithon-Kopp C, et al. Cross-sectional and 4-year longitudinal associations between brachial pulse pressure and common carotid intima-media thickness in a general population. The EVA study. Stroke 1999;30:550–555.
138. Talbot LA, Metter EJ, Fleg JL. Leisure-time physical activities and their relationship to cardiorespiratory fitness in healthy men and women 18–95 years old. Med Sci Sports Exer 2000;32:417–425.
139. Schulman SP, Fleg JL, Goldberg AP, et al. Continuum of cardiovascular performance across a broad range of fitness levels in healthy older men. Circulation 1996;94:359–367.
140. Tanaka H, DeSouza CA, Seals DR. Absence of age-related increase in central arterial stiffness in physically active women. Arterioscler Thromb Vasc Biol 1998;18:127–132.
141. Hunt BE, Farquhar WB, Taylor JA. Does reduced vascular stiffening fully explain preserved cardiovagal baroreflex function in older, physically active men? Circulation 2001;103:2424–2427.
142. Rywik TM, Blackman R, Yataco AR, et al. Enhanced endothelial vasoreactivity in endurance trained older men. J Appl Physiol 1999;87:2136–2142.
143. Avolio AP, Clyde KM, Beard TC, et al. Improved arterial distensibility in normotensive subjects on a low salt diet. Arteriosclerosis 1986;6:166–169.
144. Chen C-H, Nakayama M, Talbot M, et al. Verapamil acutely reduces ventricular vascular stiffening and improves aeerobic exercise performance in elderly individuals. J Am Coll Cardiol 1999;33:1602–1609.

145. Vaitkevicius PV, Lane M, Spurgeon H, et al. A cross-link breaker has sustained effects on arterial and ventricular properties in older rhesus monkeys. Proc Natl Acad Sci USA 2001;98:1171–1175.
146. Kass DA, Shapiro EP, Kawaguchi M, Capriotti AR, Scuteri A, deGroof RC, Lakatta EG. Improved arterial compliance by a novel advanced glycation end-product cross-link breaker. Circ 2001;104:1464–1470.
147. Levy BI, Michel JB, Salzmann JL, et al. Remodeling of heart and arteries by chronic converting enzyme inhibition in spontaneously hypertensive rats. Am J Hypertension 1991;4:240S–245S.
148. Gonzalez Bosc LV, Kurnjek ML, Muller A, Terragno NA, Basso N. Effect of chronic angiotensin II inhibition on the nitric oxide synthase in the normal rat during aging. J Hyperten 2001;19:1403–1409.
149. Moon S-K, Thompson LJ, Madamanchi N, et al. Aging, oxidative responses, and proliferative capacity in cultured mouse aortic smooth muscle cells. Am J Physiol Circ Physiol 2001;280:H2779–2788.
150. DeCavanagh EM, Fraga CG, Ferder L, Inserra F. Enalapril and captopril enhance antioxidant defenses in mouse tissues. Am J Physiol 1997;272:R514–518.
151. Inserra F, Romano L, Ercole L, deCavanagh EMV, Ferder L. Cardiovascular changes by long-term inhibition of the rennin-angiotensin system in aging. Hypertension 1995;25:437–442.
152. Ferder L, Romano LA, Ercole LB, Stella I, Inserra F. Biomolecular changes in the aging myocardium. The effect of enalapril. Am J Hyperten 1998;11:1297–1304.
153. Ferder LF, Inserra F, Basso N. Advances in our understanding of aging: role of the rennin-angiotensin system. Curr Opin Pharmacol 2002;2:189–194.
154. Alder A, Messina E, Sherman B, et al. NAD(P)H oxidase-generated superoxide anion accounts for reduced control of myocardial O2 consumption by NO inold Fisher 344 rats. Am J Physiol 2003;285:H1015–1022.
155. Benetos A, Zureik M, Morcet J, et al. A decrease in diastolic blood pressure combined with an increase in systolic blood pressure is associated with a higher cardiovascular mortality in men. J Am Coll Cardiol 2000;35:673–680.
156. Girerd X, Giannattasio C, Moulin C, et al. Regression of radial artery wall hypertrophy and improvement of carotid artery compliance after long-term antihypertensive treatment in elderly patients. J Am Coll Cardiol 1998;31:1064–1073.
157. Dart AM, Reid CM, McGrath B. Effects of ACE inhibitor therapy on derived central arterial waveforms in hypertension. Am J Hypertens 2001;14:804–810.
158. Kahonen M, Ylitalo R, Koobi T, Turjanmaa V, Ylitalo P. Influences of nonselective, beta(1)-selective and vasodilatory beta(1)-selective beta-blockers on arterial pulse wave velocity in normotensive subjects. Gen Pharmacol 2000;35:219–224.
159. Asmar RG, London GM, O'Rourke ME, Safar ME. Improvement in blood pressure, arterial stiffness and wave reflections with a very-low-dose perindopril/indapamide combination in hypertensive patient: a comparison with atenolol. Hypertension 2001;38:922–926.
160. Schulman SP, Lakatta EG, Fleg JL, et al. Age-related decline in left-ventricular filling at rest and exercise. Am J Physiol 1992;263:H1932–1938.
161. Fleg JL, Schulman SP, O'Connor F, et al. Effects of acute beta-adrenergic receptor blockade on age-associated changes in cardiovascular performance during dynamic exercise. Circulation 1994;90:2333.
162. Najjar SS, Schulman SP, Gerstenblith G, et al. Age and gender affect ventricular-vascular coupling during aerobic exercise. J Am Coll Cardiol 2004;44:611–617.
163. Nussbacher A, Gerstenblith G, O'Connor GC, et al. Hemodynamic effects of unloading the old heart. Am J Physiol 1999;277:H1863–1871.

2

Frailty

*Keystone in the Bridge
between Geriatrics and Cardiology*

William Russell Hazzard, MD

The 20th century witnessed an historical change in the landscape of human evolution as the limits of human longevity pressed ever upward in advanced cultures. At the outset of the 20th century, average longevity in America barely exceeded 48 years and only 3% of the population was over the age of 65. This reflected the underdeveloped status of our nation at that time, when public health measures were minimal, nutrition, hygiene,

From: *Contemporary Cardiology: Cardiovascular Disease in the Elderly*
Edited by: G. Gerstenblith © Humana Press Inc., Totowa, NJ

housing, and sanitation precarious, antibiotics unknown, childhood deaths from infectious diseases were frequent, and death from chronic diseases in old age uncommon. However, by the end of 20th century the picture had changed dramatically. Average American longevity exceeded 75 years, childhood deaths had declined precipitously, and survival to middle and even old age had become the norm. Now early in the 21st century, American society and the American health care system in particular is at a crossroads between opportunity and crisis: on the one hand, the prospect of extending average human longevity to its maximum draws near (85 ± 7 years has been suggested as our "barrier to immortality" [1]); on the other hand, the physician's image of their typical patient 85 or older raises the specter of an impending epidemic of sick, vulnerable, and disabled old people, frail patients who will require extraordinary levels of health and social care. This looms as a defining feature of the 21st century as members of the current wave of Americans born in the post-World War II era approach old age over the next half century: will American society become overwhelmed by the needs of aged, frail, and dependent "baby-boomers" in gradual decline, or will effective preventative public health and medical interventions succeed in prolonging their robust health and independence into advanced old age, ideally compressing their illnesses and dependency into a brief period before death?

Nowhere is the urgency to resolve this approaching dilemma more pressing than in the field of cardiovascular disease (CVD). CVD as the primary cause of death accounts for nearly half (approximately 46%) of deaths throughout middle and old age, cardiac deaths rising logarithmically with age in parallel with all-cause mortality. The prospect of facing a tsunami of aging baby-boomers who develop CVD and disability in their 70s, 80s, and 90s has spawned a new subfield, geriatric cardiology (the central subject of this entire volume). Here, as in all subspecialties of adult medicine, the special nuances of geriatrics have emerged as a focus for cardiology as it struggles to prepare for the impending surge of elderly patients in their domain.

A phenomenon of special interest to geriatricians and cardiologists (and geriatric cardiologists in particular) is the syndrome of frailty. This condition is highly prevalent among the elderly, especially the "oldest old" (those above 85). Yet it remains but vaguely defined and is often mistakenly applied interchangeably with co-morbidity and disability. This chapter is designed to persuade the critical reader that careful consideration of this syndrome as increasingly better characterized and investigated perhaps best captures the essence of the field of geriatrics and notably geriatric cardiology. Thus, systematic, serious, and critical research on the definition, diagnosis, pathophysiology, prevention, presentation, and management of this syndrome should advance the characterization of frailty well beyond its long-time status as, "You know when you see it," and the fatalistic, even nihilistic attitude that such dismissive assignment invites.

FRAILTY:
THE DEFINITION EMERGING FROM EPIDEMIOLOGY

The fields of geriatrics and chronic disease management have long struggled for a meaningful definition of "frailty" and the related condition "failure to thrive." This phenomenon is the subject of an elegant chapter by Linda Fried and Jeremy Walston in the recent, fifth edition of the *Principles of Geriatric Medicine and Gerontology (2)*. These authors suggest that frailty and failure to thrive "represent a continuum of a clinical syndrome, with Failure to Thrive being the most extreme manifestation that is associated with a low rate of recovery and presages death." In their treatise, they detail the definition and the pathophysiology of frailty, carefully dissecting its component parts before reintegrating them into a construct that comprises a complex web of the pathogenesis and clinical manifestation of this syndrome (Fig. 1).

The scientific underpinning for their definition of this syndrome has been strengthened by a series of publications from the Cardiovascular Health Study (CHS) from which the definition of frailty is largely derived *(3)*. This was a prospective, observational, community-based epidemiological study of men and women 65 years of age or older in four US communities: Sacramento County, California; Washington County, Maryland; Forsyth County, North Carolina; Allegheny County, Pennsylvania (N = 5201). This was initiated in 1989–1990, with an additional cohort of 687 African-American men and women recruited in 1992–1993 from three of these sites. Participants were recruited from age- and gender-stratified samples from the Health Care Financing Administration Medicare eligibility lists in those counties. Both cohorts received identical baseline evaluations (except for the absence of spirometry and echocardiogram at baseline in the latter cohort) and follow-up with annual in-person examinations and semi-annual telephone calls for surveillance of outcomes, including disease, hospitalization, falls, disability, and mortality.

Baseline evaluations included standardized interviews that ascertained demographics, self-assessed health, health habits, weight loss, medications used, and self-reported physician-diagnosed CVD, emphysema, asthma, diabetes, arthritis, renal disease, cancer, and hearing and visual impairment. Leisure-time activities were determined by administration of a version of the Minnesota Leisure Time Activities Questionnaire cover-

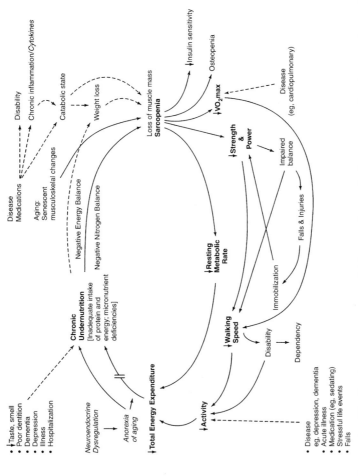

Fig. 1. The complex cycle of frailty: key components of this negative cycle that generate its phenotypic manifestations are chronic undernutrition; sarcopenia; decreases in strength, power, and exercise tolerance; and declines in activity and total energy expenditure. Factors that could precipitate or exacerbate this core cycle are indicated with dashed lines. Factors in which a relationship is hypothesized are indicated in italics. (Reproduced from ref. 2 with permission of The McGraw-Hill Companies.)

ing the 2 weeks prior to study involvement. Physical function was assessed by asking about difficulty with 15 tasks of daily life, including mobility, upper extremity function, instrumental activities of daily living (IADL) and activities of daily living (ADL). Frequency of falls during the prior 6 months was assessed by self-report. The modified 10-item Center for Epidemiological Study–Depression scale (CES–D) was used to ascertain depressive symptoms.

The presence of significant co-morbidities was also determined. These included cardiovascular diseases (myocardial infarction [MI], congestive heart failure [CHF], angina, peripheral vascular disease, and stroke). The presence of co-morbidities was validated by medications used and through standardized examinations, including echocardiogram, and the posterior tibial/brachial artery systolic (ankle-arm) blood pressure (BP) ratio. Medical records were reviewed by clinicians for consensus-based adjudication based on standardized algorithms. Other examinations measured weight, BP, maximal stenosis of internal and common carotid arteries by carotid ultrasound, and fasting blood analyses for glucose, albumin, creatinine, and fibrinogen, plus lipid analyses, with low-density lipoprotein (LDL) cholesterol estimated by calculation from total and high-density lipoprotein (HDL) cholesterol and triglyceride levels. Additional serum samples were stored for future analyses, which have notably included C-reactive protein (CRP). Cognitive function was assessed with Mini-Mental State Examination (MMSE) and the digit symbol substitution test. Standardized performance-based measures of physical function included time (in seconds) to walk 15 feet at usual pace and maximal grip strength (in kilograms) in the dominant hand using a hand-held dynamometer.

For this study, the investigators defined frailty as "a biologic syndrome of decreased reserve and resistance to stressors resulting from a cumulative decline across multiple physiologic systems, and causing vulnerability to adverse outcomes." They operationalized this definition of a frailty phenotype in the CHS according to the following criteria:

1. Shrinking: unintentional weight loss, of 10 pounds or more in the past year or, at follow-up, of at least 5% of body weight in the prior year (by direct measurement).
2. Weakness: grip strength in the lowest 20% (quintile) at baseline, adjusted for gender and body mass index.
3. Poor endurance and energy: as indicated by self-report of exhaustion, identified by two questions from the CES-D scale and associated staged exercise testing as indicator of VO_2 max.
4. Slowness: the slowest quintile of the study population, based on time to walk 15 feet, adjusting for gender and standing height.

5. Low physical activity: a weighted score of kilocalories expended per week, based on each participant's self-report, in the lowest quintile of physical activities specific to gender.

In this study, frailty was defined by the presence of three or more of these criteria. "Pre-frailty" was assigned to those participants with one or two of these attributes.

Because of possible confounding, subjects were excluded from the data analysis if they were significantly demented (with an MMSE of 18 or less) or were taking sinemet, donazepil, or antidepressants.

The 5317 people evaluated ranged from 65 to 100 years of age; 58% were female; 15% were African-American. At baseline, 7% of the cohort qualified for assignment of the frailty phenotype, 47% were pre-frail, and 46% met none of the five criteria. The prevalence of frailty increased with each advancing 5-year age group and was up to twofold higher for women than men, especially below age 80. African-Americans, especially women, had twice the prevalence of frailty as their non-African-American counterparts.

Analyses by Cox proportional hazard model models assessed the independent contribution of baseline status to major outcomes occurring over 3 and 7 years (for the two cohorts), specifically including incident frailty (including conversion from pre-frailty), falls, worsening mobility, ADL function, hospitalization, and death. Covariates were selected based on analysis of the first cohort. External validation using the second cohort showed agreement with results from the first.

In the first cohort, the 3-year incidence of frailty was 7%, with an additional 7% for the following 4 years. The second cohort (of African-American) had a 4-year frailty incidence rate of 11%. Other covariates of frailty included lower education, lower income, poorer health, and higher rates of co-morbid chronic diseases and disability. Specifically, those who became frail had significantly higher rates of CVD and pulmonary disease, arthritis, and diabetes, whereas there was no significant difference in cancer between those who became frail and those who did not. Both lower cognition and greater depressive symptomatology were associated with frailty (even after exclusion of those with MMSE <18 or who were on antidepressants at baseline).

At baseline, there was also a strong association between the frailty phenotype and self-reported disability, which was present in 76%: 72% reported difficulty in mobility tasks; 60% had difficulty with IADLs, whereas only 27% of those had difficulty in ADLs. Increasing disability paralleled increasing frailty in stepwise fashion. Viewed from a different perspective, however, among those with difficulty with ADLs, only

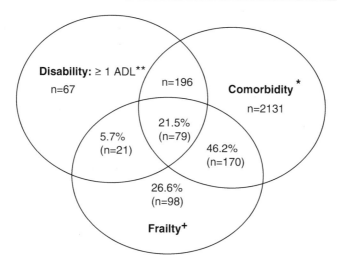

Fig. 2. Venn diagram of the relationships among frailty, disability (in activities of daily living [ADL]), and comorbidity (two or more diseases; myocardial infarction, angina, congestive heart failure, claudication, arthritis, cancer, diabetes, hypertension, chronic obstructive pulmonary disorder) in 2762 subjects in the Cardiovascular Health Study (CHS). (From ref. 3. Copyright © The Gerontological Society of America. Reproduced by permission of the publisher.)

28% were in the frail group. Thus, (Fig. 2) whereas there was substantial overlap among the three related states—disability, frailty, and co-morbidity—those domains were by no means congruent, and 26.6% of those with the phenotype of frailty reported neither disability nor co-morbidity (whereas 21.5% manifested all three concurrently).

Frailty has been widely considered clinically to predict adverse outcomes. This prediction was borne out in the CHS. Among those who met the criteria for frailty at baseline, mortality was increased by sixfold for the first 3 years and more than threefold for 7-year survival (compared with those who met none of the five criteria) (Fig. 3). After 7 years, 43% of those who were frail at baseline had died, compared to 23% of those in the intermediate category and but 12% of those in the non-frail group. Additional increases associated with baseline frailty included risk of first hospitalization (96%), first fall (41%), worsening ADL disability (63%), and worsening mobility disability (71%). In each category those who were frail experienced significantly ($p < 0.0001$) greater risk of developing the condition, with those in the intermediate category at intermediate risk. Finally, those in the intermediate group at baseline had a 4.51-fold (95% confidence interval [CI] 3.39-6.00) risk of converting to the

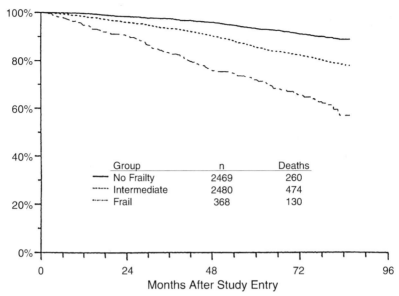

Fig. 3. Survival curve estimates (unadjusted) over 72 months of follow-up from both cohorts of the Cardiovascular Health Study by frailty status at baseline: frail (three or more criteria met); intermediate (one or two criteria met); not frail (no criteria met). (From ref. 3. Copyright © The Gerontological Society of America. Reproduced by permission of the publisher.)

frailty phenotype over the ensuing 3 years (reduced to 2.63 [1.94, 3.56] when adjusted for the co-variates of age, gender, minority status, income, smoking, brachial and tibial BP, fasting glucose, albumin, creatinine, carotid stenosis, history of CHF, cognitive function, major electrocardiogram [EKG] abnormality, use of diuretics, problems with IADLs, self-report health measures, and CES-D), relative to those in the non-frail category.

The gender-specific plight of aging women was highlighted by this study. However, whether the substantially increased risk of frailty in older women related to their lower lean body mass compared with their male counterparts or the possibility of inadequate nutrition related to living alone (or other especially prevalent female gender risks) remains a subject of speculation.

This landmark epidemiological study provides important new insights into the etiology and pathogenesis of the frailty syndrome. First, in this study frailty was strongly associated with several major chronic diseases, notably CVD, pulmonary disease, and diabetes, suggesting a possible common pathophysiological link between frailty and these disorders. However, these associations appeared to be additive: there was a greater likelihood of frailty when two or more such diseases were present than with any single one. On the other hand, the observation that a substantial subset of those who were frail reported none of those co-morbid diseases suggests perhaps two major, alternative pathways to frailty: one reflecting physiological changes of aging not related to the pathogenesis or below the threshold for diagnosis of specific diseases (e.g., aging-related sarcopenia) and the other a final common pathway of specific co-morbid diseases as more conventionally defined.

All in all this landmark study provides strong consideration of frailty as perhaps the defining syndrome of the discipline of geriatrics. The principal limitations of this study lay perhaps in the restriction of its participants to those without limitations that would preclude their living in the community as well as those with major cognitive, affective or parkinsonian disorders, a substantial proportion of those in the patient panels of geriatricians, who might well consider them frail *(4)*.

Nevertheless, this paper from the CHS by Fried et al. *(2)* especially challenges investigators to unravel the relative contributions of aging *per se* vs the development of age-associated diseases in the pathogenesis of the frailty syndrome. Moreover, it highlights the importance of developing effective strategies wherever possible to retard or reverse the downhill course leading to frailty and, at its extreme, failure to thrive. Thus, this study significantly advances definition of the clinical syndrome of frailty—including its diagnosis in a medical sense—and its associated symptoms, signs, and associated risks of adverse outcomes.

CARDIOVASCULAR DISEASE
IN THE CARDIOVASCULAR HEALTH STUDY

Given the prominent role of CVD in the aggregate burden of morbidity and mortality in the elderly, it was not surprising that CVD, both clinical and subclinical, was strongly correlated with frailty as defined in the CHS. Here the report from the CHS by Newman et al. *(5)* offers special insight. They hypothesized that the severity of frailty among subjects in this study would be related to the higher prevalence among the frail of self-reported CVD as well a greater extent of CVD as determined by standard clinical and subclinical noninvasive testing. This prediction was borne out by their analysis of the data, especially the risk of CHF in those with frailty (odds ratio [OR] 7.51, 95% CI 4.66-12.12). Furthermore, among those without a history of clinical CVD, frailty was positively asso-

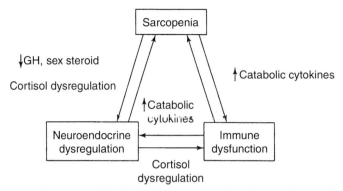

Fig. 4. Age-related physiological changes central to the syndrome of frailty. These comprise much of the basis of the poor response to stressors and vulnerability of frail persons. GH, growth hormone. (Reproduced from ref. *2* with permission of The McGraw-Hill Companies.)

ciated with several noninvasive indices of CVD: carotid stenosis greater than 75% (OR = 3.41), ankle-arm BP index less than 0.8 (OR = 3.17), major EKG abnormalities (OR = 1.58), increased left ventricular mass by echocardiography (1.16), and a higher prevalence of infarct-like lesions in the brain (OR = 1.71). Univariate analysis established significant associations between frailty and MI, angina, and claudication as well as with any CVD; on the other hand associations with transient ischemic attack, bypass surgery, and angioplasty did not reach criteria for statistical significance. Thus, whereas overt CVD was clearly associated with a higher prevalence of frailty, so was evidence of subclinical CVD in this aging cohort. This reinforces not only the centrality of CVD in its association with frailty but also perhaps shared pathophysiology in the genesis of CVD and frailty in this aging cohort.

PATHOGENESIS OF FRAILTY

Despite the prominence of CVD as well as the many other acute and chronic diseases that are so prevalent among the elderly in those defined as frail in this construct, by themselves these diseases constitute only a portion of the complex scheme depicted by Fried and Walston *(2)* as a summary of the pathogenesis of frailty (Fig. 1). In this scheme, these authors focus on three principal elements of age-related physiological changes that are central to the pathogenesis of frailty: sarcopenia (low muscle mass), neuroendocrine dysregulation, and immune dysfunction (Fig. 4).

Lean body mass—bone, muscle, other connective tissue, and major non-adipose organs—declines incrementally with advancing age, beginning on average at approximately age 35 and progressing with the passage of time to the point where, especially in those with frailty, up to 50% of lean body mass is lost (principally skeletal muscle), replaced wholly or in part by fibrotic and/or adipose tissue. Prior to old age, this decline is typically largely masked by the progressive accretion of adipose tissue as total body weight increases throughout middle age and into early old age, adiposity thought in large part to mediate the increased incidence of dyslipidemia, hypertension, and ultimately diabetes with advancing age, all consequences of the increased resistance to insulin conferred by obesity and in turn central to the pathogenesis of the metabolic syndrome and its CVD consequences that are so common in the older population. Generally in late middle age, the loss of lean body mass becomes balanced by the accretion of adipose tissue and total body mass stabilizes (typically beyond age 50 in men and age 60 in women). Ultimately, especially in old age (>75 or 80) net weight loss occurs with the incipient development, advent, and progression of frailty and the loss of both lean and fat mass as a cardinal feature of the syndrome. This catabolic spiral may be mediated by the loss of anabolic hormones, notably growth hormone (GH) and insulin-like growth factor (IGF)-1, as well as estrogen and androgen, that accompany both the aging process and the diseases of old age that perpetuate and accelerate this decline.

Ultimately, the major loss of muscle mass, defined as sarcopenia, profoundly limits functional capacity, especially in those in the oldest age group. This leads to decreased exercise (and energy expenditure), weakness and fatigue, and diminished ability to perform many ADLs, all features or strong correlates of the frailty syndrome. Other vulnerabilities also proceed from declining muscle mass; notably poor balance, slow gait, and increased risk of falls. Accompanying this decline in lean body mass is a progressive decrease in VO_2 max, which reflects both the decline in physical activity that is normative with advancing age in our society and, at a more basic level, the loss of lean body mass and its higher per kilogram basal energy metabolism that accompanies the aging process. This decreased energy expenditure is met with decreasing appetite (aggravated by the anorexia of aging and especially inflammation when present), which renders the elderly person vulnerable to both macro- and micro-nutrient deficiency, progressive weight loss and sarcopenia in a vicious spiral of decline. All of these changes contribute to the sharp decrease in exercise tolerance among older persons, particularly those who are pre-frail or frankly frail. The loss of lean body mass also contributes to the decreased tolerance to fluctuations in environmental temperatures of both heat and cold experienced by older, thinner individuals.

A second limb of this frailty scheme relates to the immune dysfunction that accompanies the aging process. This includes increased vulnerability to infections as reflected in the aging organism's diminished ability to generate T-cell proliferation in response to antigenic stimulation and the reduced ability of such T-cells to secrete interleukin (IL)-2, essential to developing appropriate hypersensitivity responses, generating cytotoxic cells, stimulating B-cell proliferation and, in turn, mounting adequate humoral immunity. As noted, this immune deficiency is also aggravated by nutritional deficiency in which inflammation often plays a central role.

Thus, an essential contribution of immune dysregulation in the genesis of frailty is suggested. This dysregulation extends to impaired maintenance of the optimal balance between pro- and anti-inflammatory forces. This has in turn generated a leading hypothesis of the pathogenesis of frailty that strongly connects CVD with frailty. This reflects the prominence of inflammation in many of the major CVDs that are so common in the elderly as well as in a general tilt of the balance toward pro-inflammation with aging, generating an increased basal degree of immune activation detectable in those destined to become frail long before they qualify for the diagnosis of frailty.

The third arm of the major triad operative in the pathophysiology of frailty emphasized by Fried and Walston focuses on the neuroendocrine dysregulation associated with aging. This includes progressive dysfunction at multiple key points of neuroendocrine regulation, including a decline with aging in the extent of the very complexity that characterizes optimal physiological control. This notably includes changes in the cardiovascular system, in which the normal and perhaps optimal variation in such parameters as the cardiac cycle declines with advancing age, for example, with loss of "sinus arrhythmia, part of the pattern of "homeostenosis" or reduced homeostatic response to environmental or internal perturbations that characterizes aging. This in turn leads to increased vulnerability of aging persons to functional impairment, a reflection of their diminished ability to response to normal stimuli and a sluggish negative feedback system.

Related to this diminished physiological complexity is increased vulnerability to stressors of a neuroendocrine nature. These include responses to physical danger, psychological distress, and pain. Diminished sensitivity to β-adrenergic receptor stimulation is a point of commonality in mediating dysfunction of this system. Moreover, the relationship between the adrenergic, cholinergic, and glucocorticoid-mediated systems appears to be altered in advanced stages of the aging process. Baseline activities of these stress-response systems appear to be elevated with advancing age, with higher baseline sympathetic nervous system activity and tone and elevated basal cortisol levels. However, tonic basal activation appears to give way to maladaptive regulation in response to stressors, both chronic and acute. In turn, chronic overproduction of cortisol may suppress immune function, as well as produce the increased insulin resistance, increased adiposity, and loss of lean body mass that parallel advancing age. Increased baseline levels of norepinephrine and epinephrine with advancing age suggest decreased tissue sensitivity to these hormones as well as a diminished secretary response to acute stimuli. In addition, in the locus ceruleus brain center, which is primarily responsible for regulation of sympathetic nervous system activity, increased concentration of corticotropin-releasing factor may in turn contribute to increasing cortisol secretion, yet another example of the vicious cycle of interactions that may accelerate the processes leading to frailty and, when irreversible, failure to thrive.

Other hormones also affected by the aging process may contribute to frailty. GH and IGF-1 are often diminished with aging, and both are clearly reduced with the chronic diseases and diminishing vitality of the frailty syndrome. Both hormones are critical to the maintenance of lean body mass, IGF-1 being secreted in response to GH and serving as an anabolic "second messenger" in regulating lean body mass. These hormones are normally secreted in pulsatile fashion; however, consistent with the general loss of complexity in biological systems with advancing age, this pulsatile secretion is progressively dampened during the aging process. In turn, through diminished IGF-1 levels, this decrease serves to reduce lean body mass of both muscle and bone. Encouragingly, supplementation of GH in older men with lower IGF-1 levels appears to produce a (small) increase in lean body mass. However, this has not been demonstrated to result in increased strength or endurance during 6-month trials, and hence GH therapy is by no means a panacea for the weakness of old age or the frailty syndrome.

Sex hormone secretion is also diminished with advancing age. This occurs most dramatically with ovarian failure across menopause in women, a sharp decrease followed by both a rapid decline in bone mineral density and also a more subtle yet clear decrease in other components of lean body mass and their replacement by adipose tissue. Males also experience diminished sex steroid secretion with aging. Although this decline is much more subtle than that in perimenopausal women, the gradual decrease in testosterone levels and increasing hypothalamic sensitivity to the negative feedback of testosterone conspire to diminish the anabolic effects of male hormone (especially free testosterone, which declines more than the total, attributable in large measure to increased secretion of sex hormone-binding globulin with advancing age). This contributes to the decrease in both bone and, especially, muscle mass in aging men.

Declining regulation of adrenocortical secretions also contributes to reduced endocrine efficiency with advancing age. Perhaps the most dramatic change in this regard is the decline in secretion of dehydroepiandrosterone. Levels of this steroid hormone peak at adolescence and decrease progressively thereafter across the remainder of the life span. The clinical significance of this decline remains controversial, however, although it has been suggested to contribute to the diminished suppression of the catabolic or inflammatory cytokines (notably IL-6, IL-1β) and increased induction of immune stimulatory cytokines such as IL-2 that accompany aging.

Other metabolic pathways whose efficiency declines with advancing age and contribute to the decrease in fine neuroendocrine regulation with advancing age include those serving other critical homeostatic functions, including regulation of body weight, appetite, thirst, and temperature.

The interaction of the three elements of this triad—lean body mass (and sarcopenia and osteopenia), immune dysfunction, and neuroendocrine dysregulation—is also critical in the complex pathogenesis of frailty. Thus, a vortex of mutually reinforcing dysregulation of these critical homeostatic systems may develop in an ever-accelerating cycle, ultimately placing the individual at grave risk for an irreversible terminal cascade. Whereas in many instances this may progress in a gradual and seemingly seamless fashion, a more dramatic cascade is perhaps more familiar to the geriatric clinician, a tragic decline initiated by a "trigger event." For convenience, such inciting stimuli have been grouped under the mnemonic of infections, infarctions, and infractions (the last including falls and fractures, other trauma including surgery, metabolic or other consequences of homeostatic collapse, and pharmacological and other iatrogenic misadventures). Alternatively, this pathogenetic scheme may be ultimately classified as attributable to "primary causes" or "secondary causes." Primary causes, currently under increasing basic investigation, focus on fundamental, time-related changes in response to the patterns of DNA that define each individual, oxidative or other changes to that DNA, and the shortening of telomeres that accompanies cellular replication to a critical point beyond which renewal through subdivision is no longer possible. Alternatively, secondary causes of frailty, more apparent clinically, include the association of frailty with the myriad of problems and diseases that are common in old age, notably including CVD and its thromboembolic or arrhythmic complications but also extending to malignancy, chronic infections, and even depression as well as vulnerability to the trigger events that are so common in the elderly and especially among those who are frail.

INFLAMMATION:
NEXUS OF THE PATHOGENESIS OF FRAILTY

As introduced previously, an altered balance between pro- and anti-inflammatory cytokine genes and levels of cytokine production during the aging process may result in a state of chronic, often subclinical inflammation in the elderly, especially those on the brink of frailty. This has been suggested explicitly in reports such as those by Hamerman *(6)*, Cohen *(7)*, and Ershler *(8)*. This central hypothesis includes the possibility that this level of smoldering inflammation results from activation of the immune system through chronic, indolent infectious processes, such as periodontal disease, chronic pulmonary disease, diverticulitis or cholecystitis, chronic renal disease, and urinary tract infection, all conditions associated with inflammation that are chronic in nature and increase in prevalence with advancing in age. Alternatively, against this perhaps more traditional, infection-driven pathogenesis of enhanced inflammation with age is the suggestion that part and parcel of the aging process is loss in fine regulation of the immune system such that the carefully modulated balance between pro- and anti-inflammatory processes maintained throughout healthy, effectively symptom-free adulthood tips toward the "pro side," resulting in subclinical chronic inflammation even in the process of "normal" aging. The markers of inflammation most studied in this respect have been the cytokine IL-6 and other cytokines even earlier in the cascade such as IL-1 and tumor necrosis factor-α. Perhaps yet more studied have been the acute phase reaction proteins, serum amyloid A (SAA), fibrinogen and, especially, CRP (Fig. 5). Indeed a number of studies have directly tied changes with aging in primary indices of physiological efficiency and vulnerability and even functional status with aging to changes in these proteins, which are essential to optimal immune regulation. Moreover, increased levels of CRP and other acute inflammatory markers are commonly seen in the other chronic diseases associated with the frailty syndrome outside of the domain of CVD, notably chronic disease of the systems noted above in the CHS, including such pervasive conditions in frail patients as depression (e.g., in the CHS, depression was associated with an increased CRP level *[9]*).

Perhaps of greatest fascination to cardiologists, however, are observations relating inflammation to the pathogenesis of the CVDs that are so

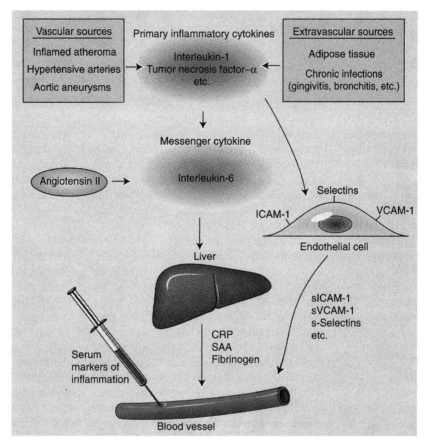

Fig. 5. Pictorial summary of the major elements of the inflammatory cascade that is hypothesized to contribute to atherothrombotic cardiovascular disease and, more generally, the pathogenesis of frailty. ICAM-1, intercellular adhesion molecule-1; VCAM-1, vascular cell adhesion molecule-1; CRP, C-reactive protein; SAA, serum amyloid A. (Reproduced with permission from ref. *8a*.)

common in the elderly and especially prevalent among the frail. Ridker *(10)* has especially championed the central role of CRP as a marker as well as, far more controversial *(11)*, perhaps even a mediator of CVD at all ages and especially among the elderly, given the exponential rise in CVD with advancing age.

CRP:
A KEY LINK BETWEEN CVD AND FRAILTY

The acute-phase response encompasses a broad array of biochemical changes mounted by endothermic organisms following various causes of tissue damage, including trauma, infections, and malignancy, all processes that generate an inflammatory response *(12)*. Cytokines present at the site of the damage upregulate the (mostly hepatic) synthesis of multiple proteins, including complement, coagulation factors, proteinase inhibitors, and transport proteins (and downregulate others, notably the apolipoproteins of LDL and HDL). The first of those proteins to be described (in 1929) and that which responds most dramatically, however, is the CRP (SAA is close to CRP in this regard).

CRP in plasma originates exclusively from the liver (although tissue CRP may arise locally), where it is under the transcriptional control principally of IL-6. The median concentration of CRP measured by the highly sensitive (hsCRP) assay in healthy young blood donors is 0.8 mg/L, with a 90th percentile at 3 mg/L and 99th percentile at 10 mg/dL. A handy rule of thumb has evolved: below 1 mg/dL is normal, between 1 and 2 borderline, and above 3 is increased. CRP levels appear remarkably constant in a given individual in a stable state of good health (comparable to the stability of cholesterol concentrations and similarly under strong but complex genetic control). Coupled with its stability during storage, this has made CRP the focus of multiple "instant" prospective studies when measured in stored samples from longitudinal epidemiological and clinical studies. This stability is all the more extraordinary given the rapidity and degree of CRP elevations following a single acute stimulus: serum levels exceed 5 mg/L within 6 hours and peak at concentrations as high as 10,000 mg/L at 48 hours. With an unvarying half-life of about 19 hours, the CRP synthesis rate alone effectively determines the plasma concentration. However, not all stimuli to CRP are acute and transient; perhaps more common and subtle are subacute or chronic inflammatory stimuli (especially relevant to gerontology and geriatrics). Therefore, investigators pursuing CRP as an index of tissue damage and inflammation following an acute insult (e.g., MI) advise waiting at least 6 weeks after such an event to judge whether CRP levels have returned to baseline and the acute inflammatory stimulus has completely abated.

The relationship between CVD and inflammation has enjoyed a crescendo of investigative and clinical interest in recent years. Historically, atherogenesis was conceptualized as a chronic, insidiously progressive process. However, the failure of standard indices of CVD risk—classically smoking, BP and cholesterol (even when fractionated into HDL, LDL, and very low-density lipoprotein)—to account for more than 50% of the risk of heart disease in a given individual has long suggested that additional pathogenic factors were at work. Atherosclerosis began to be appreciated as a more dynamic process, one under more complex regulation, in the latter third of the 20th century in the research of Ross *(13)* and

others. These researchers investigated the pathogenesis of atherosclerosis according to the "reaction-to-injury" hypothesis originally proposed
over a century earlier. The stimulus to examine CVD as a more dynamic
process in such studies received major clinical impetus from demonstration of the rapid development of new lesions on coronary angiography
repeated at relatively close intervals in patients with recurrent and progressive CVD. At a more basic level, the dynamic nature of the disease
was confirmed in studies of atherosclerosis in experimental models. Those
especially focused on the role of the arterial endothelium in modulating
both chronic atherogenesis and also the acute response to arterial ischemia and occlusive thrombosis—itself an intense stimulus to inflammation. Indeed, atherosclerosis has come to be considered an intrinsically
inflammatory disease process (13).

This hypothesis received major support in the past decade in a burst
of observational epidemiological studies, both cross-sectional and longitudinal, and even in clinical trials of anti-inflammatory agents in CVD
prevention, progress dramatically propelled by development of the hsCRP
assay. These studies included the landmark Physicians Health Study,
which disclosed an increased (2.9-fold) risk of MI and (1.9-fold) of stroke
in healthy middle-aged male doctors in the highest vs. the lowest quartile
of CRP levels (14). A similar relationship was reported in participants
in the Women's Health Study (15), in which baseline CRP levels were
linearly correlated with incident CVD (2.3-fold higher in the top vs
bottom quartile). Especially germane to this chapter on frailty, a nested
case–control study within the CHS also suggested that baseline CRP
levels predicted incident CVD, including angina, MI and death (16). Here,
however, the association of higher CRP levels with CVD events was
especially pronounced for risk of MI in those with subclinical disease
(OR 2.67 [CI = 1.04–6.81]) and notably more in women (4.50 [CI = 0.97–
20.8]) than men (1.75 [CI = 0.51–5.98]), and case–control differences
were greatest when the interval between baseline and the CVD event was
shortest (implying a more active inflammatory state at baseline).

Indeed atherogenesis has emerged as a complex, smoldering, stutter-
ing, dynamic process in which inflammation is both a cause and a result
of tissue damage. Atherogenesis may be accelerated by the release of pro-
inflammatory stimuli such as IL-6, IL-1-α, and TNFα from extravascular sites such as adipose tissue (contributing to insulin resistance) and tissue macrophages (17,18) as well as from vascular sites in the arterial wall
and the heart itself. These in turn trigger the hepatic synthesis and release
of acute phase proteins (notably CRP, fibrinogen, and SAA) that not only
signal but may also participate in the pathogenic spiral. As reported by

Lindahl et al. *(19)*, the magnitude of tissue necrosis from atherothrombotic events such as frank acute MI or even more subtle damage in patients with unstable coronary artery disease as reflected in serum troponin levels during the first 24 hours after presentation continue to predict future cardiac death for months and years. However, just as predictive are the parallel rises in CRP and fibrinogen in such patients. In a nested case–control study, these markers of inflammation also predicted future coronary events in hypercholesterolemic men in the West of Scotland Coronary (primary) Prevention Study *(20)*. A third marker, lipoprotein-associated phospholipase A_2 (platelet-activating factor acetylhydrolase) was also independently related to future risk in the same study. This enzyme, which circulates bound to both LDL and HDL, is regulated by mediators of inflammation and has been suggested to generate inflammation-promoting lysolecithin from LDL, thus inducing a direct inflammatory effect of circulating LDL *(21)*. Other factors generated by inflammatory stimuli, such as infectious diseases resulting in release of lipopolysaccharide that oxidizes LDL and increases pathogenic oxygen radicals in the vessel wall, have also been implicated in a process that not only promotes atherogenesis but also destabilizes the atherosclerotic plaque, leading to its rupture and occlusive thrombosis of the overlying lumen *(21,22)*.

Thus, a vicious cycle can be set in motion by forces that produce tissue damage, inflammation, atherogenic changes in lipoproteins and the arterial vessel wall, subclinical atherosclerosis, and atherothrombotic complications, which produce tissue damage, and so on. The major feature of this pathophysiological scheme appear now to have reached scientific consensus *(24)*, with contemporary controversy centering on whether the markers of inflammation, notably CRP, serve as mediators as well as markers of the process *(25)*.

INHIBITORS OF INFLAMMATION IN CVD PREVENTION: THE PROMISE OF HMG-CoA REDUCTASE INHIBITORS

The therapeutic implications of a central role for inflammation in atherogenesis and atherothrombotic disease have also drawn intense interest. It has been suggested that statins, hydroxymethylglutaryl-coenzyme A (HMG-CoA) reductase inhibitors, may have a dual role in CVD prevention, both by lowering LDL cholesterol through inhibition of cholesterol synthesis and also by reducing inflammation. This may directly retard the atherogenic process if indeed CRP is a mediator as well as a marker of the disease *(25)*. In support of its direct role, for

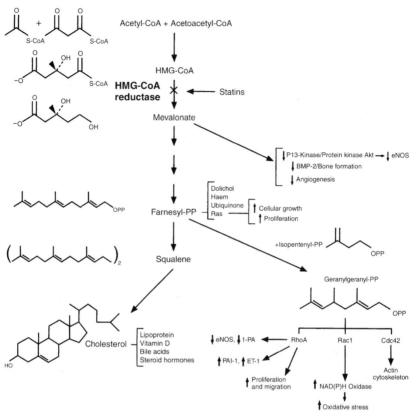

Fig. 6. Biochemical scheme of the generation of cholesterol and isoprenoids from acetyl-coenzyme A (CoA) and acetoacetyl-CoA and the changes in this complex process by inhibition of HMG-CoA reductase by statins, consequent decreases in cholesterol derivatives and signaling molecules such as Ras, Rho, and Rac, and changes in turn in the systems they modulate. (Reproduced with permission from ref. 26.)

example, CRP has been reported to bind to modified LDL in atherosclerotic plaques, in turn activating complement, which contributes to atherosclerotic lesion progression. CRP has also been reported to impair endothelial function by decreasing endothelial nitric oxide synthase (eNOS) in cultured cells, a process mediated by Rho. Here the pleiothropic potential of the HMG-CoA reductases offers special promise *(26–28)* (Fig. 6). Inhibition of HMG-CoA reductase decreases the synthesis not only of cholesterol but also the isoprenoid geranylgeranyl-pyrophosphate, which facilitates membrane lipid attachment of Rho and the membrane translocation of Rho/Rho kinase. Thus, both directly and also possibly indirectly (by decreasing inflammation and CRP synthesis) statins appear to increase eNOS expression and activity, modulating endothelial cell function in an anti-atherogenic direction. Reduction in Rho by statins also appears to enhance endothelial function by decreasing endothelin-1 and expression of the AT_1 receptor as well as decreasing thrombosis by increasing expression of tissue-type plasminogen activator and diminishing plasminogen activator inhibitor 1 (27).

Statins have also been suggested to exert primary reduction of inflammation by inhibiting production of the pro-inflammatory cytokines IL-6, IL-8, as well as the monocyte chemoattractant protein measured in peripheral blood mononuclear cells and human umbilical vein endothelial cells (29).

Additional potential for a bimodal role for statins in CVD prevention has been suggested from a growing number of studies demonstrating that hsCRP and LDL cholesterol levels contribute independently and sometimes synergistically to CVD risk (24). For example, in the AFCAPS/TexCAPS primary prevention trial, lovastatin reduced CRP levels by 15% in women, a decrease not related to their induced changes in the lipid profile. In this study, lovastatin decreased events not only in subjects at increased CVD risk by virtue of a total cholesterol/HDL cholesterol above the median (regardless of CRP level) but also in those with above median CRP (but below median total/HDL cholesterol ratios), while not reducing CVD among those with below median values for both. This led the authors to suggest that measurement of CRP in addition to lipids might permit targeting statin therapy to those most likely to benefit on either or both axes of risk (30).

However, as attractive as the simplicity, relative safety, and pleiotropic efficacy of statins in CVD prevention appears, it is important to emphasize other ways to reduce CRP that are not confined to anti-inflammatory pharmacological interventions above. Indeed simply withdrawing drugs that raise CRP levels may reduce risk: oral contraceptives and postmenopausal estrogen/progestin hormone replacement therapy (HRT) raise CRP levels (31), and HRT has been specifically associated with increased CVD risk in both secondary (Heart and Estrogen/progestin Replacement Study [32]) and primary (Women's Health Initiative [WHI; 33]) prevention trials. Hence, the plummeting use of HRT following release of the unexpected adverse results of the WHI may serve to reduce CVD risk in postmenopausal women. Interestingly, transdermal estrogen replacement therapy does not appear to increase CRP, suggesting a specific role of first-pass hepatic exposure to the estrogen–progestin combination in raising CRP levels (34) (and potentially CVD risk). Lifestyle interventions also appear to hold promise for CVD prevention via lowered inflammatory burden and reduced CRP levels: the combined effect of dietary changes and increased exercise reduces both weight and indices of inflammation, including CRP, offering promise of reduced CVD (35).

Thus interventions to reduce inflammation within the cardiovascular system offer special promise of reducing atherothrombotic disease in the elderly. However, such interventions may hold additional opportunities to reduce CVD in the elderly beyond the atherothrombotic realm. This appears especially to be the case for CHF, the most common cause for hospitalization among Medicare beneficiaries and the bane of the professional lives of so many cardiologists, geriatricians, and geriatric cardiologists. Here once again the CHS lends special insight (36). Over the average of 5.5 years of follow-up in subjects 65 to 100 (mean age 73 ± 5) the incidence of CHF was 19.3/1000 person-years, a rate that increased progressively with age and was greater in men than women. Beyond age and sex, the leading factors in the population—attributable risk of CHF in this study included a high level of CRP (9.7%) as well as prevalent CHD (13.1%) and systolic hypertension (>140).

This finding received support in a study of the incidence of CHF in more than 732 Framingham Study subjects (mean age 78, 67% women) free of prior CHF or MI (37). CHF developed in 56 subjects after a mean of 5.2 years. Three indices of inflammatory activation were measured: serum IL-6 and CRP levels and TNF-α production by peripheral blood monocytes. On multivariable analysis higher levels of each of the three predicted increased risk of CHF. CRP of at least 5 mg/dL was associated with a 2.8-fold elevation, which when combined with IL-6 and TNF-α above the respective medians was raised to 4.07 (95% CI 1.34–12.37).

Hence increased baseline indices of inflammation over and above those attributable to either clinical or subclinical atherosclerosis appear to increase risk of CHF, suggesting that this often lethal complication may reflect a more general inflection toward a pro-inflammatory status.

CVD, DISABILITY, AND FRAILTY: CLOSING THE CAUSATIVE TRIANGLE IN THE ELDERLY

Thus a prominent role of inflammation in mediating the CVD that escalates exponentially with time and aging appears increasingly clear. However, it also seems likely that inflammation plays a broader and more central role in mediating the progressive vulnerability and diminished resiliency that accompanies the aging process and leads to frailty and ultimately failure to thrive.

One index of this inflammatory burden is the gradual rise in population CRP levels (and other indices of inflammatory activation such as IL-6) seen with advancing age. Whereas this has often been attributed simply to the gradual accumulation of age-related diseases and their inflammatory pathogenesis, it appears that generally aggregate increased pro-inflammatory activation from both disease and aging per se may mediate the decline more directly at multiple points in the complex cascade of frailty illustrated in Fig. 1 and the Venn diagram that quantifies the triad of frailty, co-morbidity, and disability in the CHS depicted in Fig. 2. A growing number of epidemiological studies support this hypothesis. For example, the report by Ferrucci et al. *(38)* from the Iowa site of the Epidemiologic Studies of the Elderly (EPESE) (subjects > 71 years) suggested that participants who were in the highest (vs lowest) tertile of IL-6 levels were 1.76 times (95% CI, 1.17–2.64) more likely to develop mobility-disability and 1.62 times (1.02–2.60) more likely to develop mobility-plus-ADL disability, with a progressive rise in risk with increasing IL-6 concentrations. A decline in physical performance in subjects with higher levels of CRP and IL-6 was also seen in the MacArthur studies of Successful Aging, a subset of the EPESE populations *(39)* that included 880 high-functioning men and women. Higher levels of CRP and IL-6 were seen in less active persons, and on multivariable analysis, low levels were seen in participants with higher walking speed and greater group strength. Similar findings were reported at a more mechanistic level by Barbieri et al. *(40)*, who suggested that high circulating IL-6 levels and low IGF-1 are synergistic for poor muscle strength (IL-6 directly impairing muscle IGF-1 gene and protein expression), leading in functional terms to disability and increased mortality risk in older women *(41)*. Roubenoff et al. *(42)* came to similar conclusions from analysis of cytokines and IGF-1 and their relationship to sarcopenia and mortality in very old Framingham Study participants.

Returning to the Iowa EPESE population, the association of higher IL-6 levels with increased disability in this population also extended to an increased risk of mortality *(43)*: IL-6 in the top quartile was associated with a twofold greater risk of death compared with the lowest quartile; higher CRP levels also predicted 1.6-fold higher mortality, while elevations of both increased risk of death 2.6 times, with equivalent increases for death from cardiovascular and non-cardiovascular causes. Similar findings were reported from the Duke population within that group of studies *(44)*: the 5-year relative risk for death with IL-6 in the top quartile was 1.28 (0.98–1.69). Moreover, perhaps of special interest to cardiologists, increased coagulation diathesis as one of the cluster of factors triggered by inflammation also appeared to contribute to risk of functional decline and mortality in this population. D-dimer levels predicted a 1.53 fold higher risk of death, whereas individuals in the top quartile of both IL-6 and D-dimers had a twofold risk. Of note, the 4-year follow-up of the functional status of subjects in this population also disclosed a doubling of risk of decline in Katz ADLs and IADLs for those in the top quartiles of both indices.

A similar pattern was observed in the longitudinal data from the MacArthur Research Network on Successful Aging Community Study derivative of the EPESE study (45). This added two additional markers of inflammation to the list of such indices of frailty often noted by clinicians beside upper tertiles of IL-6 (>3.8 pg/dL) and CRP (>2.65 mg/L): a low serum albumin (<3.8 g/dL) and a low serum cholesterol (<170 mg/dL, bottom decile). In subjects with three or four (vs none) of these markers of inflammation adjusted odds ratios for 3- and 7-year mortality were 3.2 and 6.6, respectively.

Finally, to close the triangle with specific reference to the CHS in which the frailty syndrome was defined, frail (vs non-frail) subjects had increased mean levels of CRP (5.5 ± 9.8 vs 2.7 ± 4 mg/L) as well as higher levels of coagulation factors VIII and D-dimer (46), differences that remained after exclusion of diabetes and subjects with CVD and adjustment for age, sex, and race. Thus inflammation and markers of coagulation are increased in frailty even in the absence of prevalent CVD.

INFLAMMATION IN THE TRANSITION
FROM FRAILTY TO FAILURE TO THRIVE

Thus, inflammation appears to play a central role in the downward spiral from robust health to frailty to failure to thrive through its contributions to sarcopenia, neuroendocrine dysregulation, and immune dysfunction as well as CVD and the other co-morbidities and disabilities that are so prevalent among the failing elderly. For cardiologists, this is perhaps most apparent in the atherothrombotic disease so common among their clientele. But especially for those (especially geriatric) cardiologists whose patients have typically survived previous MIs, angioplasties, and coronary bypasses and now manifest heart failure and the pernicious multisystem effects of chronic inflammation and the weight loss, weakness, exhaustion, slowness, and low activity that constitute the classical pentad of frailty, understanding the pathophysiology of this syndrome is central to their practice. Such understanding also underscores the need to investigate frailty with special focus on potential intervention strategies. Here the evaluation of anti-inflammatory agents *(47)*, including statins, represents an attractive approach.

Finally, cardiologists, especially geriatric cardiologists, must learn to recognize when the downward spiral has gone beyond the point of no return and failure to thrive supervenes—and a transition to a palliative approach to care of the patient is most appropriate and humane.

REFERENCES

1. Fries JF. Aging, natural death and the compression of morbidity. N Engl J Med 1980; 303:130.
2. Fried LP, Walston J. Frailty and failure to thrive. In: Hazzard WR, Blass JP, Halter JB, Ouslander JG, Tinetti ME. (eds.), Principles of Geriatric Medicine and Gerontology, 5th ed. McGraw-Hill, New York, 2003, pp. 1487–1502.
3. Fried LP, Tangen CM, Walston J, et al. Frailty in older adults: evidence for a phenotype. J Gerontol A Biol Sci Med Sci 2001;56A(3):M146–156.
4. Gillick M. Pinning down frailty. J Gerontol A Biol Sci Med Sci 2001;56(3):M134–135.
5. Newman AB, Gottdiener JS, McBurnie MA, et al. Associations of subclinical cardiovascular disease with frailty. J Gerontol A Biol Sci Med Sci 2001;56A(3): M158–166.
6. Hamerman D. Toward an understanding of frailty. Ann Int Med 1999;130:945–950.
7. Cohen HJ. In search of the underlying mechanisms of frailty [Editorial]. J Gerontol A Biol Sci Med Sci 2000;55A(12):M706–708.
8. Ershler WB, Keller ET. Age-associated increased interleukin-6 gene expression, late-life disease, and frailty. Annu Rev Med 2000;51:245–270.
8a. Libby P, Ridker PM. Novel inflammatory markers of coronary risk: theory versus practice. Circulation 1999;100(11):1148–1150.
9. Kop WJ, Gottdiener JS, Tangen CM, et al. Inflammation and coagulation factors in persons > 65 years of age with symptoms of depression but without evidence of myocardial ischemia. Am J Cardiol 2002;89(4):419–424.
10. Ridker PM. High-sensitivity C-reactive protein and cardiovascular risk: rationale for screening and primary prevention. Am J Cardiol 2003;92(4B);17K–22K.
11. Kuller LH, Tracy RP, eds. The role of inflammation in cardiovascular disease. Arterioscler Thromb Vasc Biol 2000;20(4):901.
12. Pepys MB, Hirschfield GM. C-reactive protein: a critical update. J Clin Invest 2003; 111:1805–1812.
13. Ross R. Atherosclerosis—an inflammatory disease. N Engl J Med 1999;340(2): 115–126.
14. Ridker PM, Cushman M, Stampfer MJ, Tracy RP, Hennekens CH. Inflammation, aspirin, and the risk of cardiovascular disease in apparently healthy men. N Engl J Med 1997;336(14):973–979.
15. Ridker PM, Rifai N, Rose L, Buring JE, Cook NR. Comparison of C-reactive protein and low-density lipoprotein cholesterol levels in the prediction of first cardiovascular events. N Engl J Med 2002;347(20):1557–1565.
16. Tracy RP, Lemaitre RN, Psaty BM, et al. Relationship of C-reactive protein to risk of cardiovascular disease in the elderly. Arterioscler Thromb Vasc Biol 1997;17(6): 1121–1127.

17. Tracy RP. Inflammation, the metabolic syndrome and cardiovascular risk. Int J Clin Pract 2003;134(Suppl):10–17.
18. Yudkin JS, Kumari M, Humphries SE, Mohamed-Ali V. Inflammation, obesity, stress and coronary heart disease: is interleukin-6 the link? Atherosclerosis 1999; 148(2):209–214.
19. Lindahl B, Toss H, Siegbahn A, Venge P, Wallentin L, FRISC Study Group. Markers of myocardial damage and inflammation in relation to long-term mortality in unstable coronary artery disease. N Engl J Med 2000;343(16):1139–1147.
20. Packard CJ, O'Reilly DSJ, Caslake MJ, et al. Lipoprotein-associated Phospholipase A$_2$, as an independent predictor of coronary heart disease. N Engl J Med 2000;343 (16):1148–1155.
21. Rader DJ. Inflammatory markers of coronary risk. N Engl J Med 2000;343(16): 1179–1182.
22. Hajjar DP. Oxidized lipoproteins and infectious agents: are they in collusion to accelerate atherogenesis? Arterioscler Thromb Vasc Biol 2000;20:1421–1422.
23. Schultz D, Harrison DG. Quest for fire: seeking the source of pathogenic oxygen radicals in atherosclerosis. Arterioscler Thromb Vasc Biol 2000;20:1412–1413.
24. Taubes G. Does inflammation cut to the heart of the matter? Science 2002;296 (5566):242–245.
25. Blake GJ, Ridker PM. C-reactive protein, subclinical atherosclerosis, and risk of cardiovascular events. Arterioscler Thromb Vasc Biol 2002;22:1512–1513.
26. Liao JK. Isoprenoids as mediators of the biological effects of statins. J Clin Invest 2002;110:285–288.
27. Wolfrum S, Jensen KS, Liao JK. Endothelium-dependent effects of statins. Arterioscler Thromb Vasc Biol 2003;23:729–736.
28. Munford RS, ed. Statins and the acute-phase response. N Engl J Med 2001;344(26): 2016–2018.
29. Rezaie-Majd A, Maca T, Bucek RA, et al. Simvastatin reduces expression of cytokines interleukin-6, interleukin-8, and monocyte chemoattractant protein-1 in circulating monocytes from hyperscholesterolemic patients. Arterioscler Thromb Vasc Biol 2002;22:1194–1199.
30. Ridker PM, Rifai N, Clearfield M, et al. Measurement of C-reactive protein for the targeting of statin therapy in the primary prevention of acute coronary events. N Engl J Med 2001;344(26):1959–1965.
31. Walsh BW, Wild PS, Dean RA, Tracy RP, Cox DA, Anderson PW. The effects of hormone replacement therapy and raloxifene on C-reactive protein and homocysteine in healthy postmenopausal women: a randomized, controlled trial. J Clin Endocrinol Metab 2000;85(1):214–218.
32. Hulley S, Grady D, Bush T, et al. Randomized trial of estrogen plus progestin for secondary prevention of coronary heart disease in postmenopausal women. JAMA 1998;280:605–613.
33. Writing Group for the Women's Health Initiative. Risks and benefits of estrogen plus progestin in healthy postmenopausal women. Principal results from the Women's Health Initiative randomized controlled trail. JAMA 2002;288:321.
34. Modena MG, Bursi F, Fantini G, et al. Effects of hormone replacement therapy on C-reactive levels in healthy postmenopausal women: comparision between oral and transdermal administration of estrogen. Am J Med 2002;133:331.
35. Esposito K, Pontillo A, Di Palo C, et al. Effect of weight loss and lifestyle changes on vascular inflammatory markers in obese women: a randomized trial. JAMA 2003; 289(14):1799–1804.

36. Gottdiener JS, Arnold AM, Aurigemma GP, et al. Predictors of congestive heart failure in the elderly: the cardiovascular health study. J Am Coll Cardio 2000;35(6): 1628–1637.

37. Vasan RS, Sullivan LM, Roubenoff R, et al. Inflammatory markers and risk of health failure in elderly subjects without prior myocardial infarction: the Framingham Heart Study. Circulation 2003;107(11):1486–1491.

38. Ferrucci L, Harris TB, Guralnik JM, et al. Serum IL-6 level and the development of disability in older persons. JAGS 1999;47:639–646.

39. Taaffe DR, Harris TB, Ferrucci L, Rowe J, Seeman TE. Cross-sectional and prospective relationships of interleukin-6 and C-reactive protein with physical performance in elderly persons: MacArthur studies of successful aging. J Gerontol A Biol Sci Med Sci 2000;55A(12):M709–715.

40. Barbieri M, Ferrucci L, Ragno E, et al. Chronic inflammation and the effect of IGF-1 on muscle strength and power in older persons. Am J Physical Endocrinol Metab 2003;284:E481–487.

41. Cappolo AR, Xue QL, Ferrucci L, Guralnik JM, Valpato S, Fried LP. Insulin-like growth factor-I and interleukin-6 contribute synergistically to disability and mortality in older women. J Clin Endocrinol Metab 2003;88;2019–2025.

42. Roubenoff R, Parise H, Payette HA, et al. Cytokines, insulin-like growth factor I, sarcopenia, and mortality in very old community-dwelling men and women: the Framingham Heart Study. Am J Med 2003;115:429–435.

43. Harris TB, Ferrucci L, Tracy RP, et al. Associations of elevated interleukin-6 and C-reactive protein levels with mortality in the elderly. Am J Med 1999;106:506–512.

44. Cohen HJ, Harris T, Pieper CF. Coagulation and activation of inflammatory pathways in the development of functional decline and mortality in the elderly. Am J Med 2003;114:180–187.

45. Reuben DB, Cheh AI, Harris TB, et al. Peripheral blood markers of inflammation predict mortality and functional decline in high-functioning community-dwelling older persons. J Am Geriatr Soc 2002;50:638–644.

46. Walston J, McBurnie MA, Newman A, et al. Frailty and activation of the inflammation and coagulation systems with and without clinical comorbidities: results from the Cardiovascular Health Study. Arch Intern Med 2002;162(20):2333–2341.

47. Kuller LH, ed. Serum levels of IL-6 and development of disability in older persons. JAGS 1999;47(6):755–756.

3 Cardiovascular Risk Factors in the Elderly

Evaluation and Intervention

Susan J. Zieman, MD and Beth R. Malasky, MD

CONTENTS

INTRODUCTION

One of the most important reasons for the decline in age-adjusted cardiovascular mortality is the identification and treatment of reversible cardiac risk factors. However, until recently, most clinical studies evaluating the efficacy of these interventions excluded elderly individuals. Although the pathological process that results in coronary atherosclerosis begins with the development of fatty streaks in the arteries of children and teenagers, recent studies indicate that treatment of risk factors significantly reduces cardiovascular events, improves quality of life, and increases survival in the elderly. This chapter reviews the importance of risk-factor identification, their evaluation, and the efficacy of known interventions in the elderly. It also discusses novel, proposed risk factors because their identification allows greater insight into the pathophysiology of the disease process and can suggest the potential benefit of new risk-reduction strategies.

From: *Contemporary Cardiology: Cardiovascular Disease in the Elderly*
Edited by: G. Gerstenblith © Humana Press Inc., Totowa, NJ

CLASSICAL RISK FACTORS

Hypertension

The prevalence of hypertension increases with age and more than 60% of those 65 years or older have high blood pressure (BP) defined as a systolic blood pressure (SBP) of 140 mmHg or more, a diastolic blood pressure (DBP) of 90 mmHg or more or are currently receiving antihypertensive treatment *(1)*. In some populations (e.g., those with diabetes and known target organ damage), pharmacological treatment should be initiated at even lower levels of pressure and lifestyle measures at BPs of 120/80 or higher *(2)*. The age-associated increase in BP is owing to a decrease in total peripheral compliance resulting from increases in central vascular stiffness and peripheral resistance (*see* Chapter 1). SBP shows a continuous increase with age, whereas DBP rises early in life, plateaus, and then decreases after age 50. Data from the Framingham Heart Study suggests that an individual who is normotensive at age 55 has a 90% lifetime risk of developing hypertension *(3)*.

Although systolic hypertension in the elderly was traditionally considered a benign phenomenon, it is now recognized as one of the most potent reversible risk factors for the development of both cardiovascular and cerebrovascular events in the elderly. Thirty-year follow-up data in men and women participants in the Framingham Heart Study show a clear and almost linear association between the incidence of cardiovascular disease (CVD) and SBP, with no lower limit down to at least a systolic pressure of 120 mmHg. Event rates of angina, myocardial infarction (MI), and sudden death were associated with SBP, with higher event rates for men than women *(3)* (Fig. 1). A recent meta-analysis of more than 1 million individuals also demonstrated a logarithmic increase in vascular events, including stroke, with increases in SBP in the older, as well as younger, populations *(4)*.

Although the association between isolated systolic hypertension (ISH) and CVDs in the elderly is impressive, treatment decisions depend on the demonstration that interventions that decrease SBP prevent CVDs. The first major trial to demonstrate the benefits of pharmacological treatment for this condition was the Systolic Hypertension in the Elderly Program (SHEP), which demonstrated that first-line diuretic therapy in older individuals with an SBP of more than 160 mmHg and a DBP of less than 90 mmHg resulted in a 27% reduction in MI and coronary heart disease (CHD) mortality over a 5-year period, as compared with placebo *(5)*. The Systolic Hypertension in Europe trial in patients aged 60 or older using a long-acting dihydropyridine calcium antagonist, confirmed the find-

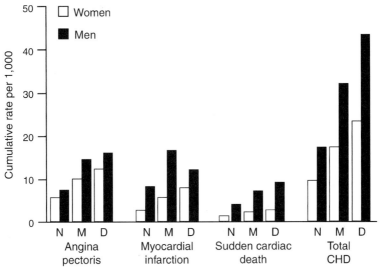

Fig. 1. Incidence of coronary heart disease (CHD) according to hypetension status over 30 years of follow-up of the Framingham Heart Study. Positive associations exist between levels of elevated blood pressure and cumulative incidence of CHD. N, normotensive (<140/90 mmHg); M, mildly hypertensive (140–159/94 mmHg); D, definitely hypertensive (≥160/95 mmHg). (Data from the National Technical Information Service; Reproduced with permission from ref. *3.*)

ings of SHEP; cardiac endpoints were decreased by 26%, strokes were decreased by 44%, and all cardiovascular endpoints were decreased by 32% *(6).* The intervention in this study was also associated with a 50% reduction in both Alzheimer's and non-Alzheimer's type dementia *(7).* A meta-analysis of more than 10 large clinical trials in more than 15,000 older individuals with DBP elevations demonstrated a 30% reduction in stroke, a 23% reduction in coronary crtery disease (CAD) events, a 26% decline in all CVD events, and an 18% decrease in cardiovascular mortality *(8).* In a meta-analysis of those participants older than 80 years of age, a 34% decrease in stroke, 22% decrease in CHD events, and 39% decrease in heart failure were present in the treatment, as compared with the control groups *(9).*

Despite overwhelming data indicating the importance of treating hypertension in the elderly, this group comprises the population with the lowest rates of BP control *(10).* The Third National Health and Nutrition Examination Survey data indicate that those over 65 constituted 44 of the hypertensive population who were unaware that they had hypertension, 33% of those who were aware they had hypertension but were not on any therapy, and 58% of those who were on therapy, but the therapy was not controlling the BP. The vast majority of these had ISH.

The evaluation of hypertension in the elderly should include an assessment for reversible, contributing factors including obstructive sleep apnea (OSA), salt-retaining medications, and renovascular disease as well as the presence of frequent concomitant risk factors, such as dyslipidemia *(2)*. The exam should include an assessment of the presence of carotid bruits as well, because the presence of significant cerebral flow obstruction might dictate the need for a relatively higher pressure and/or further therapeutic intervention. Pseudohypertension, owing to stiffness and calcification of the arteries of elderly patients, may result in falsely elevated cuff readings that do not correlate with intra-arterial measures of BP. Evaluation should also include an assessment for the presence of target organ damage because its presence increases the risk associated with hypertension and therefore the need for effective therapeutic intervention. Left ventricular hypertrophy (LVH), for example, is associated with hypertension but is also an independent risk factor for cardiovascular outcomes in the elderly. One reason may be decreased left ventricular compliance with resultant diastolic dysfunction and often, congestive heart failure (CHF). The Framingham study noted echocardiographic evidence of LVH in 33% of men older than 70 years *(11)*. In one study of older people with hypertension, 15% of whites and 20% of African-Americans had electrocardiographic (EKG) evidence of LVH and 56% of whites and 71% of African-Americans had echocardiographic evidence of LVH *(12)*. At 42-month follow-up, the odds ratio for new coronary events was 1.11 for EKG LVH and 3.12 for echocardiographic LVH. Echocardiographic evidence of LVH in that study was the most powerful independent predictor of new coronary events among older persons with hypertension. Although numerous antihypertensive therapies have been shown to result in LVH regression *(13,14)*, it is not known whether regression decreases the likelihood of these events.

Lifestyle interventions should also be stressed, as weight reduction in those overweight and a decreased sodium diet are associated with BP lowering the elderly, as well as younger, populations.

Age-associated changes in drug absorption, distribution, and metabolism (*see* Chapter 14) indicate that initiation and titration of antihypertensive therapies should be performed cautiously in the elderly. Increased vascular stiffness increases the change in pressure for any given volume change, and decreased sympathetic responsiveness may limit the cardiovascular response to hypotensive agents. Therefore, one important caveat is to determine the standing BP before deciding to initiate or increment the antihypertensive regimen. Additional considerations in the older population include the importance of long-acting agents so that the medication may be taken once daily and to decrease the likelihood of diurnal fluctuations in pressure. In older patients who may have symptoms related to transient hypotension, ambulatory monitoring may be particularly useful during the titration period.

The choice of an initial antihypertensive agent is dependent on several factors. As noted previously, a diuretic in one study and a long-acting dihydropyridine calcium antagonist in another showed superior outcomes, when compared to placebo, in the treatment of ISH in the elderly. Although it is not possible to compare newer agents with placebo, the Antihypertensive and Lipid-Lowering Treatment to Prevent Heart Attack Trial demonstrated no difference in the primary endpoint among a general hypertensive population older than 55 years of age randomized to a diuretic, an angiotensin-converting enzyme (ACE) inhibitor, or a long-acting calcium antagonist *(15)*. Joint National Committee on Prevention, Detection, Evaluation, and Treatment of High Blood Pressure (JNC-7) recommendations do note, however, that there are compelling indications for certain drugs in the presence of certain co-existing diseases including β-blockers in patients with concomitant active ischemic disease or following an MI, a diuretic in the presence of heart failure, an ACE inhibitor in patients with diabetes or systolic dysfunction, and a selective aldosterone antagonist in patients with left ventricular dysfunction following an MI. The choice of which agent to use, however, is not as important as reaching BP goal and it is important to note that most studies indicate that more than one agent is frequently required. JNC-7 guidelines suggest that therapy be initiated with two agents, in fact, when the SBP is more than 20 mmHg above goal and/or the DBP is higher than 10 mmHg above goal.

Dyslipidemia

Dyslipidemia is also a potent risk factor for the development of CVD. Although studies have found total cholesterol levels to be a risk for cardiac events in older individuals *(16,17)*, the data are confounded, in part, by some studies demonstrating an inverse relationship between cholesterol and mortality, particularly cancer death, in the very elderly. This is likely related to serum cholesterol as a marker of frailty, nutritional status, and overall health in this age group *(18–21)*. Another impediment was the exclusion of elderly from many of the early studies. The Dubbo Study of elderly Australians found total cholesterol (TC), low-density lipoprotein (LDL), apolipoprotein B and the TC/high-density lipoprotein (HDL) ratio to be significant and equivalent predictors of MI. The study also reported that low HDL was an independent and strong predictor of CVD in this elderly group as well *(22)*. Data from the Cardiovascular Health Study (CHS) and the Framingham Study report that although the association of TC and CHD risk diminishes with increasing age, low HDL levels continue to predict CHD events in those over 80 years old, particularly in women *(23,24)*.

Hydroxymethylglutaryl-coenzyme A (HMG-CoA) reductase inhibitor therapy improves clinical outcomes in older age patient subsets of large, multicenter trials and in studies confined to an older population. Primary prevention studies in patients with elevated cholesterol include the West of Scotland Coronary Prevention Study, which demonstrated a 20% decrease in primary CHD events and 20% in total mortality in those over 60 years of age treated with a statin *(25)*. In the Air Force/Texas Coronary Atherosclerosis Prevention Study, in patients with only modestly elevated TC, the reduction of MI, 40%, was similar in older and younger patients *(26,27)*, although no patients over 75 years of age were enrolled. The Anglo-Scandinavian Cardiac Outcome Trails (ASCOT) in patients with hypertension and other risk factors but without known coronary disease, and "normal" TC and LDL cholesterol levels reported that statin therapy over 3.5 years of follow-up reduced cardiovascular events and stroke in the subset over 60 years of age, 20–30%, to the same extent that it did in the entire study group *(28)*.

The results are also striking when statin therapy is used for secondary prevention. In the Scandinavian 4S study, a secondary prevention trial in patients with elevated cholesterol levels, the reduction in risk of major coronary events in those 65 years and older, 43%, was similar to that in the younger group, 42% *(29)*. As the absolute risk increases with age and as statins are effective therapies, the absolute risk reduction for all-cause and CHD mortality is greater in older patients. Subgroup analysis of older (≥65 years) participants in the Cholesterol and Recurrent Events secondary prevention trial involving patients with what was considered a normal cholesterol level of ≤240 mg/dL reported that older participants randomized to a statin as compared with those randomized to placebo had a greater reduction in major coronary events, 32% vs 19%; and in coronary mortality, 45% vs 11% *(30,31)*. The Heart Protection Study in those with and without known vascular disease reported a similar 32% decrease in the primary outcome in those enrolled at 75–80 years of age, and followed over the subsequent 5-year period, as the decrease in the rest of the enrolled population. Of note, the statin benefit was present regardless of the initial LDL cholesterol *(32)*.

The PROspective Study of Pravastatin in the Elderly at Risk evaluated statin treatment in men and women age 70 to 82 years with either known vascular disease or at increased risk owing to smoking, hypertension, or diabetes mellitus (DM) *(33)*. Overall, there was a significant 15% relative risk reduction in the primary composite end point of coronary death, nonfatal MI, and fatal or nonfatal stroke in the treatment arm. The benefit was primarily the result of a decrease in the event rate for those with known vascular disease.

Fibrate interventions designed to raise HDL and lower triglyceride also benefit the older population. The Benzafibrate Infarction Prevention (BIP) study of patients aged 45 to 74 reported a 16% reduction in cardiac mortality for a 10mg/dL increase in HDL *(34,35)*. The Veterans Affairs HDL Intervention Trial (VA-HIT) for secondary prevention achieved a 22% reduction in cardiac event rates with fibrate therapy *(36)*. These findings would suggest that the current National Cholesterol Education Guidelines that focus not only on TC and LDL but also HDL and non-LDL particles apply to the elderly as well *(37)*.

National Cholesterol Education Program- Adult Treatment Panel III (NCEP ATP-III) guidelines recommend statin therapy for patients with known vascular disease, diabetes, and those with a 10-year Framinghan risk score of more than 20% *(38)*. The Heart Protection Study and the ASCOT study noted earlier, reported after the release of these guidelines, indicate that statin therapy decreases events in important patient subsets regardless of the initial LDL level. In addition, recent studies indicate less progression of coronary atherosclerosis in patients with documented disease, and decreased coronary events in those with acute coronary syndromes, in patients randomized to intensive (i.e., LDL of 60–70 mg/dL), as compared with moderate (i.e., LDL cholesterol of 90–100 mg/dL) lipid-lowering therapies *(39,40)*.

Unfortunately, despite the very convincing data that elderly patients benefit from lipid-lowering therapy, they are markedly undertreated *(41, 42)*. The Clinical Quality Improvement Network evaluated 3304 hospitalized patients at high risk for future cardiovascular events owing to the presence of cardiac ischemia, previous MI, previous revascularization, or DM *(43)*. Only 28% had a lipid measure either in the hospital or in the 5 years prior to admission and only 8% of the patients were on lipid-lowering drug therapy. Age 70 years or older was statistically associated with a reduced likelihood of lipid determination or lipid therapy. Recent data also indicate low persistence of statin therapy in older patients. In one study of patients aged 66 years or older who were prescribed statin therapy, 2-year adherence rates were only 40.1% for those with acute coronary syndrome, 36.1% for those with chronic coronary disease, and 25.4% when statin was prescribed for primary prevention *(44)*. In another report of 345,000 patients over 65 years of age enrolled in a New Jersey assistance program, only 25% maintained greater than 80% persistence at 5 years with the greatest drop occurring within the first 6 months *(45)*. In this study, the greatest decline appeared to occur within the first 6 months. Implementation and persistent use of statin therapies known to significantly decrease cardiovascular events, including stroke and MI, in older individuals is, therefore, another significant challenge and opportunity for health care providers.

Diabetes

The incidence and prevalence of type II DM and insulin resistance increases with age; an estimated 13.2% of people 75 years and older carry the diagnosis of diabetes and another 5.7% and 14.1% of this age group have undiagnosed diabetes or impaired fasting glucose *(46,47)*. Prevalence rates vary significantly among different racial and socioeconomic groups. In Japanese-American men aged 71–93 years, the prevalence of diabetes rises to 17% with an additional 19% with undiagnosed diabetes and 32% with impaired glucose tolerance; even higher rates are estimated in non-Hispanic African-Americans and perhaps the highest rates exist in Native Americans *(1)*.

Diseases of the heart and/or blood vessels account for at least 75% of the mortality of diabetics; the risk of CHD death is two to four times higher in diabetics vs non-diabetics, this relationship is more marked in women than in men *(1,48–51)* and diabetes is a potent predictor of coronary events among older, as well as younger, people. Data from Finland demonstrate that the risk of MI is similar between patients with prior infarctions and those with diabetes but no prior infarction. Thus, diabetes is considered to impart a risk of a future coronary event similar to the risk of those with known coronary disease *(52)*. Framingham data indicate that diabetes increases the relative risk of CHD by 1.7 for men and 3.3 for women *(53)*. Strong Heart Study data assessing diabetes among Native Americans reported that the relative risk of CHD was increased by 1.8 for men and 4.6 for women *(54)*. Insulin resistance in the absence of hyperglycemia is also associated with increased cardiovascular risk, as middle aged men in the United States with the metabolic syndrome incur an added three-to fourfold risk of CHD mortality *(55)*. Diabetes is also associated with an increased likelihood for adverse outcomes following the diagnosis of coronary disease. Data from the Cooperative Cardiovascular Project evaluating Medicare patients over the age of 65 admitted with acute MI found that 30-day and 1-year mortality were significantly higher among patients with diabetes *(56)*.

Diabetes and glucose intolerance accelerate other CHD risk factors including arterial stiffening, progression of atherosclerotic lesions, and chronic kidney disease in older patients *(57–60)*. Although there are currently no data regarding the beneficial effects of tight glycemic control in elderly patients, the American Heart Association/Amercan College of Cardiology Guidelines for Preventing Heart Attack and Death in Patients with Atherosclerotic Cardiovascular Disease recommend a hemoglobin A1c level below 7% *(61)*. Efforts to control other cardiovascular risk factors in older patients with diabetes should be emphasized as treatment guidelines (NCEP-ATP3, JNC-7) suggest lower goals for BP, less than 130/80, and LDL cholesterol, less than 100 mg/dL in patients with co-existing diabetes *(2,38)*. More recent reports indicate that the routine use of statins in patients with diabetes regardless of initial LDL cholesterol decreases cardiovascular events *(32,62)*, as does the use of ACE inhibitors *(63)*. Finally, lifestyle modification should be particularly emphasized in older Americans. Exercise in older adults reduces hyperinsulinemia and improves insulin action and, when combined with dietary control, reduces the incidence of type II diabetes by 70% in those with impaired glucose tolerance *(64,65)*.

Obesity

Observational data from the Framingham cohort indicate that, on average, body mass index increases with age up to approximately age 65 years, at which point it starts to decline *(66)*. Decreases in metabolism, physical inactivity owing to sedentary lifestyle and co-morbidities such as arthritis, depression, and heart failure contribute to decreased activity levels and lean body mass.

Whether obesity, defined as a body mass index greater than 30 kg/m^2, is a risk factor for CHD in the elderly, per se, continues to be debated *(67–69)*. However, the importance of obesity in older adults is underscored by its association with other CHD risks such as hypertension and hyperlipidemia *(70,71)*. More concerning than the risk of generalized obesity in the elderly is the risk of abdominal obesity, often measured as the waist–hip ratio (WHR), and its correlation to insulin resistance *(72, 73)*. Lean body mass declines and abdominal adiposity increases in the elderly *(67,74,75)*. WHR is a CHD risk factor in the elderly, especially in women, although it is less strongly associated with CHD than in younger adults *(75,76)*. The metabolic syndrome, defined by having at least three of the following characteristics: abdominal obesity, hypertriglyceridemia,

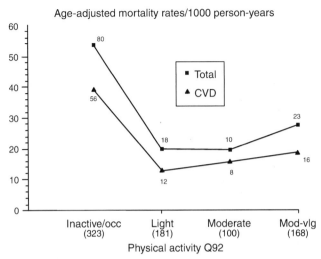

Fig. 2. Physical activity at Q92 an age-adjusted mortality rates per 1000 person-years in 772 men with diagnosed coronary heart disease (CVD in figure) excluding men reporting "poor health." Numbers indicate deaths. CVD, cardiovascular disease; vig, vigorous. (Reproduced with permission from ref. *79*.)

hypertension, low HDL and elevated fasting blood glucose, is a cluster of CHD risk factors of growing concern in older adults *(38,73)*. The prevalence of the metabolic syndrome increases with age; more than 40% of those over 60 years of age meet criteria for this CHD risk.

Exercise and weight-loss programs improve BP, cholesterol profiles, and insulin metabolism *(64,65,68,77,78)*. In the Diabetes Prevention Program, lifestyle modification including weight reduction and regular physical activity in subjects 60 years and older with elevated fasting glucose, reduced the incidence of diabetes by 71%, which was a greater reduction than in all other age groups *(68)*. In another study, physical activity in older men with established CAD was also significantly related to all cause mortality with an adjusted relative risk of 0.42 for light and 0.47 for moderate activity, as compared to inactive or only occasionally active individuals over a 5-year follow-up period (*see* Fig. 2; *79*).

Smoking

The prevalence of smoking decreases with increasing age, yet in 1998, 10.4% of men and 11.2% of people over age 65 years were current smokers *(67)*. This percentage declined to less than 5% in people over 85 years old. The increase in risk for death or MI continues to be elevated in older current smokers in comparison to age-matched former smokers (80). In the Coronary Artery Surgery Study, this elevated mortality risk was highest for those over 75 years, with a relative risk of death of 3.3 for current compared with former smokers in contrast to a relative risk of 1.5 in those aged 55–59 years. In a cohort of 7178 people over 65 years old (the Established Populations for the Epidemiologic Studies of the Elderly), the relative risks of death and cardiovascular death were 2.1 and 2.0, respectively, for current smokers compared with those who never smoked (81). In elderly patients in a long-term health care facility, cigarette smoking was associated with an increased relative risk of new coronary events by a factor of 2.2 in men and 2.0 in women.

Smoking is the second most important established risk factor, after hypertension, for stroke and it is estimated that smoking cessation could prevent approximately 60,000 strokes per year. Twenty percent of smokers over age 65 have peripheral vascular disease and continued smoking increases the risks of gangrene and limb amputation. Smoking also increases the risks of chronic obstructive pulmonary disease and lung cancer in the older population (82).

Interestingly, only 73% of smokers aged 65–75 years and 56% of smokers over age 85 years are advised to quit despite the evidence of continued, if not elevated, risk in this segment of the population (83). Smoking cessation decreases morbidity and mortality in those over age 70 who have undergone bypass surgery. In those patients with previous MI, smoking cessation reduces mortality by 25% to 50% (84–86). Reduction in relative risk of MI or death from smoking cessation was the same for those over age 70 as for those who were younger (87). Given the chronicity of the problem, cessation efforts require repeated, multiple interventions. Data on patients with MI reveal significant improvement in quit-rates when multiple providers counseled cessation while the patient was hospitalized. Efforts at behavior modification along with provision of cessation aids, such as low-dose nicotine patch or buproprion can markedly improve quit-rates (82).

Pre-Existing Atherosclerosis

The risk factor most correlated with new coronary events is known coronary disease or previous cardiac events. History of previous MI increased the risk of cardiac mortality by a factor of 2.1 in the BIP study and a prior cardiac event carried a relative risk of 2.1 for an acute MI in the Dubbo study of the elderly (22). As in the younger population, concurrent atherosclerosis evidenced by peripheral or cerebrovascular disease, increases CVD risk. In BIP, cardiac mortality was increased by a factor of 2.1 for patients with a history of a cerebrovascular accident and by 1.8 for patients with peripheral vascular disease *(34)*. Data from the Honolulu Heart Program indicated that a low ankle-brachial index was an independent risk for CHD among individuals over 70 years of age *(88)*. Particularly unique to the elderly are the high rates of silent MI, discovered by routine EKG *(89–91)*. Thirty percent of the MIs diagnosed among the Framingham cohort were discovered on routine surveillance; half of these were truly silent and half could be accounted for by very atypical symptoms *(12)*. Ten-year follow-up of the Honolulu Heart Study revealed a 33% incidence of unrecognized MI *(92)*. Aronow reported that 68% of Q-wave MIs diagnosed by EKG on nursing home admission were clinically unrecognized, yet carried the same risk for recurrent events as symptomatic MIs *(93)*. The Honolulu Heart Study 10-year mortality rates were 45% for unrecognized MI and 36% for symptomatic MI *(92)*.

Left Ventricular Hypertrophy

Probably because of an association with increased left ventricular load in older adults, the prevalence of EKG-defined LVH increases with age *(94)*. In the Framingham cohort, the prevalence of LVH on EKG was 4.2% and 4.9% for men and women, repectively, aged 75–84 years and rose rapidly to 5.9 and 9.4% for men and women, respectively, aged 85–94 years *(11)*. EKG LVH is a significant risk factor for both primary and secondary CHD events in older adults. Compared to those 65–94 year old without LVH, those with LVH in the same age cohort have an adjusted relative risk for CHD of 2.7 for men and 3.0 for women *(95,96)*. Regression of EKG LVH in the elderly can be achieved by pharmacological therapy such as ACE or blockade of angiotensin or β-adrenergic receptors; reduction with ACE inhibitor therapy is associated with reduction in the risk of death, MI, stroke and CHF *(97,98)*.

PROPOSED RISK FACTORS

Classical risk factors can be identified as those that are not only independently associated with increased risk but also those for which treatment decreases cardiovascular risk. There are also new, proposed risk factors that are associated with increased risk, but for which treatment directed at reversing the risk factor has not yet been studied, or which has not yet been proven to reverse risk. Their identification may, nevertheless, be useful because they provide prognostic information and therefore may guide the intensity of interventions for established risk factors and insight into the pathophysiology of manifestations of coronary disease, and help to direct future research.

Depression and Social Isolation

Depression, social isolation, and exhaustion are significantly associated with cardiovascular events in older individuals. Depression itself is a significant risk factor for overall mortality and for primary and secondary CHD events in the elderly *(99–101)*. The relative risks reported for those with minor and major depressive symptoms compared to nondepressed individuals for cardiac death were 1.6 and 3.0, respectively, in a cohort of 2847 men and women between the ages of 55 and 85 years old *(100)*. Loneliness and social isolation among the elderly are also associated with increased cardiovascular mortality *(102)*.

Depression is also prevalent, occurring in at least 30% of people after an MI and although often not diagnosed, clearly has a negative impact on survival *(103,104)*. Negative affectivity, overt anger, medical co-morbidities, and poor social support are risk factors for post-MI depression *(105,106)* and lack of social support increases an individual's risk of subsequent cardiac mortality almost threefold following an MI, as compared to those with adequate support systems *(107)*.

There are several potential explanations for the relationship between depression and cardiovascular outcomes. In the CHS, depression was significantly related to pro-inflammatory and and pro-thrombotic markers including high sensitivity C-reactive protein (CRP), white blood cell count, platelet count, factors VII and VIII, and to fibrinogen levels. Other possibilities include altered sympathetic/parasympathetic balance and steroid levels. In addition, depression may be related to an increased likelihood of poor health behaviors, including smoking, lack of exercise, and overeating.

The Enhancing Recovery in Coronary Heart Disease Patients trial reported the beneficial effects of a formal cognitive-behavioral intervention on reducing depression and social isolation in patients after a heart attack with these syndromes *(108)*. This study randomized 2481 post-MI patients with depression and/or low perceived social support to either cognitive-behavioral therapy with counseling and antidepressant use when indicated, or to usual care. Although formal cognitive therapy did not significantly reduce the risk of death or nonfatal MI during the 29-month follow-up period, significant improvements in depression and perceived social isolation scores were seen in the intervention, as compared with the usual care, arm as early as 6 months *(108)*. Participation in phase II cardiac rehabilitation programs also significantly reduces depressive scores in those over age 75 years *(77)*.

Newer Risk Factors

HIGH SENSITIVITY C-REACTIVE PROTEIN

High sensitivity C-reactive protein (hsCRP) is an inflammatory bio-marker that is emerging as an important CHD risk factor, especially in elderly women *(109)*. As an acute-phase reactant, hsCRP induces complement, regulates endothelial nitric oxide production and upregulates cellular adhesion molecule expression, all important steps in the atherosclerotic process. Levels of hsCRP increase with smoking, obesity, hormone replacement therapy use, hypertension, diabetes and with a low HDL level and decrease with non-steroidal anti-inflammatory and with statin therapies *(39,110)*. In case control studies, hsCRP is an independent predictor of CAD and the level reflects disease burden *(111,112)*. In comparing baseline hsCRP levels between 122 women who had a CHD event and 244 age-smoking matched controls from the Women's Health Study who did not, the relative risk of any vascular event was fivefold and for stroke or myocardial infarction was sevenfold for those women with high, as compared with a low, baseline hsCRP *(113)*. In prospective cohort studies, elevated hsCRP is associated with increased cardiovascular mortality and peripheral arterial disease CHD events, particularly in women, but the relationship between hsCRP and cardiovascular mortality may be less significant in those over 80 years of age *(109,113–115)*. In a prospective study of 27,939 participants of the Women's Health Study who were followed for a mean of 8 years, the age-adjusted relative risks for a CHD event was 3.6 in the highest quintile of hsCRP and remained 2.3 when adjusted for other traditional CHD risk factors including LDL. Thus, hsCRP levels in older women provides prognostic information which is additive to that provided by traditional CHD risk factors. Studies are ongoing as to whether the risk associated with elevated hsCRP can be lowered with therapies that reduce inflammation such as HMG-CoA reductase inhibitors *(116)*.

Coronary Artery Calcium

Coronary artery calcium (CAC), detected noninvasively by electron beam computed tomography (EBCT), is a marker of the presence and extent of atherosclerotic plaque *(117)*. With increasing age, CAC scores, on average, increase at a rate which is faster in men than in women, and which tends to be higher in Caucasians than in African-Americans, regardless of gender *(118,119)*. However, EBCT performed on 614 CHS participants of age range 67 to 99 years demonstrates that, although average CAC score increases with age, there is a wide variability including scores of no calcium *(120)*. Although those with high scores do have an increased risk of experiencing cardiovascular events, the increased calcification associated with age may decrease the discriminant value of the score itself in predicting events in the elderly. A prospective study indicates that the individual's score ranked as a percentile against published age- and gender-adjusted values is a more effective screening tool than the absolute score itself *(121)*. This may be particularly relevant in the older population, although the premise has not been separately examined in an older population.

Homocysteine

Levels of plasma homocysteine rise with increasing age and are associated with elevated risks for ISH, CAD, peripheral vascular disease, stroke, aortic atherosclerosis, MI, and both cardiovascular and overall mortality in the elderly *(122–126)*. Potential mechanisms include impaired endothelial function, increased prothrombotic state, and altered vascular smooth muscle and extracellular matrix function *(127)*. In a short-term study, 0.5 mg per day of folic acid supplementation did not reduce CHD events *(128)*, and in a more recent publication *(129)*, did not decrease re-stenosis rates following coronary angioplasty. Thus, routine screening of plasma homocysteine levels cannot be recommended in the elderly.

Carotid Intima-Media Thickness

Increased carotid intima-media thickness (IMT), as measured by high-resolution B-mode ultrasound, is associated with an increased risk for MI and stroke in older adults *(22,130,131)*. Among 5858 participants in the CHS over age 65 years, free of clinical CHD, and followed for 6.2 years, there was a progressive increase in the risk for MI and stroke as carotid IMT increased. The relative risk, after adjusting for other risk factors, for these outcomes was 3.15 for those whose baseline carotid IMT was in the highest quintile *(130)*. It is unclear whether the risk is related to the presence of subclinical atherosclerosis or increased intimal proliferation, a marker of vascular aging (*see* Chapter 1). No clinical trials assessing whether clinical events are reduced by using carotid IMT to guide pharmacological therapy have been performed. Thus, the value of carotid IMT measures in terms of therapeutic implications to decrease coronary events is not known.

Sleep Apnea

The prevalence of disordered breathing during sleep, or sleep apnea, increases with age such that in those over age 65 years, an estimated 4%

of women and 13% of men have the disorder, and up to 19% of women and 33% of men in this age group snore *(132,133)*. Sleep-disordered breathing in older adults is associated with vascular abnormalities including endothelial dysfunction and hypertension *(134,135)*. Moreover, sleep apnea is significantly correlated to abdominal fat distribution, glucose impairment and serum leptin level suggesting an association with the metabolic syndrome *(136)*. Epidemiological data as well as prospective trials confirm that sleep apnea is an independent risk factor for CHD events, cardiovascular mortality and strokes in older adults *(137–139)*. The CHS cohort demonstrate that daytime sleepiness, even more so that disrupted sleep, is associated with increased mortality and CHD events in older women more than men *(140)*. Treatment of OSA with continuous positive airway pressure is associated with significant decreases in nighttime, and 24-hour BP in hypertensive subjects *(141,142)*.

SUMMARY

The relative significance of various risk factors for CHD changes with age and is likely influenced by survival bias. Whereas some risk factors become more powerful, and treatment of these leads to a more significant CHD risk reduction in those over 65 years than they do for younger individuals, other become less significant. Lifestyle modifications such as diet, smoking, and exercise significantly impact the risk for the development and manifestations of CHD and the development of diabetes. Novel risk factors provide prognostic information, but it is not yet demonstrated that therapies based on treating these improves outcomes. Interventions should focus on initiating and maintaining treatments for known risk factors such as hypertension and hyperlipidemia, in the older population.

REFERENCES

1. American Heart Association. Heart Disease and Stroke Statistics—2005 Update. Dallas, TX, American Heart Association, 2003.
2. Chobanian AV, Bakris GL, Black HR, et al. The Seventh Report of the Joint National Committee on Prevention, Detection, Evaluation, and Treatment of High Blood Pressure: the JNC 7 report. JAMA 2003;289(19):2560–2572.
3. Wilson PW. An epidemiologic perspective of systemic hypertension, ischemic heart disease, and heart failure. Am J Cardiol 1997;80(9B):3J–8J.
4. Lewington S, Clarke R, Qizilbash N, Peto R, Collins R. Age-specific relevance of usual blood pressure to vascular mortality: a meta-analysis of individual data for one million adults in 61 prospective studies. Lancet 2002;360(9349):1903–1913.
5. SHEP Cooperative Research Group. Prevention of stroke by antihypertensive drug treatment in older persons with isolated systolic hypertension. Final results of the Systolic Hypertension in the Elderly Program (SHEP). JAMA 1991;265(24): 3255–3264.

6. Staessen J, Fagard R, Thijs L, et al. Randomised double-blind comparison of placebo and active treatment for older patients with isolated systolic hypertension. The Systolic Hypertension in Europe (Syst-Eur) Trial Investigators. Lancet 1997; 350(9080):757–764.

7. Forette F, Seux ML, Staessen JA, et al. Prevention of dementia in randomised double-blind placebo-controlled Systolic Hypertension in Europe (Syst-Eur) trial. Lancet 1998;352(9137):1347–1351.

8. Staessen J, Gasowski J, Wang J, et al. Risks of untreated and treated isolated systolic hypertension in the elderly: meta-analysis of outcome trials. Lancet 2000;355 (9207):865–872.

9. Gueyffier F, Bulpitt C, Boissel JP, et al. Antihypertensive drugs in very old people: a subgroup meta-analysis of randomised controlled trials. INDANA Group. Lancet 1999;353(9155):793–796.

10. Hyman D, Pavlik V. Characteristics of patients with uncontrolled hypertension in the United States. N Engl J Med 2001;345(7):479–486.

11. Levy D, Anderson KM, Savage DD, Kannel WB, Christiansen JC, Castelli WP. Echocardiographically detected left ventricular hypertrophy: prevalence and risk factors. The Framingham Heart Study. Ann Intern Med 1988;108(1):7–13.

12. Aronow WS. The older man's heart and heart disease. Med Clin North Am 1999; 83(5):1291–1303.

13. Kjeldsen SE, Dahlof B, Devereux RB, et al. Effects of losartan on cardiovascular morbidity and mortality in patients with isolated systolic hypertension and left ventricular hypertrophy: a Losartan Intervention for Endpoint Reduction (LIFE) substudy. JAMA 2002;288(12):1491–1498.

14. Dahlof B, Pennert K, Hansson L. Reversal of left ventricular hypertrophy in hypertensive patients. A metaanalysis of 109 treatment studies. Am J Hypertens 1992; 5(2):95–110.

15. Major outcomes in high-risk hypertensive patients randomized to angiotensin-converting enzyme inhibitor or calcium channel blocker vs diuretic: The Antihypertensive and Lipid-Lowering Treatment to Prevent Heart Attack Trial (ALLHAT). JAMA 2002;288(23):2981–2997.

16. Manolio TA, Pearson TA, Wenger NK, Barrett-Connor E, Payne GH, Harlan WR. Cholesterol and heart disease in older persons and women. Review of an NHLBI workshop. Ann Epidemiol 1992;2(1–2):161–176.

17. Sorkin JD, Andres R, Muller DC, Baldwin HL, Fleg JL. Cholesterol as a risk factor for coronary heart disease in elderly men. The Baltimore Longitudinal Study of Aging. Ann Epidemiol 1992;2(1–2):59–67.

18. Schatz IJ, Masaki K, Yano K, Chen R, Rodriguez BL, Curb JD. Cholesterol and all-cause mortality in elderly people from the Honolulu Heart Program: a cohort study. Lancet 2001;358(9279):351–355.

19. Weverling-Rijnsburger AW, Blauw GJ, Lagaay AM, Knook DL, Meinders AE, Westendorp RG. Total cholesterol and risk of mortality in the oldest old. Lancet 1997;350(9085):1119–1123.

20. Corti MC, Guralnik JM, Salive ME, et al. Clarifying the direct relation between total cholesterol levels and death from coronary heart disease in older persons. Ann Intern Med 1997;126(10):753–760.

21. Krumholz HM, Seeman TE, Merrill SS, et al. Lack of association between cholesterol and coronary heart disease mortality and morbidity and all-cause mortality in persons older than 70 years. JAMA 1994;272(17):1335–1340.

22. Simons LA, Simons J, Friedlander Y, McCallum J. Risk factors for acute myocardial infarction in the elderly (the Dubbo study). Am J Cardiol 2002;89(1):69–72.

23. Corti MC, Guralnik JM, Salive ME, et al. HDL cholesterol predicts coronary heart disease mortality in older persons. JAMA 1995;274(7):539–544.
24. Castelli WP, Garrison RJ, Wilson PW, Abbott RD, Kalousdian S, Kannel WB. Incidence of coronary heart disease and lipoprotein cholesterol levels. The Framingham Study. JAMA 1986;256(20):2835–2838.
25. Shepherd J, Cobbe S, Ford I, et al. Prevention of coronary heart disease with pravastatin in men with hypercholesterolemia. West of Scotland Coronary Prevention Study Group. N Engl J Med 1995;333[20]:1301–1307.
26. Downs J, Clearfield M, Weis S, et al. Primary prevention of acute coronary events with lovastatin in men and women with average cholesterol levels: results of AFCAPS/TexCAPS. Air Force/Texas Coronary Atherosclerosis Prevention Study. JAMA 1998;279[20]:1615–1622.
27. Whitney E, Downs J, Clearfield M. Air Force/Texas Coronary Atherosclerosis Prevention Study: extending the benefit of primary prevention to healthy elderly men and women. Circulation 1998;98:I–46.
28. Sever PS, Dahlof B, Poulter NR, et al. Prevention of coronary and stroke events with atorvastatin in hypertensive patients who have average or lower-than-average cholesterol concentrations, in the Anglo-Scandinavian Cardiac Outcomes Trial— Lipid Lowering Arm (ASCOT-LLA): a multicentre randomised controlled trial. Lancet 2003;361(9364):1149–1158.
29. Scandanavian Simvastatin Survival Study. Randomised trial of cholesterol lowering in 4444 patients with coronary heart disease: the Scandinavian Simvastatin Survival Study (4S). Lancet 1994;344:1383–1389.
30. Sacks F, Pfeffer M, Moye L, et al. The effect of pravastatin on coronary events after myocardial infarction in patients with average cholesterol levels. N Engl J Med 1996;335(14):1001–1009.
31. Lewis SJ, Moye LA, Sacks FM, et al. Effect of pravastatin on cardiovascular events in older patients with myocardial infarction and cholesterol levels in the average range. Results of the Cholesterol and Recurrent Events (CARE) trial. Ann Intern Med 1998;129(9):681–689.
32. MRC/BHF Heart Protection Study of cholesterol lowering with simvastatin in 20,536 high-risk individuals: a randomised placebo-controlled trial. Lancet 2002; 360(9326):7–22.
33. Shepherd J, Blauw GJ, Murphy MB, et al. Pravastatin in elderly individuals at risk of vascular disease (PROSPER): a randomised controlled trial. Lancet 2002;360 (9346):1623–1630.
34. Dankner R, Goldbourt U, Boyko V, Reicher-Reiss H. Predictors of cardiac and non-cardiac mortality among 14,697 patients with coronary heart disease. Am J Cardiol 2003;91(2):121–127.
35. Secondary prevention by raising HDL cholesterol and reducing triglycerides in patients with coronary artery disease: the Bezafibrate Infarction Prevention (BIP) study. Circulation 2000;102(1):21–27.
36. Rubins HB, Robins SJ, Collins D, et al. Gemfibrozil for the secondary prevention of coronary heart disease in men with low levels of high-density lipoprotein cholesterol. Veterans Affairs High-Density Lipoprotein Cholesterol Intervention Trial Study Group. N Engl J Med 1999;341(6):410–418.
37. Sprecher DL, Watkins TR, Behar S, Brown WV, Rubins HB, Schaefer EJ. Importance of high-density lipoprotein cholesterol and triglyceride levels in coronary heart disease. Am J Cardiol 2003;91(5):575–580.
38. Executive Summary of The Third Report of The National Cholesterol Education Program (NCEP) Expert Panel on Detection, Evaluation, and Treatment of High

Blood Cholesterol in Adults (Adult Treatment Panel III). JAMA 2001;285(19): 2486–2497.

39. Nissen SE, Tuzcu EM, Schoenhagen P, et al. Effect of intensive compared with moderate lipid-lowering therapy on progression of coronary atherosclerosis: a randomized controlled trial. JAMA 2004;291(9):1071–1080.

40. Cannon CP, Braunwald E, McCabe CH, et al. Intensive versus moderate lipid lowering with statins after acute coronary syndromes. N Engl J Med 2004;350(15): 1495–1504.

41. Mendelson G, Aronow WS. Underutilization of measurement of serum low-density lipoprotein cholesterol levels and of lipid-lowering therapy in older patients with manifest atherosclerotic disease. J Am Geriatr Soc 1998;46(9):1128–1131.

42. Kopjar B, Sales AE, Pineros SL, Sun H, Li YF, Hedeen AN. Comparison of characteristics of patients with coronary heart disease receiving lipid-lowering therapy versus those not receiving such therapy. Am J Cardiol 2003;91(11):1352–1354.

43. Low incidence of assessment and modification of risk factors in acute care patients at high risk for cardiovascular events, particularly among females and the elderly. The Clinical Quality Improvement Network (CQIN) Investigators. Am J Cardiol 1995;76(8):570–573.

44. Jackevicius CA, Mamdani M, Tu JV. Adherence with statin therapy in elderly patients with and without acute coronary syndromes. JAMA 2002;288(4):462–467.

45. Benner JS, Glynn RJ, Mogun H, Neumann PJ, Weinstein MC, Avorn J. Long-term persistence in use of statin therapy in elderly patients. JAMA 2002;288(4):455–461.

46. Harris MI, Flegal KM, Cowie CC, et al. Prevalence of diabetes, impaired fasting glucose, and impaired glucose tolerance in U.S. adults. The Third National Health and Nutrition Examination Survey, 1988–1994. Diabetes Care 1998;21(4):518–524.

47. Kohrt WM, Kirwan JP, Staten MA, Bourey RE, King DS, Holloszy JO. Insulin resistance in aging is related to abdominal obesity. Diabetes 1993;42(2):273–281.

48. American Heart Association. Heart and Stroke Statistics—2003 Update. 2002. Dallas, Texas, American Heart Association.

49. Natarajan S, Liao Y, Cao G, Lipsitz SR, McGee DL. Sex differences in risk for coronary heart disease mortality associated with diabetes and established coronary heart disease. Arch Intern Med 2003;163(14):1735–1740.

50. Becker A, Bos G, de Vegt F, et al. Cardiovascular events in type 2 diabetes: com-parison with nondiabetic individuals without and with prior cardiovascular disease. 10-year follow-up of the Hoorn Study. Eur Heart J 2003;24(15):1406–1413.

51. Braunstein JB, Anderson GF, Gerstenblith G, et al. Noncardiac comorbidity increases preventable hospitalizations and mortality among Medicare beneficiaries with chronic heart failure. J Am Coll Cardiol 2003;42(7):1226–1233.

52. Haffner SM, Lehto S, Ronnemaa T, Pyorala K, Laakso M. Mortality from coronary heart disease in subjects with type 2 diabetes and in nondiabetic subjects with and without prior myocardial infarction. N Engl J Med 1998;339(4):229–234.

53. Castelli WP. Epidemiology of coronary heart disease: the Framingham study. Am J Med 1984;76(2A):4–12.

54. Howard BV, Welty TK, Fabsitz RR, et al. Risk factors for coronary heart disease in diabetic and nondiabetic Native Americans. The Strong Heart Study. Diabetes 1992; 41 Suppl 2:4–11.

55. Lakka HM, Laaksonen DE, Lakka TA, et al. The metabolic syndrome and total and cardiovascular disease mortality in middle-aged men. JAMA 2002;288(21): 2709–2716.

56. Berger AK, Breall JA, Gersh BJ, et al. Effect of diabetes mellitus and insulin use on survival after acute myocardial infarction in the elderly (the Cooperative Cardiovascular Project). Am J Cardiol 2001;87(3):272–277.
57. Henry RM, Kostense PJ, Spijkerman AM, et al. Arterial stiffness increases with deteriorating glucose tolerance status: the Hoorn Study. Circulation 2003;107(16): 2089–2095.
58. Ulrich P, Cerami A. Protein glycation, diabetes, and aging. Recent Prog Horm Res 2001;56:1–21.
59. van der Meer IM, Iglesias DS, Hak AE, Bots ML, Hofman A, Witteman JC. Risk factors for progression of atherosclerosis measured at multiple sites in the arterial tree: the Rotterdam Study. Stroke 2003;34(10):2374–2379.
60. Collins AJ, Li S, Gilbertson DT, Liu J, Chen SC, Herzog CA. Chronic kidney disease and cardiovascular disease in the Medicare population. Kidney Int Suppl 2003; 87:S24–S31.
61. Smith SC Jr, Blair SN, Bonow RO, et al. AHA/ACC Scientific Statement: AHA/ACC guidelines for preventing heart attack and death in patients with atherosclerotic cardiovascular disease: 2001 update: A statement for healthcare professionals from the American Heart Association and the American College of Cardiology. Circulation 2001;104(13):1577–1579.
62. Colhoun HM, Betteridge DJ, Durrington PN, Hitman GA, Neil HA, Livingstone SJ, et al. Primary prevention of cardiovascular disease with atorvastatin in type 2 diabetes in the Collaborative Atorvastatin Diabetes Study (CARDS): multicentre randomised placebo-controlled trial. Lancet 2004;364(9435):685–696.
63. Sleight P. The HOPE Study (Heart Outcomes Prevention Evaluation). J Renin Angiotensin Aldosterone Syst 2000;1(1):18–20.
64. Knowler WC, Barrett-Connor E, Fowler SE, et al. Reduction in the incidence of type 2 diabetes with lifestyle intervention or metformin. N Engl J Med 2002;346(6): 393–403.
65. Kirwan JP, Kohrt WM, Wojta DM, Bourey RE, Holloszy JO. Endurance exercise training reduces glucose-stimulated insulin levels in 60- to 70-year-old men and women. J Gerontol 1993;48(3):M84–M90.
66. Wilson PW, Kannel WB. Obesity, diabetes, and risk of cardiovascular disease in the elderly. Am J Geriatr Cardiol 2002;11(2):119–123.
67. Poehlman ET, Toth MJ, Bunyard LB, et al. Physiological predictors of increasing total and central adiposity in aging men and women. Arch Intern Med 1995;155 (22):2443–2448.
68. Harris TB, Launer LJ, Madans J, Feldman JJ. Cohort study of effect of being overweight and change in weight on risk of coronary heart disease in old age. BMJ 1997;314(7097):1791–1794.
69. Heiat A. Impact of age on definition of standards for ideal weight. Prev Cardiol 2003;6(2):104–107.
70. Brochu M, Poehlman ET, Savage P, Ross S, Ades PA. Coronary risk profiles in men with coronary artery disease: effects of body composition, fat distribution, age and fitness. Coron Artery Dis 2000;11(2):137–144.
71. Wildman RP, Mackey RH, Bostom A, Thompson T, Sutton-Tyrrell K. Measures of obesity are associated with vascular stiffness in young and older adults. Hypertension 2003;42(4):468–473.
72. Boden G, Chen X, DeSantis RA, Kendrick Z. Effects of age and body fat on insulin resistance in healthy men. Diabetes Care 1993;16(5):728–733.
73. Park YW, Zhu S, Palaniappan L, Heshka S, Carnethon MR, Heymsfield SB. The metabolic syndrome: prevalence and associated risk factor findings in the US

population from the Third National Health and Nutrition Examination Survey, 1988–1994. Arch Intern Med 2003;163(4):427–436.

74. Williamson DF. Descriptive epidemiology of body weight and weight change in U.S. adults. Ann Intern Med 1993;119(7 Pt 2):646–649.

75. Turcato E, Bosello O, Di F, et al. Waist circumference and abdominal sagittal diameter as surrogates of body fat distribution in the elderly: their relation with cardiovascular risk factors. Int J Obes Relat Metab Disord 2000;24(8):1005–1010.

76. Ross SJ, Poehlman ET, Johnson RK, Ades PA. Body fat distribution predicts cardiac risk factors in older female coronary patients. J Cardiopulm Rehabil 1997; 17(6):419–427.

77. Lavie CJ, Milani RV. Effects of cardiac rehabilitation and exercise training programs in patients > or = 75 years of age. Am J Cardiol 1996;78(6):675–677.

78. Whelton PK, Appel LJ, Espeland MA, et al. Sodium reduction and weight loss in the treatment of hypertension in older persons: a randomized controlled trial of non-pharmacologic interventions in the elderly (TONE). TONE Collaborative Research Group. JAMA 1998;279(11):839–846.

79. Wannamethee SG, Shaper AG, Walker M. Physical activity and mortality in older men with diagnosed coronary heart disease. Circulation 2000;102(12):1358–1363.

80. Hermanson B, Omenn GS, Kronmal RA, Gersh BJ. Beneficial six-year outcome of smoking cessation in older men and women with coronary artery disease. Results from the CASS registry. N Engl J Med 1988;319(21):1365–1369.

81. LaCroix AZ, Lang J, Scherr P, et al. Smoking and mortality among older men and women in three communities. N Engl J Med 1991;324(23):1619–1625.

82. Appel DW, Aldrich TK. Smoking cessation in the elderly. Clin Geriatr Med 2003; 19(1):77–100.

83. Receipt of Advice to Quit Smoking in Medicare Managed Care—United States, 1998. MMWR 2000;49(35):797–801.

84. Sparrow D, Dawber TR. The influence of cigarette smoking on prognosis after a first myocardial infarction. A report from the Framingham study. J Chronic Dis 1978; 31(6–7):425–432.

85. Taylor CB, Houston-Miller N, Killen JD, DeBusk RF. Smoking cessation after acute myocardial infarction: effects of a nurse-managed intervention. Ann Intern Med 1990;113(2):118–123.

86. Williams MA, Fleg JL, Ades PA, et al. Secondary prevention of coronary heart disease in the elderly (with emphasis on patients > or =75 years of age): an American Heart Association scientific statement from the Council on Clinical Cardiology Subcommittee on Exercise, Cardiac Rehabilitation, and Prevention. Circulation 2002;105(14):1735–1743.

87. Messinger-Rapport BJ, Sprecher D. Prevention of cardiovascular diseases. Coronary artery disease, congestive heart failure, and stroke. Clin Geriatr Med 2002; 18(3):463–83, vii.

88. Abbott RD, Petrovitch H, Rodriguez BL, et al. Ankle/brachial blood pressure in men >70 years of age and the risk of coronary heart disease. Am J Cardiol 2000; 86(3):280–284.

89. Sheifer SE, Gersh BJ, Yanez ND, III, Ades PA, Burke GL, Manolio TA. Prevalence, predisposing factors, and prognosis of clinically unrecognized myocardial infarction in the elderly. J Am Coll Cardiol 2000;35(1):119–126.

90. Sigurdsson E, Thorgeirsson G, Sigvaldason H, Sigfusson N. Unrecognized myocardial infarction: epidemiology, clinical characteristics, and the prognostic role of angina pectoris. The Reykjavik Study. Ann Intern Med 1995;122(2): 96–102.

91. Nadelmann J, Frishman WH, Ooi WL, et al. Prevalence, incidence and prognosis of recognized and unrecognized myocardial infarction in persons aged 75 years or older: The Bronx Aging Study. Am J Cardiol 1990;66(5):533–537.
92. Yano K, MacLean CJ. The incidence and prognosis of unrecognized myocardial infarction in the Honolulu, Hawaii, Heart Program. Arch Intern Med 1989;149(7): 1528–1532.
93. Aronow WS, Starling L, Etienne F, et al. Unrecognized Q-wave myocardial infarction in patients older than 64 years in a long-term health-care facility. Am J Cardiol 1985;56(7):483.
94. De Bacquer D, De Backer G, Kornitzer M. Prevalences of ECG findings in large population based samples of men and women. Heart 2000;84(6):625–633.
95. Levy D, Salomon M, D'Agostino RB, Belanger AJ, Kannel WB. Prognostic implications of baseline electrocardiographic features and their serial changes in subjects with left ventricular hypertrophy. Circulation 1994;90(4):1786–1793.
96. Wong ND, Cupples LA, Ostfeld AM, Levy D, Kannel WB. Risk factors for long-term coronary prognosis after initial myocardial infarction: the Framingham Study. Am J Epidemiol 1989;130(3):469–480.
97. Okin PM, Devereux RB, Jern S, et al. Regression of electrocardiographic left ventricular hypertrophy by losartan versus atenolol: The Losartan Intervention for Endpoint reduction in Hypertension (LIFE) Study. Circulation 2003;108(6):684–690.
98. Mathew J, Sleight P, Lonn E, et al. Reduction of cardiovascular risk by regression of electrocardiographic markers of left ventricular hypertrophy by the angiotensin-converting enzyme inhibitor ramipril. Circulation 2001;104(14):1615–1621.
99. Cooper JK, Harris Y, McGready J. Sadness predicts death in older people. J Aging Health 2002;14(4):509–526.
100. Penninx BW, Beekman AT, Honig A, et al. Depression and cardiac mortality: results from a community-based longitudinal study. Arch Gen Psychiatry 2001;58(3): 221–227.
101. Luukinen H, Laippala P, Huikuri HV. Depressive symptoms and the risk of sudden cardiac death among the elderly. Eur Heart J 2003;24(22):2021–2026.
102. Inouye SK, Peduzzi PN, Robison JT, Hughes JS, Horwitz RI, Concato J. Importance of functional measures in predicting mortality among older hospitalized patients. JAMA 1998;279(15):1187–1193.
103. Luutonen S, Holm H, Salminen JK, Risla A, Salokangas RK. Inadequate treatment of depression after myocardial infarction. Acta Psychiatr Scand 2002;106(6): 434–439.
104. Shiotani I, Sato H, Kinjo K, et al. Depressive symptoms predict 12-month prognosis in elderly patients with acute myocardial infarction. J Cardiovasc Risk 2002; 9(3):153–160.
105. Frasure-Smith N, Lesperance F. Depression and other psychological risks following myocardial infarction. Arch Gen Psychiatry 2003;60(6):627–636.
106. Watkins LL, Schneiderman N, Blumenthal JA, et al. Cognitive and somatic symptoms of depression are associated with medical comorbidity in patients after acute myocardial infarction. Am Heart J 2003;146(1):48–54.
107. Berkman LF, Leo-Summers L, Horwitz RI. Emotional support and survival after myocardial infarction. A prospective, population-based study of the elderly. Ann Intern Med 1992;117(12):1003–1009.
108. Berkman LF, Blumenthal J, Burg M, et al. Effects of treating depression and low perceived social support on clinical events after myocardial infarction: the Enhancing Recovery in Coronary Heart Disease Patients (ENRICHD) Randomized Trial. JAMA 2003;289(23):3106–3116.

109. Ridker PM. High-sensitivity C-reactive protein and cardiovascular risk: rationale for screening and primary prevention. Am J Cardiol 2003;92(4B):17K–22K.
110. Harris TB, Ferrucci L, Tracy RP, et al. Associations of elevated interleukin-6 and C-reactive protein levels with mortality in the elderly. Am J Med 1999;106(5):506–512.
111. Haidari M, Javadi E, Sadeghi B, Hajilooi M, Ghanbili J. Evaluation of C-reactive protein, a sensitive marker of inflammation, as a risk factor for stable coronary artery disease. Clin Biochem 2001;34(4):309–315.
112. Tracy RP, Lemaitre RN, Psaty BM, et al. Relationship of C-reactive protein to risk of cardiovascular disease in the elderly. Results from the Cardiovascular Health Study and the Rural Health Promotion Project. Arterioscler Thromb Vasc Biol 1997; 17(6):1121–1127.
113. Ridker PM, Buring JE, Shih J, Matias M, Hennekens CH. Prospective study of C-reactive protein and the risk of future cardiovascular events among apparently healthy women. Circulation 1998;98(8):731–733.
114. Ridker PM, Stampfer MJ, Rifai N. Novel risk factors for systemic atherosclerosis: a comparison of C-reactive protein, fibrinogen, homocysteine, lipoprotein(a), and standard cholesterol screening as predictors of peripheral arterial disease. JAMA 2001;285(19):2481–2485.
115. Strandberg TE, Tilvis RS. C-reactive protein, cardiovascular risk factors, and mortality in a prospective study in the elderly. Arterioscler Thromb Vasc Biol 2000;20(4): 1057–1060.
116. Ridker PM. Rosuvastatin in the primary prevention of cardiovascular disease among patients with low levels of low-density lipoprotein cholesterol and elevated high-sensitivity C-reactive protein: rationale and design of the JUPITER trial. Circulation 2003;108(19):2292–2297.
117. Raggi P. Coronary calcium on electron beam tomography imaging as a surrogate marker of coronary artery disease. Am J Cardiol 2001;87(4A):27A–34A.
118. Hoff JA, Chomka EV, Krainik AJ, Daviglus M, Rich S, Kondos GT. Age and gender distributions of coronary artery calcium detected by electron beam tomography in 35,246 adults. Am J Cardiol 2001;87(12):1335–1339.
119. Newman AB, Naydeck BL, Whittle J, Sutton-Tyrrell K, Edmundowicz D, Kuller LH. Racial differences in coronary artery calcification in older adults. Arterioscler Thromb Vasc Biol 2002;22(3):424–430.
120. Newman AB, Naydeck BL, Sutton-Tyrrell K, Feldman A, Edmundowicz D, Kuller LH. Coronary artery calcification in older adults to age 99: prevalence and risk factors. Circulation 2001;104(22):2679–2684.
121. Raggi P, Callister TQ, Cooil B, et al. Identification of patients at increased risk of first unheralded acute myocardial infarction by electron-beam computed tomography. Circulation 2000;101(8):850–855.
122. Sutton-Tyrrell K, Bostom A, Selhub J, Zeigler-Johnson C. High homocysteine levels are independently related to isolated systolic hypertension in older adults. Circulation 1997;96(6):1745–1749.
123. Ridker PM, Manson JE, Buring JE, Shih J, Matias M, Hennekens CH. Homocysteine and risk of cardiovascular disease among postmenopausal women. JAMA 1999;281(19):1817–1821.
124. Kark JD, Selhub J, Adler B, et al. Nonfasting plasma total homocysteine level and mortality in middle-aged and elderly men and women in Jerusalem. Ann Intern Med 1999;131(5):321–330.
125. Bostom AG, Rosenberg IH, Silbershatz H, et al. Nonfasting plasma total homocysteine levels and stroke incidence in elderly persons: the Framingham Study. Ann Intern Med 1999;131(5):352–355.

126. Aronow W, Ahn C. Increased plasma homocysteine is an independent predictor of new coronary events in older persons. Am J Cardiol 2000;86:346–347.
127. Woo KS, Chook P, Lolin YI, et al. Hyperhomocyst(e)inemia is a risk factor for arterial endothelial dysfunction in humans. Circulation 1997;96(8):2542–2544.
128. Liem A, Reynierse-Buitenwerf GH, Zwinderman AH, Jukema JW, van Veldhuisen DJ. Secondary prevention with folic acid: effects on clinical outcomes. J Am Coll Cardiol 2003;41(12):2105–2113.
129. Lange H, Suryapranata H, De Luca G, et al. Folate therapy and in-stent restenosis after coronary stenting. N Engl J Med 2004;350(26):2673–2681.
130. O'Leary DH, Polak JF, Kronmal RA, et al. Thickening of the carotid wall. A marker for atherosclerosis in the elderly? Cardiovascular Health Study Collaborative Research Group. Stroke 1996;27(2):224–231.
131. Cao JJ, Thach C, Manolio TA, et al. C-reactive protein, carotid intima-media thickness, and incidence of ischemic stroke in the elderly: the Cardiovascular Health Study. Circulation 2003;108(2):166–170.
132. Shochat T, Pillar G. Sleep apnoea in the older adult: pathophysiology, epidemiology, consequences and management. Drugs Aging 2003;20(8):551–560.
133. Enright PL, Newman AB, Wahl PW, Manolio TA, Haponik EF, Boyle PJ. Prevalence and correlates of snoring and observed apneas in 5,201 older adults. Sleep 1996;19(7):531–538.
134. Nieto FJ, Harrington DM, Redline S, Benjamin EJ, Robbins JA. Sleep apnea and markers of vascular endothelial function in a large community sample of older adults. Am J Respir Crit Care Med 2003.
135. Peppard PE, Young T, Palta M, Skatrud J. Prospective study of the association between sleep-disordered breathing and hypertension. N Engl J Med 2000;342(19): 1378–1384.
136. Schafer H, Pauleit D, Sudhop T, Gouni-Berthold I, Ewig S, Berthold HK. Body fat distribution, serum leptin, and cardiovascular risk factors in men with obstructive sleep apnea. Chest 2002;122(3):829–839.
137. Young T, Peppard P. Sleep-disordered breathing and cardiovascular disease: epidemiologic evidence for a relationship. Sleep 2000;23 Suppl 4:S122–S126.
138. Schafer H, Koehler U, Ewig S, Hasper E, Tasci S, Luderitz B. Obstructive sleep apnea as a risk marker in coronary artery disease. Cardiology 1999;92(2):79–84.
139. Bassetti C, Aldrich MS. Sleep apnea in acute cerebrovascular diseases: final report on 128 patients. Sleep 1999;22(2):217–223.
140. Newman AB, Spiekerman CF, Enright P, et al. Daytime sleepiness predicts mortality and cardiovascular disease in older adults. The Cardiovascular Health Study Research Group. J Am Geriatr Soc 2000;48(2):115–123.
141. Hla KM, Skatrud JB, Finn L, Palta M, Young T. The effect of correction of sleep-disordered breathing on BP in untreated hypertension. Chest 2002;122(4):1125–1132.
142. Sanner BM, Tepel M, Markmann A, Zidek W. Effect of continuous positive airway pressure therapy on 24-hour blood pressure in patients with obstructive sleep apnea syndrome. Am J Hypertens 2002;15(3):251–257.

4 Stable Coronary Artery Disease in the Elderly

Beth R. Malasky, MD and Joseph S. Alpert, MD

CONTENTS

EVALUATION
THERAPEUTIC INTERVENTIONS
CONCLUSIONS
REFERENCES

EVALUATION

History and physical examination as well as an electrocardiogram (EKG) should be obtained in all patients with suspected coronary artery disease (CAD). American College of Cardiology/American Heart Association (ACC/AHA) guidelines also recommend checking hemoglobin, fasting blood glucose, and a fasting lipid panel in new patients presenting with angina *(1)*. Co-morbid conditions that may precipitate functional angina should be considered (i.e., anemia, hyperthyroidism, tachyarrhythmias, heart failure, uncontrolled hypertension, etc.). One study in the elderly revealed a significantly elevated risk of cardiovascular disease (CVD) events in patients with subclinical hypothyroidism evidenced by an elevated thyrotropin and normal thyroid function tests *(2)*.

Given the high prevalence of CAD in this group, a classic anginal story most likely represents coronary atherosclerosis. Assessment of the patient's functional status, mental acuity, and overall physical health are all important in determining the extent of further evaluation *(3)*. Geriatric literature supports the accuracy of physician assessments ("the eyeball test") of functional status and predicted survival *(4)*. Is the patient an active

From: *Contemporary Cardiology: Cardiovascular Disease in the Elderly*
Edited by: G. Gerstenblith © Humana Press Inc., Totowa, NJ

and hearty 80-year-old or frail and homebound? Because evaluation for coronary ischemia is likely to disclose ischemia, is the patient a candidate for invasive evaluation? Would referral for bypass surgery or angioplasty be appropriate? Aggressive medical therapy and symptomatic improvement may be the most appropriate goals in those elderly people with limited life expectancy resulting from poor functional status or co-morbidity. In those with good baseline status, invasive evaluation and intervention may be most appropriate. If the patient has heart failure symptoms, evaluation of left ventricular function with echocardiography, prior to ischemia evaluation, can be helpful in directing the next test because CAD is a common reversible etiology of left ventricular dysfunction. If symptoms are not clear, as is often the case in the elderly, stress testing can be helpful in assessing the presence of CAD, the likelihood of left main or triple vessel disease (5), the extent to which it limits exercise, functional status, risk of future events, and the efficacy of medical therapy. In an elderly population with a high prevalence of disease, however, a diagnostic test does not significantly increase the yield of undiagnosed disease and is associated with a high false-negative rate. The ACC/AHA guidelines rely heavily on initial clinical assessment and data regarding disease prevalence in different populations to guide further testing in individual patients.

Exercise Stress Testing

Stress testing can be used to diagnose disease and gauge the severity of CAD, measure functional capacity and the efficacy of medical therapies, and assess the presence of significant stress-induced arrhythmias. The diagnostic test of choice is usually an exercise stress test with EKG monitoring. Treadmill testing is most often used and exercise capacity can be uniformly assessed by the use of metabolic equivalents (MET) (1 MET = 3.5 mL/kg per minute of oxygen uptake) to describe workload performed on various protocols. A positive test is defined as 1 mm or more of horizontal or downsloping ST depressions 60 ms to 80 ms after the J-point of the QRS in three consecutive beats during exercise or in recovery. It is important to remember that ST depression in stress testing does not localize ischemic territory.

During stress testing, important information is obtained from monitoring blood pressure (BP), exercise tolerance, ability to attain target heart rate (HR) and the occurrence of any symptoms. Exercise tolerance is a very important prognosticator, and, in a number of studies, mortality rate is associated with exercise duration and the ability to achieve target HR (6,7). In some studies, a low exercise workload, secondary to symptoms or ischemia, was the most important variable associated with increased cardiac mortality in patients treated with medical therapy. Moreover, good exercise tolerance is associated with better outcomes, regardless of whether the test is positive or the patient has CAD; patients able to exercise for 10 minutes of a Bruce protocol to a workload of 13 METS have a very good prognosis for long-term survival. A markedly positive EKG response (>2.0 mm of downsloping or horizontal depression), fall in systolic BP of 10 mmHg or more, a prolonged positive response (persistent depressions for more than 8 minutes into recovery), exercise-induced ST elevation (in leads without pathological Q waves), and/or exercise-induced malignant ventricular arrhythmias are all signs of extensive CAD and identify a high-risk patient.

In elderly patients, the treadmill test may be associated with technical difficulties owing to unfamiliarity with or fear of how to properly use the machine. Imbalance or physical disability may be prohibitive. The percentage of people able to successfully complete a treadmill test decreases with age; only 26% of those over age 75, without other co-morbidities, achieved maximal predicted effort (8). Assessment of functional status at home is essential in deciding the appropriateness for the treadmill. Gentler, more graded protocols that allow the patient to warm up and achieve an appropriate cardiac workload before they stop from muscle fatigue are helpful. Decreased β-adrenergic responsiveness, conduction disease, other medications, and decreased vascular compliance may limit the ability of the patient to achieve target HR. Adequate staff must be available to initiate the test and ensure that the patient is not injured during the test. Unless the patient is an active cyclist, bicycle protocols are usually difficult.

Sensitivity of the stress EKG increases with age from 56% for those under age 40 to 84.4% in those older than 60; specificity, on the other hand, declines, from 84 to 70% in the older patients (7). Improved sensitivity is the result of the high prevalence of severe disease; the low specificity among the elderly likely relates to the high rates of other conditions, e.g. left ventricular hypertrophy that may result in false-positive readings, as well as inadequacies of the test itself. Evaluation of the Duke Treadmill Score revealed no significant predictive value for either cardiac mortality or events in those 75 years old and older (9). Exercise tolerance still carries prognostic significance in this population, if technical aspects do not prohibit appropriate evaluation (10). If there are baseline EKG abnormalities, an imaging study may be required.

Screening Asymptomatic Individuals

Given the increased likelihood of silent ischemia and infarction in the elderly, should noninvasive screening be performed routinely in this high-risk population? Whereas the ACC/AHA guidelines do not recommend screening all high-risk, asymptomatic populations *(1)*, there are several circumstances under which such screening might be appropriate. The guidelines recommend stress testing, for example, for patients over the age of 45 years who wish to engage in an exercise program. The prevalence of silent exercise-induced ischemia increases with age. Of participants in the Baltimore Longitudinal Study of Aging, 26% had asymptomatic ST-segment changes on treadmill testing and a positive test was associated with a threefold increased event rate at follow-up *(11)*.

For the purpose of diagnosing the presence of significant coronary disease, it is preferred that β-blocker therapy be discontinued for four to five half-lives or 48 hours *(1)*. β-Blocker therapy may attenuate the ischemic response on the EKG and limit the ability to achieve the target HR, i.e., β-blockers decrease the sensitivity of the stress EKG for the purpose of detecting the presence of significant disease. If the purpose of the testing is to assess the ischemic threshold on medical therapy, then it is appropriate to test patients on their usual drug regimen. Acute nitrate therapy also alters the ischemic response and decreases the sensitivity of stress testing for detection of CAD. It should be noted that a negative test at a submaximal HR has a much lower ability to predict the absence of disease (negative predictive value) than a negative test at the target HR ([220 – age] × >1.85). In the absence of a medication effect, the inability to achieve the target HR is a poor prognosticator and may result from deconditioning, dyspnea related to poor left ventricular compliance, chronic lung disease, chronotropic incompetence, peripheral vascular disease, or other co-morbidties.

Stress Imaging

Imaging modalities used for the diagnosis, localization, and quantification of coronary ischemia include echocardiography and nuclear studies. The most common imaging technique is single-photon computed tomography (SPECT) imaging in association with either treadmill or pharmacological stress. SPECT imaging is performed primarily with thallium-201 or technetium-99m *(12)*. Thallium, which has a significantly longer half-life, tends to give more physiological information because it moves in and out of cells through potassium channels, giving it the unique characteristic of redistribution. Technetium binds to mitochondria and so does not wash-in and wash-out; it is a higher energy emitter, however, and decreases the effects of attenuation from breast shadow, diaphragm, or fat. Technetium studies can be gated to assess wall motion during stress because of higher count rates than thallium. The sensitivity for SPECT imaging with either agent is higher than stress EKG alone, approaching 89%. Sensitivity also increases with extent of disease. Specificity is in the range of 76%. Technetium is often the agent of choice in women because there is less breast attenuation artifact and, in conjunction with gating, has a specificity of 92% as compared with 67% for thallium. SPECT imaging is most often used to assess ischemia, as evidenced by a defect present at stress but not at rest. The durability of a normal nuclear stress test in predicting low event rates is time-dependent and limited in those with diabetes and known coronary disease *(13)*. Thus in an older patient who has a normal nuclear study, recurrence, or change in symptoms should prompt another evaluation.

The sensitivity of pharmacological stress echocardiography is similar to that of SPECT imaging, 85% and 82%, respectively. Stress echocardiography enables the physician to evaluate regional wall motion at baseline and with stress; the finding of one or more stress-induced regional wall motion abnormalities is consistent with CAD. Specificity for stress echocardiography approximates 86%, which is better than SPECT imaging. In both imaging modalities, sensitivity was increased for multivessel disease. A serious flaw associated with SPECT imaging is evaluation of "balanced three-vessel disease," which may result in a false-negative study owing to software manipulation required to make two sets of images comparable. For stress echocardiography, imaging of the lateral wall is relatively insensitive and may result in a false-negative exam. In all circumstances, the best imaging technique may be the technique with which the physicians at a given institution have the most comfort, experience, and skill.

Pharmacological Stress Testing

The most common pharmacological stress agents are dipyridamole, adenosine, and dobutamine. Dipyridamole and adenosine are potent vasodilators and are most commonly used in conjunction with nuclear imaging. The ability of a diseased artery to dilate is limited and when a vasodilator is administered, blood flow to areas supplied by normal or less obstructed arteries will increase relative to areas supplied by diseased arteries resulting in a differential in counts from the nuclear perfusion agent. Both agents are counteracted by caffeine and so the agents are ineffective if given after caffeine consumption. Beverages containing caffeine should be avoided for at least 18 hours prior to administration of either dipyridamole or adenosine. Although there is some uncertainty regarding the response to these agents, the original studies suggest that an appropriate hemodynamic response is either a 10 beat per minute increase in HR or a 10 mmHg change in BP from baseline to peak infusion. A negative study in the absence of these hemodynamic changes may be inadequate to rule out the presence of disease. Adenosine protocols are usually significantly quicker than dipyridamole protocols because the half-life of adenosine is only about 30 seconds, allowing for rapid cessation of drug effect once the infusion is terminated. Dipyridamole has a significantly longer half-life and can be reversed with aminophylline, an agent that blocks adenosine receptors in the coronary arteries. Both agents can result in significant bronchospasm and are contraindicated in patients with a current history of reactive airway disease. Adenosine is associated with a higher rate of heart block and should be used cautiously in patients with EKG evidence of significant baseline conduction disease. Intense emotional reactions have been described with both agents, but tend to occur more frequently with adenosine.

Dobutamine is a β-agonist that increases HR and contractility and although it is most often used in conjunction with echocardiographic imaging, it can be used with nuclear imaging if traditional agents are contraindicated and echocardiographic imaging is not feasible. Traditional dobutamine echocardiography protocols have the disadvantage of being long and arduous. A baseline study is performed and then the dobutamine dose is increased gradually, with repeat imaging at the end of each stage, up to 40 μg/kg per minute. If the target HR or positive test is not achieved at this point, atropine is administered to increase HR. Final imaging is then performed after the HR has returned to baseline. The study is then processed to provide gated images at each stage, side-by-side, enabling comparison that improves the ability to detect subtle wall motion abnormalities. It is preferred that patients not take β-blockers prior to dobutamine echocardiography because β-blockers counteract the dobutamine and increase the need to administer atropine to achieve target HR. Dobutamine protocols, with administration of atropine if necessary, are quite successful in achieving HR goals in the elderly. The oldest patients actually achieve target HRs at a lower dobutamine dose and are less likely to require atropine. In the elderly, it has been noted that dobutamine increases the amount of ventricular ectopy and asymptomatic hypotension, but these side effects rarely required premature cessation of the test *(14,15)*. Baseline use of β-blockers is associated with an increased risk of ventricular arrhythmias during dobutamine stress testing, both in younger and older patients *(15)*. Newer accelerated dobutamine protocols *(16)* have not been tested in the elderly and given unique pharmacological effects of dobutamine in the elderly, the accelerated regimen cannot be recommended without safety data in this population. If the patient is very large or does not have adequate acoustic windows, echocardiography is not a suitable imaging modality. The sensitivity of the test is also dependent on the skill of both the sonographer and the echocardiographer.

Other Noninvasive Modalities

Less common modalities for evaluation of CAD include positron emission tomography (PET) scanning, transesophageal pacing stress echocardiography, electron beam computed tomography (EBCT or Ultrafast CT), and cardiac magnetic resonance imaging (MRI). PET scanning is a very sensitive and specific modality for assessing coronary ischemia; it is a nuclear imaging technique using nitrogen-13-ammonia or rubidium-82 as high-energy emitters coupled with pharmacological stress, usually either dipyridamole or adenosine. The image has much better spatial resolution and higher count rates than SPECT imaging; attenuation artifact is corrected and hence the scans provide a more accurate picture of relative distribution of myocardial blood flow. However, PET scanners are not commonly available, require an onsite generator or cyclotron for production of the imaging agent, and are relatively expensive, although some cost analyses suggest that this might be the most cost-effective approach for the evaluation of coronary disease *(17)*.

EBCT enables the physician to detect and quantify coronary calcification, which correlates with the amount of coronary artery calcium and atherosclerosis. However, the study does not provide a functional evaluation of ischemia *(16)*. Significant differences in calcium scores exist between men and women of the same age group, likely related to differences in prevalence of CAD but possibly related to differences in the characteristics of the coronary atherosclerosis and sensitivity of the test in different populations *(12)*. Age-dependent calcium scores have been proposed to help the specificity of the test in this population.

Cardiac MRI is still in development and its utility has yet to be determined. Special software packages that allow for reconstruction of images of the coronary arteries and stress imaging are being evaluated *(18)*. At the present time, however, it is not readily available. Transesophageal pacing stress echocardiography may be a promising option, although again it is not readily available, requires an invasive procedure that may not be well tolerated by the patient, and has not been fully compared with other stress techniques *(19)*.

Ambulatory holter monitoring for arrhythmias and ST-segment deviation has been evaluated in older patients. One study reported the predictive value of ST-segment deviation, defined as depression or elevation of at least 1 mm for more than 60 seconds using a two-lead monitoring system in 277 patients with chest pain sent for angiography. Of the patients, 145 were older than 70 years. In both the younger and older groups, the specificity (91% and 90%, respectively) and positive predictive values (86% and 95%) for coronary disease were high, but the diagnostic accuracy was low (34% and 32%) in both groups *(20)*. Aronow and Epstein reported that 21% of nursing home patients with underlying heart disease had silent ischemia on holter and, of these, 65% had cardiac events in the 26-month follow-up *(21)*. Among older Scandinavian men, ischemia on holter in those without CAD predicted a fourfold increased risk of coronary events and in those with documented CAD, the relative risk for coronary events increased to 16 *(22)*. Holter-identified arrhythmias also have prognostic significance in the elderly. In older patients with known CAD, especially those unable to exercise on a treadmill, ambulatory holter with ST analysis may be helpful in risk stratification. Among an elderly cohort in Finland, daytime sinoatrial pauses of longer than 1.5 seconds were associated with a fourfold excess cardiac mortality and multifocal ventricular ectopic beats of more than 100 beats during the night was associated with a cardiac mortality odds ratio of 2.7, independent of age or clinical CVD *(23)*, Thus, in older patients with known CAD, particularly in those unable to exercise, ST-segment and arrhythmia analysis performed on ambulatory holter data obtained during daily activities may be helpful in risk stratification.

Coronary Angiography

Coronary angiography remains the gold standard for the evaluation of CAD. Use of coronary angiography in patients with suspected CAD is indicated for those patients with abnormal noninvasive testing suggesting a high-risk profile, abnormal but nondiagnostic noninvasive test results, and patients with chest pain but who are unable to undergo any of the available noninvasive testing modalities. Patients with known or possible angina who have survived sudden death should also undergo diagnostic angiography. Not clearly addressed in the ACC/AHA guidelines are patients with decreased left ventricular function and risk factors for CAD because there is clear evidence that mortality is improved in patients with decreased left ventricular function and triple-vessel, two-vessel CAD involving the proximal left anterior descending artery, or significant left main disease. Angiography would also be appropriate if coronary artery bypass surgery is a consideration. Contraindications to angiography include the presence of prohibitive co-morbidities.

Coronary angiography enables the physician to estimate coronary stenoses, evaluate calcification, assess coronary anatomy including presence of coronary anomalies, and evaluate left ventricular pressures and function. Angiography alone does not allow assessment of the functional significance of lesions. A number of adjuncts have been developed to allow for functional assessment of coronary artery stenoses in the catheterization laboratory—these include use of Doppler flow wires to assess adenosine-induced coronary flow reserve across a stenosis and pressure wires to assess pressure gradients across stenoses during adenosine infusion. Intravascular ultrasound allows for quantification of stenoses and identification of normal vessels, as well as characterization of plaque structure (i.e., presence of thrombus, calcium, and dissection). Although these techniques improve the accuracy of cardiac angiography, they are not commonly necessary, not commonly available except at tertiary care centers, and increase the costs and risks of an already expensive procedure. In unusual cases where a stenosis is of borderline significance and the patient's symptoms are unclear, these adjuncts can be very helpful in determining whether coronary revascularization is indicated.

THERAPEUTIC INTERVENTIONS

Pharmacological Agents

The goals of medical therapy are to improve survival, decrease cardiac events and improve symptoms. The relative importance of these goals and the risk–benefit evaluation for each approach may change with increasing age. Aspirin is indicated in patients with known or probable coronary atherosclerosis. In numerous studies, aspirin in doses ranging from 75 to 325 mg daily is associated with a reduction in adverse coronary events and in some studies with a decreased risk of sudden death. The Swedish Angina Pectoris Trial of older patients with stable angina, mean age 67, reported a 34% reduction in first myocardial infarction (MI) or sudden death and a 32% reduction in first MI, stroke, or vascular death *(24)*, The Physicians Health Study cohort of 333 men with chronic angina randomized to alternate-day aspirin at 325 mg or placebo showed a significant decrease in risk of first MI at 5-year follow-up *(25)*. The Benzafibrate Infarction Prevention study revealed a 39% reduction in cardiovascular mortality among women receiving aspirin, with the greatest benefit seen among those who were older, diabetic, symptomatic, or with previous MI *(26)*. Given the increased risks of bleeding and cerebrovascular bleeds at higher doses, without known added benefit, current recommendations are to treat stable coronary syndromes with low-dose daily aspirin (75 to 81 mg). In patients with a contraindication to aspirin, clopidogrel, which inhibits adenosine diphosphate-mediated platelet aggregation, may be used.

Lipid-lowering agents also decrease the risk of adverse events in patients with coronary disease. Data suggest that for every 1% reduction in total cholesterol there is a 2% reduction in coronary events. There is clear evidence that in patients with CAD, lowering low-density lipoprotein cholesterol to less than 100 mg/dL improves survival and reduces major coronary events. (*See* Chapter 3 for a complete discussion of lipid-lowering therapies.)

β-Blockers are an important component of anti-anginal therapy *(27)*. They decrease angina by decreasing myocardial oxygen demand by reducing HR and contractility, and improve supply by prolonging diastole, when most of coronary flow occurs. Doses can be titrated to a reduction in HR, particularly the HR during activity. Medicare data on elderly diabetic patients who have suffered an MI, revealed a significant improvement in survival with β-blocker therapy for insulin-treated diabetics, non-insulin-treated diabetics, and non-diabetics, compared to those not discharged on β-blockers *(28)*. β-Blockers also decrease anginal episodes, ventricular arrhythmias, sudden death, and silent ischemia and prolong exercise duration in patients with coronary heart disease *(29–31)*. Aronow reported a 47% reduction in sudden cardiac death and a 37% reduction in total cardiac death with propranolol compared to placebo in the treatment of elderly patients with heart disease, complex ventricular arrhythmias, and left ventricular ejection fractions of 40% or more *(30,31)*. Although β-blockers provide significant therapeutic benefits in the elderly, they are often underutilized in this age group *(32,33)*.

In the elderly, particular attention should be paid to the risk of bradycardia and conduction delay. Ophthalmologic β-blockers are partially absorbed and are associated with bradycardia; care should be taken in the co-administration of systemic and ophthalmic β-blockers. Orthostatic hypotension and fatigue, along with confusion, depression, and incontinence, may be other complications of β-blocker therapy in elderly.

Calcium channel blockers are also effective in relieving angina and delaying onset of ischemia *(34)*. They are also the drugs of choice for vasospastic angina. Calcium antagonists cause vasodilation of the coronary arteries and decrease myocardial oxygen demand by decreasing BP and lowering coronary and systemic vascular resistances. Some agents also decrease HR and contractility, thereby decreasing demand. The use of short-acting dihydropyridine calcium antagonists in the absence of β-blockade is associated with an increase in ischemic events and should be avoided. Long-acting calcium antagonists are very effective anti-anginals and can be added to β-blocker therapy if additional therapy is indicated, or substituted if β-blockers are contraindicated or if the patient develops unacceptable side effects. Concomitant nitrate and long-acting dihydropyriding calcium channel blocker therapy can be more effective than single agents alone *(35)*.

Nitrates are coronary and peripheral vasodilators and through this mechanism improve myocardial oxygen supply and decrease demand. They also have antithrombotic and antiplatelet effects. Nitrates clearly improve symptoms and exercise tolerance and raise the ischemic threshold. Their efficacy is enhanced when they are combined with either β-blockers or calcium antagonists. They also have particular efficacy in the treatment of vasospasm. In patients who are continuing to experience anginal episodes despite other therapies, intermittent or planned sublingual use of nitroglycerin may be necessary. If the patient's anginal pattern is predictable and associated with certain activities, prophylactic use of sublingual nitroglycerin prior to engaging in these activities may provide symptomatic relief and improved functional status. As with all vasodilators, orthostatic hypotension, syncope, and falls are risks with nitrate use, especially in the elderly.

Patients with CAD should be educated extensively regarding the signs of instability, such as increasing frequency of angina, angina occurring at lower workloads, angina occurring at rest, and persistent pain that does not resolve after a few minutes. These patients should be instructed on the appropriate use of sublingual nitroglycerin in these circumstances, and when to seek immediate medical attention.

Lifestyle Modifications

Lifestyle modification is an important component of angina therapy *(36)*. Patients should be counseled to stop smoking, adhere to dietary recommendations, engage in regular exercise, and lose weight if indicated. Treadmill testing and clinical symptoms can guide exercise regimens.

Aging results in decreased muscle mass and strength and a relative increase in body fat. CAD and angina are major predictors of disability and activity limitations in older patients. Eighty percent of women and 55% of men with CAD and symptoms of angina or heart failure, over age 70, reported activity limitations *(37,38)*. Aerobic training in older patients results in improved cardiovascular fitness as measured by maximal oxygen consumption, improved endurance, and a decrease in mobility limitations and disability *(39–41)*. Increased physical activity and walking in women, aged 65 to 75, resulted in a 36% reduction in cardiovascular mortality and a 48% reduction in all-cause mortality, compared to sedentary women; however, the association of exercise with improved outcome decreased in those over 75 years of age *(42)*. Among older men, light or moderate physical activity was associated with a 36% decrease in cardiovascular mortality and a 52% decrease in noncardiovascular mortality *(43)*. After major cardiac events, cardiac rehabilitation in the elderly improves exercise capacity, quality of life, and risk profiles, and decreases depression *(44,45)*.

The benefits of diet modification in the elderly are not well defined. Some cardiovascular benefits may not be evident for several years and it may be more appropriate to counsel dietary modification in a 65-year-old than in an 80-year-old. Dietary restrictions should be avoided in the approximately 12% of elderly who are undernourished and underweight because this state is associated with increased mortality *(46)*. Increased intake of dietary fiber and omega-3 fatty acids and decreased intake of saturated and *trans*-fatty acids are likely to be beneficial *(47)*. Modest alcohol intake is protective and not associated with increases in coronary events or heart failure in the elderly *(48,49)*. Modest restriction of salt intake to less than 5 g of sodium has a BP-lowering effect equivalent to hydrochlorthiazide in the elderly *(50,51)*. Observational data indicate that high dietary consumption of carotenoids and the lipid-soluble antioxidants present in green and yellow fresh fruits and vegetables, are associated with significantly lower cardiovascular mortality and event rates *(52)*. Weight loss should be encouraged in all obese older individuals to improve mobility and BP control, and to decrease co-morbidities, such as sleep apnea and diastolic dysfunction, which are associated with increased cardiovascular risk.

Revascularization

Revascularization is another therapeutic option for elderly patients with chronic stable angina. More than half of the coronary artery bypass operations in this country are performed on patients 65 years and older. Bypass mortality increases significantly in those over age 75 and 80 *(53–55)*. Although the elderly tend to be excluded from clinical trials, there is a large body of data regarding outcomes from surgical and interventional databases and institutional reports. Although the very elderly suffer increased mortality and morbidity risks from both percutaneous and surgical revascularization compared to younger populations, significant symptomatic relief occurs following these procedures.

Decision making may be more driven by quality-of-life issues than by survival statistics in this population. In general, functional status and co-morbidities play an important role in assessing the patient's physiological reserve and ability to tolerate surgical revascularization *(56)*. Percutaneous revascularization has the benefits of avoiding surgical morbidity and recovery, but may results in incomplete revascularization in a population likely to have multivessel disease *(57–60)*. Vascular and other complications from percutaneous procedures also occur more frequently in this high-risk population. Restenosis rates may be higher if vessel size is small or disease is diffuse.

The Trial of Invasive versus Medical therapy in Elderly patients (TIME) compared invasive and medical strategies for the treatment of chronic symptomatic CAD in patients aged 75 and older with persistent angina despite standard pharmacological therapy *(61)*. In the TIME study, 150 patients were randomized to receive a more aggressive medical therapy, with anti-anginal, antiplatelet, and lipid-lowering agents and close monitoring and 155 patients were randomized to an invasive strategy involving angiography, with revascularization by either percutaneous coronary intervention or bypass surgery. Angina severity, quality-of-life measures, and major cardiac events were then monitored based on treatment strategy. Notably, of the group who underwent angiography, 79% had multivessel disease and only 7% had no significant stenoses. Of the invasive group, 26% crossed over to medical therapy because they could not be revascularized. At 6 months, improvements in angina severity and health status were greater in the invasive group. Although there were no significant differences in mortality or MI rates between the strategies, there were significantly fewer readmissions for acute coronary syndromes in the invasive strategy group. At 1 year of follow-up, 71.6% of those in the medical therapy arm had been hospitalized with uncontrolled symptoms compared with 18.3% in the invasive arm ($p < 0.001$) *(61)*. Of those randomized to optimal medical therapy, 46% required revascularization within the 1-year period compared with only 10% of those who had initially been randomized to an invasive strategy ($p < 0.001$). Major adverse clinical events occurred significantly more often in the medical therapy group as well. At 1 year, using an intention-to-treat model, there was no statistically significant difference between the groups, with regard to symptoms or quality of life. The conclusions from this trial seem sensible —the elderly patient can be offered "early" revascularization if medical therapy fails to control anginal episodes, with the benefits of good symptom relief and a decreased likelihood of rehospitalization, at the price of a small excess in mortality. They can, alternatively, have their medical therapy advanced with the understanding that this approach will be ineffective in the majority of patients and may ultimately require revascularization.

If medical therapies are not controlling symptoms and patients are not candidates for revascularization, enhanced external counterpulsation may be attempted *(62,63)*, although results in the elderly are not reported.

CONCLUSIONS

The prevalence of CAD increases with age, as do the risk factors for coronary events. The elderly shoulder the greatest burden of coronary atherosclerosis and coronary events. Unfortunately, the likelihood of silent ischemia also increases in the elderly, making identification of those at high risk for events more difficult. The utility of various noninvasive techniques in assessing coronary risk decrease in the elderly owing to the high prevalence of disease. Risk-factor modification, medical therapy, and revascularization, if indicated, can improve outcomes and quality of life. Attention must be paid to the unique socioeconomic, psychological, and physical co-morbidities of the elderly. In the elderly, mortality benefits of various interventions may be difficult to prove given co-morbidities and limited life expectancy. For those patients, therapeutic goals often shift toward improved symptoms and enhanced quality of life.

REFERENCES

1. Gibbons RJ, Chatterjee K, Daley J, et al. ACC/AHA/ACP-ASIM guidelines for the management of patients with chronic stable angina: a report of the American College of Cardiology/American Heart Association Task Force on Practice Guidelines (Committee on Management of Patients With Chronic Stable Angina). J Am Coll Cardiol 1999;33(7):2092–2197.
2. Parle JV, Maisonneuve P, Sheppard MC, Boyle P, Franklyn JA. Prediction of all-cause and cardiovascular mortality in elderly people from one low serum thyrotropin result: a 10-year cohort study. Lancet 2001;358(9285):861–865.
3. Inouye SK, Peduzzi PN, Robison JT, Hughes JS, Horwitz RI, Concato J. Importance of functional measures in predicting mortality among older hospitalized patients. JAMA 1998;279(15):1187–1193.
4. Batchelor WB, Jollis JG, Friesinger GC. The challenge of health care delivery to the elderly patient with cardiovascular disease. Demographic, epidemiologic, fiscal, and health policy implications. Cardiol Clin 1999;17(1):1–15, vii.
5. Blumenthal DS, Weiss JL, Mellits ED, Gerstenblith G. The predictive value of a strongly positive stress test in patients with minimal symptoms. Am J Med 1981; 70(5):1005–1010.
6. Morris CK, Ueshima K, Kawaguchi T, Hideg A, Froelicher VF. The prognostic value of exercise capacity: a review of the literature. Am Heart J 1991;122(5):1423–1431.
7. Marolf GA, Kuhn A, White RD. Exercise testing in special populations: athletes, women, and the elderly. Prim Care 2001;28(1):55–72.
8. Gill TM, DiPietro L, Krumholz HM. Role of exercise stress testing and safety monitoring for older persons starting an exercise program. JAMA 2000;284(3):342–349.
9. Kwok JM, Miller TD, Hodge DO, Gibbons RJ. Prognostic value of the Duke treadmill score in the elderly. J Am Coll Cardiol 2002;39(9):1475–1481.
10. Goraya TY, Jacobsen SJ, Pellikka PA, et al. Prognostic value of treadmill exercise testing in elderly persons. Ann Intern Med 2000;132(11):862–870.
11. Josephson RA, Shefrin E, Lakatta EG, Brant LJ, Fleg JL. Can serial exercise testing improve the prediction of coronary events in asymptomatic individuals? Circulation 1990;81(1):20–24.
12. Hoff JA, Chomka EV, Krainik AJ, Daviglus M, Rich S, Kondos GT. Age and gender distributions of coronary artery calcium detected by electron beam tomography in 35,246 adults. Am J Cardiol 2001;87(12):1335–1339.
13. Hachamovitch R, Hayes S, Friedman JD, et al. Determinants of risk and its temporal variation in patients with normal stress myocardial perfusion scans: what is the warranty period of a normal scan? J Am Coll Cardiol 2003;41(8):1329–1340.

14. Elhendy A, van Domburg RT, Bax JJ, et al. Safety, hemodynamic profile, and feasibility of dobutamine stress technetium myocardial perfusion single-photon emission CT imaging for evaluation of coronary artery disease in the elderly. Chest 2000;117(3):649–656.

15. Hiro J, Hiro T, Reid CL, Ebrahimi R, Matsuzaki M, Gardin JM. Safety and results of dobutamine stress echocardiography in women versus men and in patients older and younger than 75 years of age. Am J Cardiol 1997;80(8):1014–1020.

16. Shavelle DM, Budoff MJ, Lamont DH, Shavelle RM, Kennedy JM, Brundage BH. Exercise testing and electron beam computed tomography in the evaluation of coronary artery disease. J Am Coll Cardiol 2000;36(1):32–38.

17. Patterson RE, Horowitz SF, Eisner RL. Comparison of modalities to diagnose coronary artery disease. Semin Nucl Med 1994;24(4):286–310.

18. Nagel E, Lehmkuhl HB, Bocksch W, et al. Noninvasive diagnosis of ischemia-induced wall motion abnormalities with the use of high-dose dobutamine stress MRI: comparison with dobutamine stress echocardiography. Circulation 1999;99(6): 763–770.

19. Atar S, Cercek B, Nagai T, et al. Transthoracic stress echocardiography with transesophageal atrial pacing for bedside evaluation of inducible myocardial ischemia in patients with new-onset chest pain. Am J Cardiol 2000;86(1):12–16.

20. Nair CK, Khan IA, Mehta NJ, Ryschon KL. Comparison of diagnostic and prognostic implications of ST-segment changes on ambulatory holter monitoring in patients aged >70 years with those aged <70 years. Am J Cardiol 2002;90(9):1002–1005.

21. Aronow WS, Epstein S. Usefulness of silent myocardial ischemia detected by ambulatory electrocardiographic monitoring in predicting new coronary events in elderly patients. Am J Cardiol 1988;62(17):1295–1296.

22. Hedblad B, Juul-Moller S, Svensson K, et al. Increased mortality in men with ST segment depression during 24 h ambulatory long-term ECG recording. Results from prospective population study "Men born in 1914," from Malmo, Sweden. Eur Heart J 1989;10(2):149–158.

23. Raiha IJ, Piha SJ, Seppanen A, Puukka P, Sourander LB. Predictive value of continuous ambulatory electrocardiographic monitoring in elderly people. BMJ 1994;309 (6964):1263–1267.

24. Juul-Moller S, Edvardsson N, Jahnmatz B, Rosen A, Sorensen S, Omblus R. Double-blind trial of aspirin in primary prevention of myocardial infarction in patients with stable chronic angina pectoris. The Swedish Angina Pectoris Aspirin Trial (SAPAT) Group. Lancet 1992;340(8833):1421–1425.

25. Ridker PM, Manson JE, Gaziano JM, Buring JE, Hennekens CH. Low-dose aspirin therapy for chronic stable angina. A randomized, placebo-controlled clinical trial. Ann Intern Med 1991;114(10):835–839.

26. Harpaz D, Benderly M, Goldbourt U, Kishon Y, Behar S. Effect of aspirin on mortality in women with symptomatic or silent myocardial ischemia. Israeli BIP Study Group. Am J Cardiol 1996;78(11):1215–1219.

27. Heidenreich PA, McDonald KM, Hastie T, et al. Meta-analysis of trials comparing beta-blockers, calcium antagonists, and nitrates for stable angina. JAMA 1999;281 (20):1927–1936.

28. Chen J, Marciniak TA, Radford MJ, Wang Y, Krumholz HM. Beta-blocker therapy for secondary prevention of myocardial infarction in elderly diabetic patients. Results from the National Cooperative Cardiovascular Project. J Am Coll Cardiol 1999;34(5):1388–1394.

29. Pepine CJ, Cohn PF, Deedwania PC, et al. Effects of treatment on outcome in mildly symptomatic patients with ischemia during daily life. The Atenolol Silent Ischemia Study (ASIST). Circulation 1994;90(2):762–768.

30. Aronow WS, Ahn C, Mercando AD, Epstein S, Kronzon I. Decrease in mortality by propranolol in patients with heart disease and complex ventricular arrhythmias is more an anti-ischemic than an antiarrhythmic effect. Am J Cardiol 1994;74(6): 613–615.

31. Aronow WS, Frishman WH, Cheng-Lai A. Cardiovascular drug therapy in the elderly. Heart Dis 2000;2(2):151–167.

32. Wang TJ, Stafford RS. National patterns and predictors of beta-blocker use in patients with coronary artery disease. Arch Intern Med 1998;158(17):1901–1906.

33. Mendelson G, Aronow WS. Underutilization of beta-blockers in older patients with prior myocardial infarction or coronary artery disease in an academic, hospital-based geriatrics practice. J Am Geriatr Soc 1997;45(11):1360–1361.

34. Deanfield JE, Detry JM, Lichtlen PR, Magnani B, Sellier P, Thaulow E. Amlodipine reduces transient myocardial ischemia in patients with coronary artery disease: double-blind Circadian Anti-Ischemia Program in Europe (CAPE Trial). J Am Coll Cardiol 1994;24(6):1460–1467.

35. Pehrsson SK, Ringqvist I, Ekdahl S, Karlson BW, Ulvenstam G, Persson S. Monotherapy with amlodipine or atenolol versus their combination in stable angina pectoris. Clin Cardiol 2000;23(10):763–770.

36. Blumenthal RS, Cohn G, Schulman SP. Medical therapy versus coronary angioplasty in stable coronary artery disease: a critical review of the literature. J Am Coll Cardiol 2000;36(3):668–673.

37. Pinsky JL, Jette AM, Branch LG, Kannel WB, Feinleib M. The Framingham Disability Study: relationship of various coronary heart disease manifestations to disability in older persons living in the community. Am J Public Health 1990;80(11): 1363–1367.

38. Ades PA. Cardiac rehabilitation in older coronary patients. J Am Geriatr Soc 1999; 47(1):98–105.

39. Aggarwal A, Ades PA. Exercise rehabilitation of older patients with cardiovascular disease. Cardiol Clin 2001;19(3):525–536.

40. Stahle A, Nordlander R, Bergfeldt L. Aerobic group training improves exercise capacity and heart rate variability in elderly patients with a recent coronary event. A randomized controlled study. Eur Heart J 1999;20(22):1638–1646.

41. Dionne IJ, Ades PA, Poehlman ET. Impact of cardiovascular fitness and physical activity level on health outcomes in older persons. Mech Ageing Dev 2003;124(3): 259–267.

42. Gregg EW, Cauley JA, Stone K, et al. Relationship of changes in physical activity and mortality among older women. JAMA 2003;289(18):2379–2386.

43. Wannamethee SG, Shaper AG, Walker M. Changes in physical activity, mortality, and incidence of coronary heart disease in older men. Lancet 1998;351(9116):1603–1608.

44. Lavie CJ, Milani RV. Effects of cardiac rehabilitation programs on exercise capacity, coronary risk factors, behavioral characteristics, and quality of life in a large elderly cohort. Am J Cardiol 1995;76(3):177–179.

45. Milani RV, Lavie CJ. Prevalence and effects of cardiac rehabilitation on depression in the elderly with coronary heart disease. Am J Cardiol 1998;81(10):1233–1236.

46. Peddi R. Dietary prescription in atherosclerosis. Clin Geriatr Med 2002;18(4):819–826.

47. Oomen CM, Ocke MC, Feskens EJ, Erp-Baart MA, Kok FJ, Kromhout D. Association between trans fatty acid intake and 10-year risk of coronary heart disease in the Zutphen Elderly Study: a prospective population-based study. Lancet 2001;357 (9258):746–751.

48. Lindeman RD, Romero LJ, Allen AS, et al. Alcohol consumption is negatively associated with the prevalence of coronary heart disease in the New Mexico Elder Health Survey. J Am Geriatr Soc 1999;47(4):396–401.
49. Valmadrid CT, Klein R, Moss SE, Klein BE, Cruickshanks KJ. Alcohol intake and the risk of coronary heart disease mortality in persons with older-onset diabetes mellitus. JAMA 1999;282(3):239–246.
50. Appel LJ, Champagne CM, Harsha DW, et al. Effects of comprehensive lifestyle modification on blood pressure control: main results of the PREMIER clinical trial. JAMA 2003;289(16):2083–2093.
51. Whelton PK, Appel LJ, Espeland MA, et al. Sodium reduction and weight loss in the treatment of hypertension in older persons: a randomized controlled trial of non-pharmacologic interventions in the elderly (TONE). TONE Collaborative Research Group. JAMA 1998;279(11):839–846.
52. Gaziano JM, Manson JE, Branch LG, Colditz GA, Willett WC, Buring JE. A prospective study of consumption of carotenoids in fruits and vegetables and decreased cardiovascular mortality in the elderly. Ann Epidemiol 1995;5(4):255–260.
53. Alexander KP, Peterson ED. Coronary artery bypass grafting in the elderly. Am Heart J 1997;134(5 Pt 1):856–864.
54. Hirose H, Amano A, Yoshida S, Takahashi A, Nagano N, Kohmoto T. Coronary artery bypass grafting in the elderly. Chest 2000;117(5):1262–1270.
55. Akins CW, Daggett WM, Vlahakes GJ, et al. Cardiac operations in patients 80 years old and older. Ann Thorac Surg 1997;64(3):606–614.
56. Rumsfeld JS, MacWhinney S, McCarthy M Jr, et al. Health-related quality of life as a predictor of mortality following coronary artery bypass graft surgery. Participants of the Department of Veterans Affairs Cooperative Study Group on Processes, Structures, and Outcomes of Care in Cardiac Surgery. JAMA 1999;281(14):1298–1303.
57. Peterson ED, Batchelor WB. Percutaneous intervention in the very elderly: weighing the risks and benefits. Am Heart J 1999;137(4 Pt 1):585–587.
58. Alfonso F, Azcona L, Perez-Vizcayno MJ, et al. Initial results and long-term clinical and angiographic implications of coronary stenting in elderly patients. Am J Cardiol 1999;83(10):1483–1487, A7.
59. Jackman JD Jr, Navetta FI, Smith JE, et al. Percutaneous transluminal coronary angioplasty in octogenarians as an effective therapy for angina pectoris. Am J Cardiol 1991;68(1):116–119.
60. Wennberg DE, Makenka DJ, Sengupta A, et al. Percutaneous transluminal coronary angioplasty in the elderly: epidemiology, clinical risk factors, and in-hospital outcomes. The Northern New England Cardiovascular Disease Study Group. Am Heart J 1999;137(4 Pt 1):639–645.
61. Pfisterer M, Buser P, Osswald S, et al. Outcome of elderly patients with chronic symptomatic coronary artery disease with an invasive vs optimized medical treatment strategy: one-year results of the randomized TIME trial. JAMA 2003;289(9):1117–1123.
62. Lawson WE, Hui JC, Zheng ZS, et al. Three-year sustained benefit from enhanced external counterpulsation in chronic angina pectoris. Am J Cardiol 1995;75(12):840–841.
63. Holubkov R, Kennard ED, Foris JM, et al. Comparison of patients undergoing enhanced external counterpulsation and percutaneous coronary intervention for stable angina pectoris. Am J Cardiol 2002;89(10):1182–1186.

5

Age and Mortality and Morbidity in ST-Segment Elevation Myocardial Infarction

Steven P. Schulman, MD
and Gary Gerstenblith, MD

CONTENTS

Advanced age is a powerful independent predictor of in-hospital and subsequent mortality and morbidity in patients following an ST-elevation myocardial infarction (MI) *(1–4)*. Randomized studies including thousands of patients with ST-segment elevation MI indicate 10-fold increases in death, clinical heart failure, and cardiogenic shock following either thrombolytic or primary angioplasty as age increases from younger than 60 to older than 85 years, with an exponential rise in both in-hospital and 6-month post-discharge mortality *(1–4)*. Public health data indicate that nearly 85% of all deaths from coronary disease in the

From: *Contemporary Cardiology: Cardiovascular Disease in the Elderly*
Edited by: G. Gerstenblith © Humana Press Inc., Totowa, NJ

United States occur in individuals older than 65 years of age *(5)*, and that cardiac disease is the leading cause of death in older Americans, which is the most rapidly growing segment of the US population.

The most likely cause for the age-associated increase in mortality and morbidity in the setting of an MI is progressive left ventricular dysfunction. An analysis of the Gruppo Italiano per lo Studio della Sopravvivenza nell'Infarto Miocardico-2 data, in patients with a first ST-segment elevation MI all of whom were treated with thrombolytic therapy, indicates that deaths in the older patients were primarily related to myocardial dysfunction resulting from the infarct, with a surprisingly high incidence of rupture, clinical heart failure, and impaired left ventricular function; despite no age-associated increase in the clinical markers of infarct size itself and no increase in the extent of fixed coronary atherosclerotic disease *(1)*. Although age differences in complications and mortality may relate in part to delayed and atypical presentations and the increased likelihood of contraindications and complications from thrombolytic and β-blocker therapies *(2)*, the pre-existing age-associated changes in vascular and ventricular properties alter the substrate upon which the infarction occurs and likely play a critical role in the poor prognosis of the elderly patient with acute ST-segment elevation MI.

CARDIOVASCULAR CHANGES WITH PHYSIOLOGICAL AGING

As discussed in Chapter 1, there are several myocardial and vascular changes associated with physiological aging that may be responsible for the poor prognosis in older patients with acute ST-segment elevation MI. These include decreased β-adrenergic sympathetic responsiveness *(6,7)*, slowed and delayed early diastolic filling *(8,9)*, increased vascular stiffness *(10,11)*, and endothelial dysfunction *(12,13)*.

Decreased inotropic β-adrenergic responsiveness may affect cardiovascular function post-infarction by limiting contractile reserve in the region remote from the infarct and thereby the ability of that myocardium to compensate for the contractile performance lost as the result of the infarct itself. Age-associated decreased early filling, on the order of 6%–7% per decade *(9)*, increases the dependence of end-diastolic volume on atrial contraction and is thought to result in higher left atrial and pulmonary pressures for any given stroke volume *(14)*. Higher left ventricular pressures in diastole may also impair coronary perfusion at that time, when most of coronary flow occurs. Thus, age-associated changes in filling properties may also contribute to adverse outcomes post-infarction in older patients.

The age-associated increased arterial stiffness results from several factors, including fragmentation of the elastic membrane, intimal thickening, increases in collagen content and linking, decreased baroreflex sensitivity, and diminished endothelium-dependent vasorelaxation *(6)*. These changes increase the vascular load on the left ventricle and exert a significant influence on cardiovascular performance in healthy subjects *(15–17)*. A relationship between arterial stiffness, as indexed by sphygmomanometry-determined pulse pressure and increased risk of future coronary heart disease, congestive heart failure (CHF), and death has been demonstrated in elderly populations previously free of symptomatic heart disease *(18–20)*. In addition, elevated pulse pressure is an independent predictor of mortality in patients with chronic heart failure and left ventricular dysfunction following an MI *(21,22)*. The increased vascular load likely contributes to the high risk of heart failure in the elderly following acute MI.

Aging is also associated with endothelial dysfunction. Studies in subjects free of coronary artery disease and the classic risk factors for atherosclerosis demonstrate a significant inverse linear relationship between age and percent change in coronary and brachial arterial dimensions and blood flow responses to the intra-arterial (IA) administration of the endothelial-dependent vasodilator acetylcholine *(12,13)*. There is no effect of age on the vasodilator responses to IA papaverine and nitroprusside, endothelial-independent vasodilators. Furthermore, inhibition of nitric oxide (NO) synthase with NG-monomethyl L-arginine reduces forearm blood flow significantly less in older compared to younger subjects *(23)*. These studies suggest that in healthy subjects, the basal release of NO from vascular endothelium is reduced in the elderly, and the age-associated reduction in the vascular responsiveness to endothelium-dependent vasodilatation in both the coronary and forearm circulation suggests a general diminution in NO-induced vasodilatation in all vascular beds *(24)*. Because endothelial dysfunction affects conduit as well as arteriolar vessels, endothelial dysfunction of these vessels would be expected to significantly contribute to decreased arterial compliance and increased vascular load *(25)*. Thus, endothelial dysfunction in the elderly can contribute to the age-associated increase in peripheral vascular resistance, arterial stiffness, and vascular load.

In addition to increased vascular load, age-associated endothelial dysfunction negatively impacts older patients with acute MI by contributing to impaired collateral blood vessel growth *(26)*. In a recent study, angiographic collateral blood flow was assessed in 1934 patients with acute MI and an occluded infarct vessel. The presence of collaterals decreased progressively with increasing age of the patient and on multivariate analysis, age was independently associated with a lower prevalence of angiographic collaterals. In older patients, the lack of angiographic collaterals to the infarct vessel was an independent predictor of mortality.

Although the primary stimulus for collateral growth is controversial, angiogenesis requires the proliferation and migration of endothelial cells (27,28). With increasing age in animal models, endothelial dysfunction in collateral arterioles caused by a reduction in endothelial NO synthase expression contributes to a decline in angiogenesis (28–30). In addition to endothelial dysfunction, there is an age-related decrease in bone marrow-derived endothelial progenitor cells (31) that likely limits the ability to form new blood vessels in response to ischemia.

Another important link between age-associated endothelial dysfunction and impaired collateral vessel growth is decreased endothelial release of growth factors critical for angiogenesis (29,32,33), including platelet-derived growth factor-B (PDGF-B). Release of this growth factor stimulates the endothelial expression of several other growth factors, including vascular endothelial-derived growth factor (VEGF) (32). Animal models show that the endothelial expression of PDGF-B is downregulated in the senescent heart, which also reduces VEGF expression (32). In animal models of ischemia, VEGF mRNA and protein are reduced in aged animals, and this may contribute to significantly lower perfusion pressure, and decreased angiographic collateral vessel development and capillary density as compared to young animals (29). Pretreating aged ischemic animals with VEGF protein, PDGF-AB, or bone marrow-derived endothelial precursor cells from young animals results in an increase in angiographically visible collaterals, improved perfusion pressure, improved angiogenesis, and reduced MI size (29,32,33). These studies suggest that age-associated endothelial dysfunction results in reduced elaboration of endothelial-derived growth factors in response to ischemia and impaired angiogenesis.

The excess morbidity and mortality in older patients with acute MI is an increasing challenge as the population ages and suggest that establishment of normal coronary and myocardial blood flow in an expeditious fashion is particularly important in the older patient with acute MI as the infarct vessel is less likely to receive collateral flow compared to younger patients. Furthermore, initiation of therapies that in large, randomized, placebo-controlled trials reduce morbidity and mortality in the elderly is critical to optimizing outcomes in this high-risk group of ST-segment elevation MI patients.

All of these factors favor the potential benefits of an aggressive approach. Although randomized trials of thrombolytic vs placebo therapy clearly show a benefit in the general population, subset analyses of the older enrolled patients demonstrate only nonsignificant trends. Thus, although there was an absolute benefit in the Fibrinolytic Therapy Trialists' Collaborative Group's Trial metanalysis, which included 5800 patients over age 75 (34), the difference did not reach statistical significance. Subsequent personal communication data indicate a significant benefit in more recent data from the Fibrinolytic Therapy Trialists' Group that included elderly patients with ST-segment elevation on the electrocardiogram (35). It should be noted, however, that outcomes of enrolled patients in clinical trials may be better than those in the general population because the former usually have less co-morbidities and more frequently receive guideline-directed therapies. A retrospective analysis from the Comparative Cardiovascular Project in 7864 Medicare beneficiaries aged 65–86 years with ST-elevation MI, demonstrated a significant interaction between age and the effect of thrombolytic therapy on 30-day survival (Fig. 1) (36). There was a significant survival advantage for those aged 65–75, years which was comparable to that reported in the randomized studies of younger patients; but a survival disadvantage, with a 30-day mortality hazard ratio of 1.38 for those over 75 years of age.

Limitations of thrombolytic therapy in the elderly include an increased likelihood for relative or absolute contraindications, including hypertension and prior cerebrovascular accident; lower Thrombolysis in Myocardial Infarction grade flow following therapy; and an increased likelihood for intracranial hemorrhage. In the general population, flow is restored in only about 85% of patients, and a significant number experience recurrent ischemia. In an attempt to overcome the latter limitations, investigators have examined the utility of combining low-dose thrombolytics with more aggressive antiplatelet therapy in patients with ST-elevation MI. This approach was supported by angiographic studies demonstrating earlier and more complete reperfusion with the combination (37). The strategy was evaluated in the Global Use of Strategies to Open Occluded Coronary Arteries (GUSTO) V trial of 16,588 patients enrolled within the first 6 hours of an ST-elevation infarction who were randomized to standard-dose reteplase, two 10 U boluses 30 minutes apart, or to the combination of half-dose reteplase, two boluses of 5 U, 30 minutes apart, plus a standard abciximab infusion of 0.25 mg/kg bolus and 0.125 µg/kg per minute for 12 hours (38). All patients received aspirin and heparin was administered, with a lower initial dose in the combined group, so as to achieve an activated partial thromboplastin time of 50 to 70 seconds. In the overall population, there was no significant difference in the primary endpoint of 30-day mortality. In the 2237 patients 75 years or older, mortal-

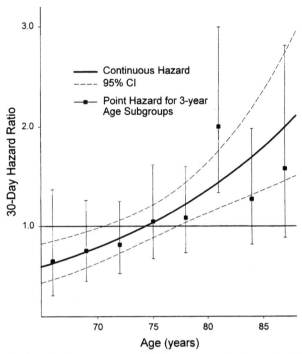

Fig. 1. The relationship between age and 30-day mortality hazard ratios in 7864 Medicare beneficiaries with ST-elevation myocardial infarction and no contraindications to thrombolytic therapy from the Cooperative Cardiovascular Project. The points are hazard ratios calculated from 3-year age subgroups. There is a survival benefit for the younger age groups, but an increase in the hazard ratios after age 75 years. (From ref. *36*.)

ity was 18.3% in the combination group and 17.9% in the reteplase alone group. Moreover, there was a significant interaction between age and the effect of treatment of intracranial hemorrhage *(39)*. Although the risk of intracranial hemorrhage increased with age in both groups, it was lower with the combination therapy than that with reteplase alone up to age 55 years and thereafter increased, reaching significantly higher values after age 80 years *(see* Fig. 2).

The limitations of thrombolytic therapy are overcome to a significant extent with primary angioplasty therapy. In a large review of 23 randomized trials, primary angioplasty significantly reduced short-term mortality and the combined outcome of death, nonfatal MI, and stroke when compared with thrombolytic therapy *(40)*. The benefit appears to be particularly significant in the elderly population. In a trial confined to patients

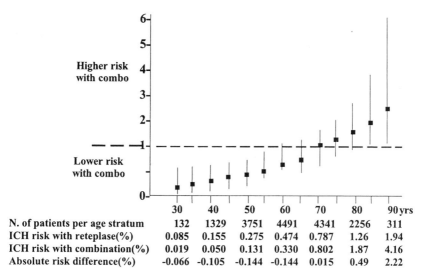

Fig. 2. The relationship between age and the relative risk of intracranial hemorrhage with reteplase alone and with reteplase plus abciximab in the GUSTO-5 trial. The risk with thrombolytic therapy increases from 0.085% for those aged 30 years to 1.94 for those 90 years. It is significantly higher after age 70 in those who received combination therapy. (From ref. *39*.)

over age 75 years with ST-elevation infarction, the participants were randomized to primary angioplasty or intravenous streptokinase *(41)*. At 30 days, the composite of death, re-infarction, or stroke occurred in 9% of patients in the angioplasty and 29% of patients in the thrombolysis group ($p = 0.01$). At 1 year, the composite endpoint was reached in 13% of the angioplasty and 44% of the thrombolytic group. Furthermore, in a retrospective analysis from the Medicare Cooperative Cardiovascular Project, those who underwent angioplasty had lower 30-day and 1-year mortality. After adjusting for baseline characteristics, the 30-day hazard ratio was 0.74 and the 1-year hazard ratio 0.88 for primary angioplasty *(42)*.

Cardiogenic shock is the most frequent cause of in-hospital mortality in patients with acute MI and as noted previously, older patients are more likely to experience this complication. The SHOCK (SHould we emergently revascularize Occluded Coronaries for cardiogenic shocK) trial randomized 300 individuals with acute MI and who were within 12 hours of the onset of cardiogenic shock to revascularization within 6 hours of randomization or to late or no revascularization *(43)*. Age, older or younger than 75 years, was a prespecified subgroup. Among those older than 75 years, mortality at 1 month, the primary outcome variable, did not differ in the two randomized groups, although it trended higher in the early re-vascularization group. At 1 year as well, there was no significant benefit of early revascularization in the older group *(44)*. However, in the accom-panying SHOCK Registry, covariate adjusted analysis showed that eld-erly patients selected for early revascularization had a lower mortality than those who were not *(45)*. The older patients were more likely than the younger patients to have a history of prior MI, heart failure, and renal insufficiency and were more likely to have a lower mean diastolic pres-sure and cardiac index as well as triple-vessel and left main coronary dis-ease. The elderly group were also less likely to have Swan-Ganz catheters and intra-aortic balloon pumps placed and to undergo coronary angiog-raphy, percutaneous transluminal coronary angioplasty, and bypass sur-gery. The differences between the trial and registry results likely reflect selection bias but nevertheless indicate that not all elderly patients with cardiogenic shock should be denied revascularization if they are viewed as appropriate candidates. It should also be noted that routine stent and glycoprotein-IIb/IIIa inhibitors were not in use at the time of the study.

Although early angioplasty improves outcomes in elderly patients, there is still a marked age effect on mortality risk and the risk of other post-infarction complications. In a pooled analysis of three primary angio-plasty trials, Second Primary Angioplasty in Myocardial Infarction Trial (PAMI-2), Stent PAMI, and PAMI No Surgery, consisting of 3032 patients, 452 of whom were 75 years or older, in hospital mortality significantly increased with age from 0.6% for those under 60 years, to 11.5% for those older than 79 years (Fig. 3) *(4)*. Those 75 years and older also had higher rates of other post-MI complications including renal failure requir-ing dialysis (3.9% vs 0.9%), stroke or transient ischemia attack (2.9% vs 0.8%), mitral regurgitation (6.6% vs 2.6%), and CHF (21.9% vs 8.0%). On multivariable analysis, the only in-hospital factors that predicted mor-tality in the over-75 age group were arrhythmias requiring treatment (with an odds ratio [OR] 5.0) and left ventricular ejection fraction (EF) less than 40% (OR 3.9).

An important limitation of angioplasty is that relatively few hospitals have surgical backup. To some extent the requirement for emergency surgery availability is lessened by the use of coronary artery stents, which decrease the incidences of, and can be used to treat, abrupt closure and dissection. A randomized trial of primary angioplasty vs thrombolytic therapies in 451 patients performed in hospitals without surgical backup demonstrated that short- and long-term outcomes were improved with angioplasty, although results in the older patients were not reported sep-arately *(46)*. Perhaps a more attractive option is to transfer patients to facilities where primary angioplasty is frequently performed. In a meta-

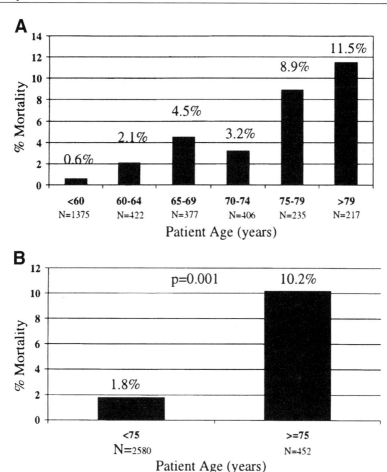

Fig. 3. A meta-analysis of the relationship between age and in-hospital mortality in 3032 patients from three primary angioplasty trials. (From ref. 4.)

analysis of six randomized trials evaluating the feasibility, safety, and efficacy of transfer for angioplasty compared with thrombolysis in the first admitting hospital, death, re-infarction or stroke were reduced by 42% in the transfer for angioplasty group (47). The Danish Multicenter Randomized study separately reported the results in the subset of those over 63 years, with a hazard ratio of 0.54, p = 0.002 for the composite of death, re-infarction or disabling stroke at 30-day follow-up (48). However, data from one of the studies indicate equivalent outcomes, that is, no difference between thrombolysis and transfer, if the patient presents within 3 hours of symptom onset (49). The addition of abciximab at the time of angioplasty in patients with acute transmural infarction is associated with improved survival at 1 year (95% vs 88%), in the entire patient population, although results were not separately reported for the older subsets *(50)*. The addition of lytic therapy to glycoprotein-IIb/IIIa treatment, on the other hand, was not associated with decreased infarct size, the primary outcome, and was associated with an increased risk of major bleeding *(51)*.

ASPIRIN

The large, randomized International Study of Infarct Survival-2 conducted in more than 17,000 patients with suspected MI, the majority presenting with ST-segment elevation, demonstrated that aspirin therapy reduces mortality in these patients *(52)*. Compared to placebo, aspirin reduced 35-day mortality by approximately 23%, from 13% to 10%. This study included 3411 patients with MI over 70 years of age. In this important subgroup, aspirin therapy decreased mortality by 22.3% compared to placebo. Chronic aspirin therapy also reduces recurrent MI, stroke, or cardiovascular death in older subjects who have experienced an MI *(53)*. In the Cooperative Cardiovascular Project review of more than 10,000 MI patients 65 years of age and older, aspirin use reduced 30-day mortality by 22% *(54)*. Despite these overwhelming data for the use of aspirin therapy in acute MI, up to one-third of older patients with no contraindication do not receive aspirin at the time of their infarct *(55)*. All older patients without contraindications should receive aspirin therapy on admission to the hospital with acute MI and chronically thereafter.

β-BLOCKERS

β-Blocker use following acute MI is greatly underutilized in the elderly, despite overwhelming data that show significant survival advantage with this therapy. In the large, randomized trials, the majority of long-term benefit of β-blockers was driven by the benefit in those patients over 65 years of age *(56)*. In the large Cooperative Cardiovascular Project database of more than 200,000 patients with MIs 65 years of age and older, only 37% of all patients and 50% of "ideal" β-blocker therapy candidates were discharged from the hospital on a β-blocker *(57)*. Of ideal candidates among the older post-MI patient with no contraindication to β-blocker therapy, only 50% leave the hospital on this life-saving therapy. In this large observational database, discharge on β-blocker resulted in a 40% relative, and nearly 10% absolute, reduction in 2-year mortality *(57)*. This large survival benefit extends to all subgroups analyzed in this large database, including all age groups from under 70 to older than 80 years, Q-wave and non-ST-segment elevation MI, EF from less than 20% to more than 50%, and regardless of other treatments received, including angioplasty, coronary artery bypass surgery, and thrombolytic therapy. Paradoxically, older patients who are less likely to receive β-blocker therapy post-MI are those at highest risk for morbidity and mortality and thus, would benefit most from this therapy. β-Blocker use in the older post-MI patient is also beneficial long-term, particularly for those with left ventricular dysfunction. In an analysis of the Metoprolol CR/XL Randomized Interventional Trial in Heart Failure, that included patients with symptomatic heart failure and an EF of 40% or lower, 1926 patients had a prior MI *(58)*. The mean age of this cohort was over 65 years, with nearly all subjects on an angiotensin-converting enzyme (ACE) inhibitor or an angiotensin receptor blocker (ARB). The mean EF was 28%. This older cohort of post-MI patients with heart failure and left ventricular dysfunction tolerated randomization to a β-blocker very well with fewer study drug discontinuations in the β-blocker, compared to the placebo, group. Eighteen-month mortality was reduced by 40%, sudden death by 50%, and death from worsening heart failure by 49%. These data suggest that chronic β-blocker administration results in a significant survival advantage over and above that afforded by standard ACE-inhibitor therapy in older patients with heart failure and ischemic left ventricular dysfunction.

Randomized, placebo-controlled β-blocker trials have also evaluated the short-term benefits of acute intravenous β-blockade. The majority of patients enrolled into these trials suffered acute, transmural MIs. An important mechanism of death in older patients with ST-segment elevation MI is myocardial rupture *(1)* and age is an important predictor of myocardial rupture following transmural MI. Because one of the benefits of acute intravenous β-blockade is a reduction in left ventricular wall stress, and thereby a decreased risk of rupture, older patients with acute ST-segment elevation MI would be expected to benefit from intravenous β-blockade in the acute MI setting as well. Although less than 10% of older patients with an ST-segment elevation MI receive acute intravenous β-blockade, data from large, randomized placebo-controlled trials indicate that this therapy significantly reduces short-term mortality in those patients above the age of 65 years *(59)*.

There are probably several reasons why providers are reluctant to prescribe β-blockers despite their proven benefit in post-MI older patients. These include perceived increased risk of side effects and lack of benefit. Cardiologists are most likely to prescribe β-blockers to older post-infarction patients, whereas family practitioners are least likely *(57)*. Efforts at educating health care providers and providing feedback at discharge to practitioners can improve the use of proven therapies in this age group *(60)*. In the thousands of older patients with MI who have been evaluated in randomized trials, there does not appear to be any subgroup that does not benefit from β-blocker treatment.

INHIBITION OF THE RENIN–ANGIOTENSIN–ALDOSTERONE SYSTEM

Similar to β-blockers, ACE inhibitor therapy offers a significant benefit to the older, post-infarction patient, particularly those with left ventricular dysfunction or heart failure. A meta-analysis of the four randomized, placebo-controlled trials evaluating the effects of ACE inhibitor therapy on early post-infarction mortality (primarily ST-segment elevation MIs) in 100,000 patients randomized to an ACE inhibitor showed a significant reduction in 30-day mortality *(61)*. These trials did not mandate left ventricular dysfunction or heart failure as entry criteria. Of this population, 30% was aged 65–74 years and 15% of the cohort was aged 75 years and older. In the former age group, 30-day mortality was nearly 11% lower in the ACE inhibitor group compared to the placebo group. In patients 75 years of age and older, 30-day mortality was similar in both groups. Importantly, the lack of benefit in those over 75 years of age was related to excess mortality in older patients who developed hypotension with intravenous ACE inhibitor therapy *(62)*, particularly early in the hospital course. Therefore, ACE inhibitors must be initiated at a low dose and titrated based on hemodynamic stability of the patient.

There is a large benefit associated with ACE inhibitor therapy in higher risk patients with left ventricular dysfunction or clinical heart failure while in the coronary care unit. A meta-analysis of three randomized, placebo-controlled trials involving 5966 patients with left ventricular dysfunction (EF < 40%) or heart failure was reported *(63)*. The mean age of the cohort was 63 years. After a mean follow-up of 31 months, patients randomized to the ACE inhibitor experienced a 26% reduction in mortality, a 27% decrease in heart failure hospitalizations, and a 20% decrease in recurrent MI *(63)*. There was no statistical heterogeneity on the ACE inhibitor effect by age less than 55 years, 55–75 years, or older than 75 years and in each of the individual studies of high-risk patients, patients over the age of 65 years and randomized to the ACE inhibitor arm had a larger survival advantage vs placebo compared to the younger subjects *(64–66)*. These data suggest that ACE inhibitor therapy is an important therapy for older post-MI patients with left ventricular dysfunction or heart failure. Despite these data, only 58% of Medicare recipients without any contraindications to ACE inhibitors were prescribed this medication at hospital discharge following an MI *(67)*. Discharge programs need to be initiated to ensure appropriate post-infarct therapies are administered to the elderly.

Although ACE inhibitor therapy saves lives in patients post-MI with left ventricular dysfunction and heart failure, angiotensin II and aldosterone levels, initially inhibited by high-dose ACE inhibitor therapy, eventually rise to pretreatment levels despite continued therapy *(68,69)*. There are several potential mechanisms including incomplete inhibition of the renin–angiotensin–aldosterone system (RAAS) at maximally tolerated doses of ACE inhibitors and enzymatic pathways other than ACE that may contribute to angiotensin II and aldosterone production *(70)*. These findings have prompted more recent post-infarction studies evaluating the use of additional agents to further inhibit the RAAS.

The Valsartan in Acute Myocardial Infarction (VALIANT) trial tested the hypothesis that treatment with the ARB valsartan, alone or in combination with the ACE inhibitor, captopril, would result in improved survival compared with an ACE inhibitor alone in post-infarction patients with left ventricular dysfunction (EF $\leq$ 35%), clinical heart failure, or both *(71)*. This large trial randomized 14,703 patients to high-dose captopril, high-dose valsartan, or a combination of the two. The median duration of follow-up was almost 25 months. The majority of patients had Q-wave infarcts and more than 70% of patients were on β-blocker therapy. The primary outcome of mortality (19.3% to 19.9%) did not differ among the three randomized groups. The secondary outcome of cardiovascular mortality, recurrent MI, or heart failure hospitalization was also similar in the three groups. Patients randomized to the captopril plus valsartan group were more likely to experience hypotension and renal dysfunction compared to the ACE inhibitor or ARB-only groups. The mean age of this large cohort was about 65 years. Group comparisons in patients 65 years of age and older also showed no difference in mortality or cardiovascular mortality and morbidity among the randomized groups. The VALIANT trial therefore demonstrates that an ACE inhibitor or ARB are equally beneficial. The clinical experience with ACE inhibitor therapy is more extensive, but ARBs may be used in those patients who cannot tolerate ACE inhibitor therapy. The combination, however, should not be part of routine therapy owing to an increased risk of side effects without any additional benefit.

Aldosterone production is stimulated in the setting of left ventricular dysfunction and heart failure, and hepatic clearance of aldosterone is impaired. This results in a 20-fold increase in aldosterone levels in heart failure patients *(72)*. Elevated aldosterone levels not only promote salt and water retention, but also stimulate inflammation and fibroblast growth and synthesis of collagen *(73)*. This results in myocardial fibrosis and probably contributes to adverse left ventricular remodeling following MI *(73)*. Adding an aldosterone receptor antagonist to an ACE inhibitor in animal models of acute MI improves left ventricular remodeling with decreases in left ventricular volumes and pressures, catecholamine levels, collagen gene expression and left ventricular collagen content *(73)*. These animal data were followed by the Eplerenone Post-Acute Myocardial Infarction Heart Failure Efficacy and Survival Study (EPHESUS) trial, which tested whether eplerenone, an aldosterone antagonist which selectively blocks the mineralocorticoid receptor, when added to standard post-infarction therapy reduces mortality among patients with acute MI complicated by left ventricular dysfunction and heart failure *(74)*. In this study, 6642 post-infarction patients were enrolled with EF of 40% or less and clinical heart failure or with a low EF and diabetes. The majority of patients suffered a Q-wave MI. Eighty-seven percent of the patients received an ACE inhibitor, whereas 75% were on β-blockers. Potassium levels were carefully followed with dose adjustments or discontinuation of the study drug if potassium levels became elevated. Mortality, the primary outcome, was reduced 15%, from 16.7% to 14.4%, over a mean follow-up of 16 months. Cardiovascular mortality or cardiovascular hospitalizations were also significantly reduced in the eplerenone arm. There was also a significant reduction in sudden cardiac death and heart failure admissions in the eplerenone group. There was no statistical heterogeneity of benefit between subjects less than 65 years or 65 years or older. These data indicate that in older patients with left ventricular dysfunction and heart failure following a large transmural MI, the addition of eplerenone to standard post-infarction therapy should be considered if renal function is not impaired and potassium levels are carefully monitored.

HMG-CoA REDUCTASE INHIBITORS

Hydroxymethylglutaryl-coenzyme A (HMG-CoA) reductase inhibitors also reduce cardiovascular events in the older post-infarction patient, and are also usually under prescribed. The Cholesterol and Recurrent Events trial randomized patients with a recent MI (60% Q-wave), total cholesterol levels less than 240 mg/dL and low-density lipoprotein cholesterol levels between 115 and 174 mg/dL to a statin or placebo. Twelve hundred and eighty three patients in this trial were between 65 and 75 years of age. Five-year cardiovascular event rates in this older cohort were reduced a relative 32% and absolute 9% (19.7% vs 28.1%) with active therapy compared with placebo *(75)*. Secondary outcomes of coronary death and stroke were also significantly reduced with statin therapy compared to placebo in the elderly. The number of older post-infarct patients needed to treat with statin therapy to prevent one major cardiovascular event was 11, and the number needed to treat to prevent one coronary death was 22.

These impressive beneficial results of statin therapy in older post-infarction patients are mirrored in other large trials of secondary prevention. In the Heart Protection Study, 5806 subjects enrolled were 70 years of age or older and a large number of these had a history of a prior MI *(76)*. Similar to the total study population, the older subjects, including those 75 to 80 years at the time of enrollment, experienced a significant reduction in cardiovascular events over the 5-year study period. In a large observational study of more than 7000 patients with angiographic coronary disease (30% with an MI), statin therapy prescribed at discharge decreased significantly as the age of the patient increased *(77)* with fewer than one in five patients with coronary disease over 80 years of age discharged on statin therapy. After 3.3 years of observational follow-up, patients discharged on statin therapy had a significantly lower mortality irregardless of age. Importantly, the small number of side effects from statin therapy was not age-related. Nevertheless, only a minority of older post-infarct patients leaves the hospital on statin therapy, and a large number discontinue statin therapy soon after hospital discharge *(78)*. Education of physicians and older patients of the benefit of risk-factor modification after an MI, including statin therapy, will improve outcomes in these high-risk patients.

SUMMARY

Increased age is a powerful predictor of short- and long-term morbidity and mortality following acute MI. This increase in mortality exists even in older patients with a first ST-segment elevation MI. The increase probably results from important age-associated changes in the cardiovascular system, including impaired early diastolic filling, decreased β-adrenegic response, increased vascular stiffness, and impaired endothelial function. The latter age-associated change may explain why older patients with acute ST-segment elevation MI are less likely to have collateral blood flow to the occluded infarct vessel.

These findings mandate an aggressive approach to the older patient with an ST-segment elevation MI. Angioplasty of the infarct vessel decreases morbidity and mortality. Furthermore, large, randomized, placebo-controlled trials that included older subjects demonstrate that aspirin, β-blockers, ACE inhibitors, and HMG-CoA reductase inhibitors should be standard post-MI therapy in the older post-infarct patient. Physician and patient education are critical to implementing the findings from these clinical trials into routine provider practice.

REFERENCES

1. Maggioni AP, Maseri A, Fresco C, Franzosi MG, Mauri F, Santoro E, Tognoni G, on behalf of the investigators of the Gruppo Italiano per lo Studio della Sopravvivenza nell Infarto Miocardico (GISSI-II). Age-related increase in mortality among patients with first myocardial infarctions treated with thrombolysis. N Engl J Med 1993;329:1442–1448.
2. White HD, Barbash GI, Califf RM, et al. Age and outcome with contemporary thrombolytic therapy. Results from the GUSTO-I trial. Circulation 1996;94:1826–1833.
3. Aguirre FV, McMahon RP, Mueler H, et al. Impact of age on clinical outcome and postlytic management strategies in patients treated with intravenous thrombolytic therapy. Results from the TIMI II study. Circulation 1994;90:78–86.
4. DeGeare VS, Stone GW, Grines L, et al. Angiographic and clinical characteristics associated with increased in-hospital mortality in elderly patients with acute myocardial infarction undergoing percutaneous interventions (a pooled analysis of the primary angioplasty in myocardial infarction trials). Am J Cardiol 2000;86:30–34.
5. American Heart Association. Heart Disease and Stroke Statistics—2005 Update. Dallas, TX, American Heart Association; 2003.
6. Lakatta EG. Cardiovascular regulatory mechanisms in advanced age. Physiol Rev 1993;73:413–467.
7. Lakatta EG, Gertenblith G, Angell CS, Shock NW, Weisfeldt ML. Diminished inotropic response of aged myocardium to catecholamines. Circ Res 1975;36:262–269.
8. Lakatta EG, Gerstenblith G, Angell CS, Shock NW, Weisfeldt ML. Prolonged contraction duration in aged myocardium. J Clin Invest 1975;55:61–68.
9. Schulman SP, Lakatta EG, Fleg JL, Lakatta L, Becker LC, Gerstenblith G. Age-related decline in left ventricular filling at rest and exercise. Am J Physiol 1992;263 (Heart Circ Physiol):H1932–H1938.
10. Yin FCP, Weisfeldt ML, Milnor WR. The role of aortic input impedance and the decreased cardiovascular response to exercise with aging in the dog. J Clin Invest 1981;68:28–38.
11. Nichols WW, O'Rourke MF, Avolio AP, Yaginuma T, Murgo JP, Pepine CV, Conti CR. Effects of age on ventricular–vascular coupling. Am J Cardiol 1985;55:1179–1184.
12. Taddei S, Virdis A, Mattei P, et al. Aging and endothelial function in normotensive subjects and patients with essential hypertension. Circulation 1995;91:1981–1987.
13. Celermajer DS, Sorensen KE, Spiegelhalter DJ, Georgakopoulos D, Robinson J, Deanfield JE. Aging is associated with endothelial dysfunction in healthy men years before the age-related decline in women. J Am Coll Cardiol 1994;24:471–476.
14. Arora R, Machac J, Goldman ME, Butler RN, Gorlin R, Horowitz SF. Atrial kinetics and left ventricular diastolic filling in the healthy elderly. J Am Coll Cardiol 1987; 9:1255–1260.
15. Vaitkevicius PV, Fleg JL, Engel JH, et al. Effects of age and aerobic capacity on arterial stiffness in healthy adults. Circulation 1993;88:1456–1462.
16. Lakatta EG, Levy D. Arterial and cardiac aging: Major shareholders in cardiovascular disease enterprises. Part I. Circulation 2003;107:139–146.

17. Lakatta EG, Levy D. Arterial and cardiac aging: Major shareholders in cardiovascular disease enterprises. Part II. Circulation 2003;107:346–354.
18. Franklin SS, Khan SA, Wong ND, Larson MG, Levy D. Is pulse pressure useful in predicting risk for coronary heart disease? The Framingham Heart Study. Circulation 1999;100:354–360.
19. Chae CU, Pfeffer MA, Glynn RJ, Mitchell GF, Taylor JO, Hennekens GH. Increased pulse pressure and risk of heart failure in the elderly. JAMA 1999;281: 634–639.
20. Glynn RJ, Chae CU, Guralnik JM, Taylor JO, Hennekens CH. Pulse pressure and mortality in older people. Arch Intern Med 2000;160:2765–2772.
21. Domanski MJ, Mitchell GF, Norman JE, Exner DV, Pitt B, Pfeffer MA. Independent prognostic information provided by sphygmomanometrically determined pulse pressure and mean arterial pressure in patients with left ventricular dysfunction. J Am Coll Cardiol 1999;33:951–958.
22. Mitchell GF, Moye LA, Braunwald E, et al. Sphygmomanometrically determined pulse pressure is a powerful independent predictor of recurrent events after myocardial infarction in patients with impaired left ventricular function. Circulation 1997; 96:4254–4260.
23. Lyons D, Roy S, Patel M, Benjamin N, Swift CG. Impaired nitric oxide-mediated vasodilatation and total body nitric oxide production in healthy old age. Clin Sci 1997;93:519–525.
24. Drexler H. Endothelial dysfunction. Prog in Cardiovasc Dis 1997;39:287–324.
25. Vallance P, Collier J, Moncada S. Effects of endothelium-derived nitric oxide on peripheral arteriolar tone in man. Lancet 1989;ii:997–1000.
26. Kurotobi T, Sato H, Imai K, et al. Reduced collateral circulation to the infarct related artery in elderly patients with acute myocardial infarction. J Am Coll Cardiol 2004; 44:28–34.
27. D'Amore PA, Thompson RW. Mechanisms of angiogenesis. Ann Rev Physiol 1987; 9:453–464.
28. Tuttle JL, Hahn TL, Sanders BM, et al. Impaired collateral development in mature rats. Am J Physiol Heart Circ Physiol 2002;283;H146–H155.
29. Rivard A, Fabre JE, Silver M, et al. Age-dependent impairment of angiogenesis. Circulation 1999;99:111–120.
30. Csiszar A, Ungvari Z, Edwards JG, et al. Aging-induced phenotypic changes and oxidative stress impair coronary artteriolar function. Circ Res 2002;90:1159–1166.
31. Rauscher FM, Goldschmidt-Clermont PJ, Davis BH, et al. Aging, progenitor cell exhaustion, and atherosclerosis. Circulation 2003;108:457–463.
32. Edelberg JM, Lee SH, Kaur M, et al. Platelet-derived growth factor-AB limits the extent of myocardial infarction in a rat model. Circulation 2002;105:608–613.
33. Edelberg JM, Tang L, Hattori K, Lyden D, Rafii S. Young adult bone marrow-derived endothelial precursor cells restore aging-impaired cardiac angiogenic function. Circ Res 2002;90:e89–e93.
34. Fibrinolytic Therapy Trialists' (FFT) Collaborative Group. Indications for fibrinolytic therapy in suspected acute myocardial infarction: Collaborative overview of early mortality and major morbidity from all randomised trials of more than 1000 patients. Lancet 1994;343:311–322.
35. White HD. Debate: Should the elderly receive thrombolytic therapy or primary angioplasty? Current Controlled Trials in Cardiovascular Medicine 2000:1:150–154.
36. Thiemann DR, Coresh J, Schulman SP, Gerstenblith G, Oetgen WJ, Powe NR. Lack of benefit for intravenous thrombolysis in patients with myocardial infarction who are older than 75 years. Circulation 2000;101:2239–2246.

37. The SPEED Group. Randomized trial of abciximab with and without low-dose reteplase for acute myocardial infarction. Circulation 2000;101:2788–2794.
38. The GUSTO V Investigators. Reperfusion therapy for acute myocardial infarction with fibrinolytic therapy or combination reduced fibrinolytic therapy and platelet glycoprotein IIb/IIIa inhibition: the GUSTO V randomised trial. The Lancet 2001; 357:1905–1914.
39. Savonitto S, Armstrong PW, Lincoff AM, et al. Risk of intracranial hemorrhage with combined fibrinolytic and glycoprotein IIb/IIIa inhibitor therapy in acute myocardial infarction: Dichotomous response as a function of age in the GUSTO V trial. European Heart Journal 2003;24:1807–1814.
40. Keeley EC, Boure JA, Grines CL. Primary angioplasty versus intravenous thrombolytic therapy for acute myocardial infarction: a quantitative review of 23 randomised trials. Lancet 2003;361:13–20.
41. De Boer M-J, Ottervanger J-P, van't Hof, AWJ, et al. Reperfusion therapy in elderly patients with acute myocardial infarction. A randomized comparison of primary angioplasty and thrombolytic therapy. J Am Coll Cardiol 2002;39:1723–1728.
42. Berger AK, Schulman KA, Gersh BJ, et al. Primary coronary angioplasty vs thrombolysis for the management of acute myocardial infarction in elderly patients. JAMA 1999;282:341–348.
43. Hochman JS, Sleeper LA, Webb JG, et al. Effect of early revascularization on mortality in cardiogenic shock complicating acute myocardial infarction. N Engl J Med 1999;341:625–634.
44. Hochman JS, Sleeper LA, White HD, et al. One-year survival following early revascularization for cardiogenic shock. JAMA 2001;285:190–192.
45. Dzavik V, Sleeper LA, Cocke TP, et al. Early revascularization is associated with improved survival in elderly patients with acute myocardial infarction complicated by cardiogenic shock: a report from the SHOCK Trial Registry. Eur Heart J 2003;24: 828–837.
46. Aversano T, Aversano LT, Passamani E, et al. Thrombolytic therapy vs primary percutaneous intervention for myocardial infarction in patients presenting to hospitals without on-site cardiac surgery. JAMA 2002;287:1943–1951.
47. Dalby M, Bouzamondo A, Lechat P, Montalescot G. Transfer for primary angioplasty versus immediate thrombolysis in acute myocardial infarction. A Meta-Analysis. Circulation 2003;108:1809–1814.
48. Andersen HR, Nielsen TT, Rasmussen K, et al. A comparison of coronary angioplasty with fibrinolytic therapy in acute myocardial infarction. N Engl J Med 2003; 349:733–742.
49. Widimsky P, Budesinsky T, Vorac D, et al. Long distance transport for primary angioplasty vs immediate thrombolysis in acute myocardial infarction. Final results of the randomized national multicentre trial—Prague 2. Eur Heart J 2003;24:94–104.
50. Antoniucci D, Migliorini A, Parodi G, et al. Abciximab-supported infarct artery stent implantation for acute myocardial infarction and long-term survival. A prospective, multicenter, randomized trial comparing infarct artery stenting plus abciximab with stenting alone. Circulation 2004;109:1704–1706.
51. Kastrati A, Mehilli J, Schlotterbeck K, et al. Early administration of reteplase plus abciximab vs abciximab alone in patients with acute myocardial infarction referred for percutaneous coronary intervention. A randomized controlled trial. JAMA 2004; 291:947–968.
52. International Study of Infarct Survival-2 (ISIS-2) Investigators. Randomised trial of intravenous streptokinase, oral aspirin, both or neither among 17,187 cases of suspected myocardial infarction. Lancet 1988;ii:349–360.

53. Antithrombotic Trialists' Collaboration. Collaborative meta-analysis of randomized trials of antiplatelet therapy for prevention of death, myocardial infarction, and stroke in high risk patients. BMJ 2002;324:71–86.
54. Krumholz H, Radford M, Ellerbeck E, Hennen J, Meehan T, Petrillo M. Aspirin in the treatment of acute myocardial infarction in elderly Medicare beneficiaries: patterns of use and outcomes. Circulation 1995;92:2841–2847.
55. Krumholz H, Radford M, Ellerbeck E, et al. Aspirin for secondary prevention after acute myocardial infarction in the elderly: prescribed use and outcomes. Ann Intern Med 1996;124:292–298.
56. Gottlieb SS, McCarter RJ, Vogel RA. Effect of beta-blockade on mortality among high-risk and low-risk patients after myocardial infarction. N Engl J Med 1998;339: 489–497.
57. Krumholz HM, Radford MJ, Wang Y, Chen J, Heiat A, Marciniak TA. National use and effectiveness for the treatment of elderly patients after acute myocardial infarction. JAMA 1998;280:623–629.
58. Janosi A, Ghali JK, Herlitz J, et al. Metoprolol CR/XL in postmyocardial infarction patients with chronic heart failure: Experiences from MERIT-HR. Am Heart J 2003; 146:721–728.
59. ISIS-1 (First International study of Infarct Survival) Collaborative Group. Mechanisms for the early mortality reduction produced by beta-blockade started early in acute myocardial infarction: ISIS-1. Lancet 1988;I:921–923.
60. Rochon PA, Gurwitz JH. Prescribing for seniors. JAMA 1999;281:113–115.
61. ACE Inhibitor Myocardial Infarction Collaborative Group. Indications for ACE inhibitors in the early treatment of acute myocardial infarction. Circulation 1998;97: 2202–2212.
62. Swedberg K, Held P, Kjekshus J, et al. Effects of the early administration of enalapril on mortality in patients with acute myocardial infarction: results of the Cooperative New Scandinavian Enalapril Survival Study II (CONSENSUS II). N Engl J Med 1992;327:678–684.
63. Flather MD, Yusuf S, Køber L, et al. Long-term ACE-inhibitor therapy in patients with heart failure or left-ventricular dysfunction: a systematic overview of data from individual patients. Lancet 2000; 355:1575–1581.
64. Pfeffer MA, Braunwald E, Moye L, et al. Effect of captopril on mortality and morbidity in patients with left ventricular dysfunction after myocardial infarction-results of the Survival and Ventricular Enlargement Trial. N Engl J Med 1992;327:669–677.
65. Kober L, Torp-Pedersen C, Carlsen J, et al. A clinical trial of the angiotensin-converting enzyme inhibitor trandolapril in patients with left ventricular dysfunction after myocardial infarction. N Engl J Med 1995;333:1670–1676.
66. Acute Infarction Ramipril Efficacy (AIRE) Study Investigators. Effect of ramapril on mortality and morbidity of survivors of acute myocardial infarction with clinical evidence of heart failure. Lancet 1993; 342:821–825.
67. Krumholz H, Chen YT, Wang Y, Radford M. Aspirin and angiotensin-converting enzyme inhibitors among elderly survivors of hospitalization for an acute myocardial infarction. Arch Inter Med 2001;161:538–544.
68. Pitt B. "Escape" of aldosterone production in patients with left ventricular dysfunction treated with an angiotensin-converting enzyme inhibitor: implications for therapy. Cardiovasc Drugs Ther 1995;9:145–149.
69. Jorde UP, Ennezat PV, Lisker BA, et al. Maximally recommended doses of angiotensin-converting enzyme (ACE) inhibitors do not completely prevent ACE-medicated formation of angiotensin II in chronic heart failure. Circulation 2000;101: 844–846.

70. Mann DL, Deswal A, Bozkurt B, Torre-Amione G. New therapeutics for chronic heart failure. Ann Rev Med 2002;53:59–74.
71. Pfeffer MA, McMurray JJV, Velazquez EJ, et al. Valsartan, captopril, or both in myocardial infarction complicated by heart failure, left ventricular dysfunction, or both. N Engl J Med 2003;349:1893–1906.
72. Weber KT. Aldosterone in congestive heart failure. N Engl J Med 2001;345:1689–1697.
73. Fraccarollo D, Galuppo P, Hildemann S, Christ M, Ertl G, Bauersachs J. Additive improvement of left ventricular remodeling and neurohormonal activation by aldosterone receptor blockade with eplerenone and ACE inhibition in rats with myocardial infarction. J Am Coll Cardiol 2003;42:1666–1673.
74. Pitt B, Remme W, Zannad F, et al. Eplerenone, a selective aldosterone blocker, in patients with left ventricular dysfunction after myocardial infarction. N Engl J Med 2003;348:1309–1321.
75. Lewis SJ, Moye LA, Sacks FM, et al. Effect of pravastatin on cardiovascular events in older patients with myocardial infarction and cholesterol levels in the average range. Results of the Cholesterol and Recurrent Events (CARE) Trial. Ann Intern Med 1998;129:681–689.
76. Heart Protection Study Investigators. MRC/BHF Heart Protection Study of cholesterol lowering with simvastatin in 20536 high-risk individuals: a randomized placebo-controlled trial. Lancet 2002;360:7–22.
77. Maycock CA, Muhlestein JB, Carlquist JF, et al. Statin therapy is associated with reduced mortality across all age groups of individuals with significant coronary disease, including very elderly patients. J Am Coll Cardiol 2002;40:1777–1785.
78. Applegate WB. Elderly patients' adherence to statin therapy. JAMA 2002;288:495–497.

6

Unstable Angina/Non-ST-Elevation Myocardial Infarction in the Elderly

Stephen D. Wiviott, MD and Christopher P. Cannon, MD

INTRODUCTION

Ischemic heart disease is the leading cause of morbidity and mortality for adults in the Western world. Approximately 1.4 million patients are admitted to US hospitals for unstable angina and non-ST-elevation myocardial infarction (UA/NSTEMI) *(1)*. Of patients admitted to US hospitals for MI, 37% are 75 years of age or older *(2)*. When compared to younger patients with acute coronary syndrome (ACS), elderly patients are more likely to have medical and cardiac co-morbidities and atypical symptoms complicating initial diagnosis. Elderly patients are more likely to have adverse outcomes associated with ACS, with 60% of MI-related deaths occurring in the population 75 years of age or older *(2)*. Despite the

From: *Contemporary Cardiology: Cardiovascular Disease in the Elderly*
Edited by: G. Gerstenblith © Humana Press Inc., Totowa, NJ

burden of risk in elderly patients, evidence-based therapies are under-used in this age group *(3–5)*.

Significant improvements in the care of patients with UA/NSTEMI have resulted from the introduction and evaluation of new pharmacological and interventional therapies. However, elderly patients are severely underrepresented in clinical trials for ACS *(2)*. As a result of this under-representation and physiological differences among age groups, recommendations for treatment of elderly patients often rely on subgroup analyses of major trials and extrapolation based on physiological differences.

DEFINITIONS AND PATHOGENESIS

UA/NSTEMI comprises a pathophysiological syndrome, characterized by an imbalance between myocardial oxygen supply and demand (Fig. 1). The most common cause is decreased myocardial perfusion resulting from coronary narrowing caused by nonocclusive thrombus formation following disruption of an atherosclerotic plaque. Resultant microembolization of platelet aggregates causes small vessel occlusion. Elderly patients are more likely than younger patients to have hypertension, myocardial hypertrophy and diastolic dysfunction as contributing mechanisms to ACS *(6)*. Additional pathophysiological differences include reduced hepatic and renal function resulting in impaired metabolism and clearance of therapeutics. Elderly patients tend to have decreased arterial compliance resulting in increased cardiac afterload and to have diminished β-sympathetic responses. These factors combined with more frequent medical co-morbidities and polypharmacy in the elderly increase the risk of drug–drug interactions and side effects. Risk factors for coronary artery disease (CAD) differ among elderly and non-elderly patients. In the Thrombolysis In Myocardial Infarction (TIMI)-III registry, elderly patients were more likely than non-elderly to have systemic hypertension, and a prior history of MI, but less likely to have hypercholesterolemia, a family history of CAD and to smoke *(5)*.

To help standardize the assessment and treatment of patients with UA/ NSTEMI the American Heart Association (AHA) and American College of Cardiology (ACC) convened a task force to produce guidelines for the management of UA/NSTEMI. The original document was published in 2000 *(1)*, and as a result of significant advances in the field, an update was published in 2002 *(7)*. Elderly patients are discussed in this document as a "special group," recognizing physiological differences from younger populations *(7)*. This recognition of the importance of the care of elderly patients with UA/NSTEMI, the underutilization of secondary preventive measures and potential differences in response to therapies led to the

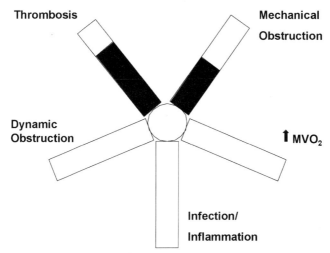

Fig. 1. Schematic of the causes of unstable angina/non-ST-evaluation myocardial infarction (UA/NSTEMI). Each of the five bars represents an etiological mechanism and the filled portion of the bar represents the extent to which this mechanism is operative. This figure represents the most common form of UA/NSTEMI in which an underlying plaque (mechanical obstruction) combined with acute thrombosis causes severe obstruction. (Modified from ref. *5a*.)

Table 1
American College of Cardiology/American Heart Association
Classification of Evidence Used in Unstable Angina/Non-ST-Evaluation
Myocardial Infarction Guidelines

Class I:	Conditions for which there is evidence and/or general agreement that a given procedure is useful and effective
Class II:	Conditions for which there is conflicting evidence and/or a divergence of opinion about the usefulness/efficacy of a procedure or treatment
Class IIa:	Weight of evidence/opinion is in favor of usefulness/efficacy
Class IIb:	Usefulness/efficacy is less well established by evidence/opinion
Class III:	Conditions for which there is evidence and/or general agreement that a given procedure is not useful/effective and in some cases may be harmful

From ref. *7*.

publication of an AHA scientific statement on the secondary prevention of coronary heart disease in the elderly in 2002 *(8)*. When possible, strength of recommendations (Table 1) will be referred to in the text of this chapter.

DIAGNOSIS AND EARLY MANAGEMENT
OF UA/NSTEMI

Two important issues arise in the initial evaluation of any patient with a suspected ACS; the likelihood that the clinical presentation represents true ACS, and the risk of adverse outcomes. The initial clinical evaluation to address both of these issues should include history, physical examination, electrocardiogram (EKG), and cardiac biomarkers including a cardiac-specific troponin and/or creatine kinase MB iso-enzyme. Both of these initial goals are modified by the evaluation of elderly patients. Elderly patients are more likely to present with atypical symptoms of UA/NSTEMI, including shortness of breath and congestive heart failure (CHF). These symptoms are thought to result from exaggerated increases in ventricular pressures resulting from the combination of ischemia and a noncompliant left ventricle (9). As a result of these atypical features, a high index of suspicion is necessary in the evaluation of elderly patients and a lower threshold for ordering diagnostic testing should be maintained. In addition, advanced age alone places patients in a higher clinical risk category prior to assessment of other factors.

The use of a risk prediction rule for early assessment of patients with UA/NSTEMI can help clinical decisions regarding level of monitoring, pharmacological therapies and use of an early catheterization strategy. Multiple risk scores have been developed from large clinical trials to assess risk of adverse outcomes in patients presenting with unstable angina and NSTEMI (10–12). One example is the TIMI risk score for UA/NSTEMI (10), a seven-point risk score (Fig. 2) integrating historical factors, tempo of presentation, EKG findings, and cardiac biomarkers into an integer score. Increasing scores are associated with an increased risk of developing adverse outcomes including death, (re)infarction, and recurrent ischemia requiring revascularization. The risk of developing these outcomes ranged from 5% to 41% with increasing scores. Importantly, this risk score may be used to help guide therapeutic decisions. Patients with higher risk scores derive greater benefit from specific pharmacological therapies (enoxaparin [10], or glycoprotein [GP] IIb/IIIa inhibitors [13]) and an early cardiac catheterization (early invasive) strategy (14). Elderly patients tend to have higher risk score values than younger patients as a result of age being one component of the score, and a greater likelihood of co-morbidities and severity of CAD. Some controversy exists regarding the applicability of these risk scores to elderly populations (15), although the utility of using these scores as an intellectual framework to understand contributors to adverse outcomes remains.

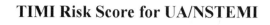

TIMI Risk Score for UA/NSTEMI

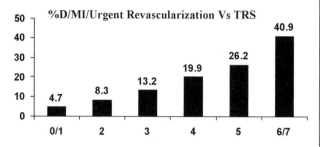

One Point for each of:
•Age ≥ 65 y
•≥ 3 CAD Risk Factors
•Prior Stenosis > 50 %
•ST deviation
•≥ 2 Anginal events ≤ 24 h
•ASA in last 7 days
•Elevated Cardiac Markers

Fig. 2. Thrombolysis In Myocardial Infarction (TIMI) risk score for unstable angina/ non-ST-evaluation myocardial infarction (UA/NSTEMI). A single point is assigned for each of the risk factors present at the time of presentation. The risk score is the total number of risk factors present. D, death; MI, myocardial infarction; TRS, TIMI Risk Score; CAD, coronary artery disease; ASA, acetyl salacytic acid (aspirin). (Adapted from ref. *10*.)

HOSPITAL CARE

General Principles

Patients with UA/NSTEMI should be admitted to an in-patient unit and undergo continuous monitoring for arrhythmia and monitoring for recurrent ischemia. Patients with high-risk indicators such as recurrent pain or hemodynamic disturbance should be admitted to a unit, such as a coronary care unit, capable of intensive monitoring. The main considerations for treatment include anti-ischemic agents, antiplatelet agents, anti-thrombotic agents and a strategy of care with consideration of an early invasive strategy. Elderly patients are less likely to receive evidence-based therapies for the management of UA/NSTEMI, despite being at higher risk for adverse outcomes *(5)*. General recommendations for the pharmacological treatment of elderly patients with UA/NSTEMI is to follow accepted treatment for younger patients with recognition and anticipation of increased side-effect profiles of therapeutics in this population *(7,16)*.

Anti-Ischemic Therapy

ACC/AHA class I anti-ischemic interventions for all patients include supplemental oxygen, nitroglycerin sublingually or intravenously for relief of recurrent ischemia and associated symptoms, and β-blocker intravenously for ongoing chest pain followed by oral administration in the absence of contraindications.

Nitroglycerin acts as a venous and arterial vasodilator and reduces myocardial oxygen demand by decreasing both afterload and preload, and increases oxygen supply by direct vasodilation of coronary arteries. Nitrates given sublingually, orally, topically, or intravenously are indicated for symptomatic relief of angina in patients with UA/NSTEMI. There are no large-scale, randomized controlled trials of nitrates in UA/NSTEMI, thus recommendations are based on extrapolation from physiological principles. Elderly patients are more prone to exaggerated hypotensive effects of nitroglycerin (17), thus cautious dose escalation and careful monitoring should be employed with these agents.

β-Adrenergic receptor blockers, a cornerstone of treatment of patients with UA/NSTEMI, act by competitively inhibiting catecholamine action at β-1 adrenergic receptors on cell surfaces. They act by reducing heart rate, contractility, and systemic blood pressure and decreasing myocardial oxygen demand. β-blockers should be administered intravenously and then by orally in high-risk patients or patients with ongoing anginal symptoms or orally in low to intermediate risk patients (7). These agents reduce subsequent infarctions in patients with UA/NSTEMI (18), and reduce mortality in acute MI (19,20), including the elderly (4). Elderly patients have diminished responsiveness to β-adrenergic stimuli and decreased atrioventricular (AV) nodal conduction, thus the response to these agents may not be entirely predictable. Despite these concerns, the use of β-adrenergic receptor blockers is recommended in all elderly patients with special attention to pharmacological response and careful use of other agents that also may affect AV nodal conduction.

Antiplatelet Therapy

Three classes of antiplatelet agents have important roles in the management of UA/NSTEMI: aspirin, thienopyridines, and GP IIb/IIIa inhibitors. Aspirin is a cornerstone of the management of ACS, and has been shown to reduce recurrent ischemic events by 50%–70% (21), and in patients older than 65 with acute MI, it is associated with a 22% lower mortality (3). For these reasons, aspirin should be used in all patients with suspected, likely, or definite ACS in the absence of known contraindication. For patients who cannot take aspirin because of intolerance, the thienopyridine antiplatelet agent clopidogrel should be substituted.

Clopidogrel is a potent thienopyridine antiplatelet agent that acts by irreversibly blocking the P2Y12 receptor on the platelet surface and thereby inhibiting platelet activation and aggregation. In the care of the patient with UA/NSTEMI, clopidogrel in addition to aspirin is now considered a class I recommendation *(7)* by the ACC/AHA. Recent publication of major clinical trials studying this agent has increased indications for its use. Clopidigrel in Unstable Angina to prevent Recurrent Ischemic Events (CURE) *(22)* randomized more than 12,000 patients with UA/ NSTEMI to clopidogrel or placebo in addition to aspirin. Patients were followed for 3 to 12 months. Those assigned to clopidogrel experienced a 20% reduction in the composite of death, MI, and stroke. This improvement was accompanied by a small, but significant increase in bleeding, especially in patients who underwent coronary artery bypass grafting (CABG) within 5 days of the discontinuation of clopidogrel. Among 6208 patients in the CURE study older than 65, there was a statistically significant 14% reduction in the primary endpoint. In an analysis of patients in this study undergoing percutaneous coronary intervention (PCI-CURE) *(23)*, patients were pretreated with clopidogrel or placebo for a median of 10 days. After PCI, patients received open-label clopidogrel for 4 weeks followed by study drug for an average of 8 months. Patients treated with clopidogrel had a 30% reduction in both early (30-day) and long-term cardiovascular events. As a result of these studies, clopidogrel is recommended in addition to aspirin for the treatment of UA/NSTEMI *(7)*. Treatment is recommended for at least 1 month and up to 9 months, as supported by the Clopidogrel for the Reduction of Events During Observation (CREDO) trial *(24)*. For patients in whom elective CABG is planned, the drug should be withheld for 5 to 7 days. There have been no specific studies of clopidogrel limited to the elderly, although nearly half of the patients enrolled in CURE were older than 65 years. Thus, for elderly patients with ACS without contraindication, clopidogrel should be used in addition to aspirin.

A third class of agents to be considered during hospitalization for UA/ NSTEMI is the intravenous GP IIb/IIIa inhibitors. GP IIb/IIIa inhibitors bind to the GP IIb/IIIa receptor on the platelet surface and interfere with platelet aggregation by interrupting the formation of fibrin crosslinks. There are three agents currently available for clinical use, abciximab, a monoclonal antibody, and the "small-molecule" GP IIb/IIIa inhibitors eptifibatide (a peptide) and tirofiban (a synthetic non-peptide). Clinical trials of the small-molecule GP IIb/IIIa inhibitors indicate that these agents benefit selected patients with UA/NSTEMI *(25)*. The Platelet Glycoprotein IIb/IIIa in Unstable Angina: Receptor Suppression Using Integrilin Therapy (PURSUIT) trial compared eptifibatide vs placebo in combination with heparin and aspirin in 10,948 patients with UA/NSTEMI, and showed a 9.5% overall reduction in the composite endpoint of death and nonfatal MI at 30 days *(26)*. In subgroup analyses among patients 65 years and older, a nonsignificant benefit was observed, and there was no age-treatment interaction, suggesting that benefit was similar regardless of age *(27)*. The Platelet Receptor Inhibition in Ischemic Syndrome Management in Patients Limited by Unstable Signs and Symptoms (PRISM-PLUS) study evaluated the combination of tirofiban with heparin vs heparin alone in patients with UA/NSTEMI *(28)*. The group assigned the combination of heparin and tirofiban experienced a 32% reduction in the primary endpoint of death, MI, or refractory ischemia at 7 days. In the subgroup of patients older than 65, a significant 24% reduction in the primary endpoint was seen. Among patients receiving GP IIb/IIIa inhibitors for UA/NSTEMI, there appears to be a greater benefit for patients who are undergoing a subsequent early invasive strategy (cardiac catheterization with planned PCI) *(25,29)*, and for those with elevated cardiac troponins *(30)*, or other high-risk indicators such as elevated TIMI risk score *(13)*. Global Use of Strategies to Open Occluded Arteries in Acute Coronary Syndromes (GUSTO IV-ACS showed no benefit for abciximab as compared to placebo *(31)* in patients for whom an early conservative (noninterventional) strategy was chosen, including the over 65 subgroup. As a result of these findings, GP IIb/IIIa inhibitors are recommended for patients in whom catheterization and PCI are planned and the small-molecule inhibitors are recommended for high-risk patients regardless of treatment strategy. Among elderly patients, the results appear to be consistent with the overall trial results and it is reasonable to follow similar recommendations. Specific attention should be given to renal function as the small-molecule GP IIb/IIIa inhibitors are cleared by the kidney and impaired renal function may result in higher drug levels and an increased likelihood of bleeding complications.

Anti-Thrombin Therapy

Activation of thrombin plays an important role in the pathophysiology of ACS, and blockade of this pathway is an important target in the therapeutic strategy. Two classes of agents, unfractionated heparin (UFH) and low-molecular-weight heparins (LMWHs) should be considered. UFH dosing is usually performed by weight-based algorithms, however owing to decreased protein levels and renal function, these may overestimate the dosing needed to achieve therapeutic levels in elderly patients *(32)*. Advanced age is also associated with higher heparin levels, higher partial thromboplastin times, and an increased bleeding risk *(33)*. LMWHs are relatively more potent inhibitors of factor Xa, and have more predictable pharmacology *(34)*. A major advantage of these compounds is this predictability, removing the need for laboratory monitoring of anticoagulation status.

UFH and aspirin are superior to aspirin alone for the treatment of patients with UA/NSTEMI *(35)*, and therefore anticoagulation with a heparin has a class I indication in the ACC/AHA guideline *(7)*. Limited data are available from randomized trials regarding the outcomes of this therapy in elderly patients with UA/NSTEMI, however, data from studies of other disease states suggest that the elderly are more likely to have bleeding complications *(36)* and cautious dosing and monitoring should be followed.

Recent trial data have shown superiority of the LMWH enoxaparin when compared to UFH for patients with UA/NSTEMI *(37)*, resulting in a class IIa recommendation for enoxaparin as a preferred anticoagulant over UFH in patients with UA/NSTEMI *(7)*.

Coronary Revascularization

In addition to the medical management of patients with UA/NSTEMI, important decisions regarding a strategy of coronary angiography and subsequent revascularization must be made. An early conservative strategy refers to initial medical management of patients without intent to perform coronary angiography unless there is evidence of recurrent ischemia at rest (or with minimal activity) or a strongly positive noninvasive test for ischemia. An early invasive strategy refers to the planned use of coronary angiography and revascularization early in the hospital course in patients without contraindications.

Several clinical trials have been performed to evaluate the question of which strategy is superior in the treatment of patients with UA/NSTEMI. Early trials including TIMI-III B *(38)* and VA Non-Q Wave Infarction Strategies in-Hospital (VANQUISH) *(39)* showed similar clinical outcomes overall regardless of treatment strategy. However, more recent trials employing more modern medical and procedural techniques including Fragmin during Instability in Coronary Artery Disease (FRISC)–II *(40)* and Treat angina with Aggrastat and determine Cost of Therapy with Invasive or Conservative Strategy (TACTICS)-TIMI 18 *(41)* have shown a significant benefit for an early invasive strategy. The benefits were strongest in patients with indicators of high-risk including ST-segment deviation and elevated cardiac troponins. In accord with these results, the 2002 ACC/AHA guideline recommends an early invasive strategy in patients with UA/NSTEMI and high-risk indicators including recurrent angina/ischemia at rest or with low-level activities despite intensive anti-ischemic therapy, elevated cardiac troponins, ST-segment depression, CHF, depressed left ventricular function (ejection fraction [EF] <40%), sustained ventricular tachycardia, PCI within 6 months or prior coronary bypass surgery.

As with medical therapy, characteristics of elderly patients including a greater likelihood of severe CAD and medical co-morbidities affect decisions regarding interventional strategy. Observational studies indicate that elderly patients are much less likely than are younger patients to undergo coronary angiography and revascularization *(5,42)*. Several studies examining the procedural success rates in elderly patients have shown results similar to younger patients in carefully chosen subjects *(43)*. However, some studies show decreased procedural success rates and increased complications in the oldest groups *(44,45)* including an increase in peri-procedural MI *(46)*. Predictors of adverse outcomes in PCI such as CHF, renal impairment, and diabetes apply to both in younger and older patients, but more likely to be present in elderly patients *(47)*.

Most clinical trials have not specifically addressed the issue of invasive vs conservative management of the elderly. One prospective randomized trial of invasive vs conservative therapy in patients older than 75 years with chronic CAD (at least Canadian Cardiovascular Society [CCS] II), the Trial of Invasive Versus Medical Therapy in Elderly Patients With Chronic Symptomatic Coronary-Artery Disease (TIME) trial has been published *(48)*. Patients undergoing revascularization had a lower rate of major adverse cardiac events (26% vs 65%, $p < 0.0001$) at 6 months and improved symptomatic status compared to patients assigned to an initial conservative management strategy. In an analysis of the TACTICS-TIMI 18 trial *(49)*, an enhanced benefit was seen in elderly patients treated with an invasive strategy for UA/NSTEMI. Among 962 patients 65 years or older, an early invasive strategy was associated with a 4.1% absolute and 44% relative reduction in the incidence of death or nonfatal MI at 30 days (5.7% vs 9.8%, $p = 0.018$), and a 4.8% absolute and 39% relative reduction at 6 months. Among patients younger than 65 years old the benefit was not significant at 30 days (6.1% vs 6.5%, $p = 0.79$) or 6 months. This analysis showed that the number needed to treat to prevent one event was 21 among the elderly, compared to 250 among patients younger than 65. The results in this trial were even more striking for the patients older than 75 years, with an absolute benefit of 10.8% and a relative benefit of 56% at 6 months (10.8% vs 21.6%). These benefits in clinical endpoints were somewhat offset by an increased rate of hemorrhage in patients older than 75 years treated with the invasive strategy (16.5% vs 6.5% TIMI major bleeding, $p = 0.009$). A similar pattern was present in the FRISC-II trial, with the majority of the benefit of early invasive therapy occurring in patients 65 years or older *(40)*.

The results of these trials suggest that similar to other high-risk patient subsets, the elderly may derive particular benefit from an invasive strategy, although the risk of adverse events may also be increased. Although patients in clinical trials tend to have less severe co-morbidities than the general population, these data suggest that well-chosen elderly patients are likely to derive an important benefit from this strategy, and that in the absence of significant medical co-morbidities, that advanced age should be considered an indication for, rather than a contraindication to, an invasive approach.

If an invasive strategy is pursued, indications for type of revascularization in UA/NSTEMI are similar to those for patients with chronic stable angina *(50)*. The mode of revascularization (PCI vs CABG) is dependent on the extent and location of atherosclerotic lesions, left ventricular function and co-morbidities. CABG is recommended for patients with left main CAD. CABG is also recommended for patients with three-vessel CAD or two-vessel CAD including proximal left-anterior descending coronary involvement with either decreased left ventricular function or diabetes mellitus. The rates of important adverse outcomes including cerebrovascular events is significantly increased in elderly patients *(51)*, however, observational studies showed improved clinical outcomes among octogenarians undergoing CABG compared to patients with similarly severe CAD who do not undergo CABG *(7)*. When examined over time, outcomes seem to be improving *(52)*, and when adjusted for risk factors such as left ventricular dysfunction, repeat CABG, peripheral vascular disease, and diabetes, age *per se* was not a significant predictor of outcome *(52)*. Because of the increased risk of adverse events, careful consideration of operative risk and benefit must be considered in the decision for surgical revascularization in the elderly. As noted previously, recent data suggest that these procedures are of benefit in well-chosen patients, however, in patients with considerable medical comorbidities, PCI may be an important option for patients who would otherwise have "surgical" CAD.

SECONDARY PREVENTION

Discharge Medications and Risk-Factor Modification

In addition to anti-ischemic medications in incompletely revascularized patients, the ACC/AHA guidelines list five medications as class I recommendations for long-term treatment of patients following UA/NSTEMI. These agents include aspirin, clopidogrel in addition to aspirin for 9 months, a β-blocker, an angiotension-convering enzyme (ACE) inhibitor for patients with CHF, EF less than 40%, hypertension, or diabetes, and a hydroxymethylglutaryl-coenzyme A (HMG-CoA) reductase inhibitor for patients with low-density lipoprotein (LDL) greater than130 or greater than 100 after diet intervention. More recent guidelines suggest a goal LDL of less than 70 mg/dL in patients with unstable angina *(52a)*. The benefits of aspirin, clopidogrel, and β-blockers as well as the risks associated with their use in the elderly were discussed previously in this chapter. In addition to considerable clinical trial data regarding the benefit of ACE inhibitors in CHF, information from the Heart Outcomes Prevention and Evaluation *(53)* has shown a benefit of long-term use of ACE inhibitors in patients with CAD (or patients at risk for development of CAD). In the subgroup of patients at least 65 years old, there was a consistent and significant benefit for ACE inhibitor use. The use of HMG-CoA reductase inhibitors for secondary prevention of CAD is well established *(54)*. In the Cholesterol and Recurrent Events study, the subset of patients over age 60 derived a 27% relative reduction in death, MI, or need for subsequent revascularization *(54)*. The Pravastatin or Atorvastatin Evaluation and Infection Therapy-TIMI 22 trial compared early intensive treatment with 80 mg of atorvastatin with moderate intensity therapy with 40 mg of pravastatin in 4162 patients stabilized following ACS *(55)*. The intensive lowering arm achieved a median LDL cholesterol of 62 mg/dL, whereas the moderate therapy group achieved a median LDL cholesterol of 95 mg/dL. The overall trial demonstrated a 16% relative reduction in the composite of death, MI, rehospitalization for ACS, and revascularization with a mean follow-up period of 24 months. In the subgroup of patients 65 or older (30%) there was a nonsignificant 5% reduction in the primary endpoint for intensive therapy, although there was no significant interaction between age and treatment suggesting the main results can be applied to the elderly *(55)*. As a result of these studies, it can be recommended that following ACS, patients without contraindications, including the elderly, should be treated with an HMG-CoA reductase inhibitor, regardless of their LDL level. Careful monitoring for side effects including myositis and liver function abnormalities should be performed on a regular basis.

In addition to medical treatment for secondary prevention, control of known risk factors for CAD is an important goal for post-ACS treatment *(8)*. These risk factors include smoking, hypertension, hypercholesterolemia, obesity, diabetes mellitus, and sedentary lifestyle. Extensive data exist for the benefits of exercise training following hospitalization in the elderly in terms of improvement of functional capacity *(8)*. A greater level of physical activity among patients with and without heart disease is associated with improved outcomes *(56,57)*, although causality has not been established. Clinical studies of cardiac rehabilitation are lacking in the elderly population, but these interventions may be of particular benefit to elderly patients who are more likely to become deconditioned during hospital stays for UA/NSTEMI *(58)*.

SUMMARY AND CONCLUSIONS

UA/NSTEMI represents a clinical syndrome that affects more than 1 million patients annually, with a significant proportion of these patients being elderly. Important medical advances in the care of these patients have improved outcomes. The elderly represent a subset of patients who are at high risk for adverse events. Because of differences in physiology and pathophysiology, co-morbidities and polypharmacy, the elderly also are at increased risk for side effects from medications and complications of interventions. However, despite these risks, available data suggests that elderly patients tend to have similar or greater benefit from established therapies. Unfortunately, the elderly are still less likely to receive proven therapies. In conclusion, the care of elderly patients presents particular difficulties in risk stratification and choice of therapies, but a remarkable opportunity to improve both single-patient and population outcomes with evidence-based therapies.

REFERENCES

1. Braunwald E, Antman EM, Beasley JW, et al. ACC/AHA guidelines for the management of patients with unstable angina and non-ST-segment elevation myocardial infarction. A report of the American College of Cardiology/American Heart Association Task Force on Practice Guidelines (Committee on the Management of Patients With Unstable Angina). J Am Coll Cardiol 2000;36:970–1062.
2. Lee PY, Alexander KP, Hammill BG, et al. Representation of elderly persons and women in published randomized trials of acute coronary syndromes. JAMA 2001; 286:708–713.
3. Krumholz HM, Radford MJ, Ellerbeck EF, et al. Aspirin in the treatment of acute myocardial infarction in elderly Medicare beneficiaries. Patterns of use and outcomes. Circulation 1995;92:2841–2847.
4. Krumholz HM, Radford MJ, Wang Y, et al. National use and effectiveness of beta-blockers for the treatment of elderly patients after acute myocardial infarction: National Cooperative Cardiovascular Project. JAMA 1998;280:623–629.
5. Stone PH, Thompson B, Anderson HV, et al. Influence of race, sex, and age on management of unstable angina and non-Q-wave myocardial infarction: the TIMI III registry. JAMA 1996;275:1104–1112.
5a. Braunwald E. Unstable angina; an etiologic approach to management. Circulation 1998;98:2219–2222.
6. Lakatta E, Gerstenblith G, Weisfeldt M. The aging heart: structure, function and disease. In: Braunwald E (ed.), Heart Disease. WB Saunders, Philadelphia, 1997, pp. 1687–1703.

7. Braunwald E, Antman EM, Beasley JW, et al. ACC/AHA guideline update for the management of patients with unstable angina and non-ST-segment elevation myocardial infarction—2002: summary article: a report of the American College of Cardiology/American Heart Association Task Force on Practice Guidelines (Committee on the Management of Patients With Unstable Angina). Circulation 2002; 106:1893–1900.

8. Williams MA, Fleg JL, Ades PA, et al. Secondary prevention of coronary heart disease in the elderly (with emphasis on patients > or =75 years of age): an American Heart Association scientific statement from the Council on Clinical Cardiology Subcommittee on Exercise, Cardiac Rehabilitation, and Prevention. Circulation 2002; 105:1735–1743.

9. Lernfelt B, Wikstrand J, Svanborg A, et al. Aging and left ventricular function in elderly healthy people. Am J Cardiol 1991;68:547–549.

10. Antman EM, Cohen M, Bernink PJ, et al. The TIMI risk score for unstable angina/non-ST elevation MI: A method for prognostication and therapeutic decision making. JAMA 2000;284:835–842.

11. Boersma E, Pieper KS, Steyerberg EW, et al. Predictors of outcome in patients with acute coronary syndromes without persistent ST-segment elevation. Results from an international trial of 9461 patients. The PURSUIT Investigators. Circulation 2000; 101:2557–2567.

12. Jacobs DR Jr, Kroenke C, Crow R, et al. PREDICT: A simple risk score for clinical severity and long-term prognosis after hospitalization for acute myocardial infarction or unstable angina: the Minnesota heart survey. Circulation 1999;100:599–607.

13. Morrow DA, Antman EM, Snapinn SM, et al. An integrated clinical approach to predicting the benefit of tirofiban in non-ST elevation acute coronary syndromes. Application of the TIMI Risk Score for UA/NSTEMI in PRISM-PLUS. Eur Heart J 2002;23:223–229.

14. Cannon CP, Weintraub WS, Demopoulos LA, et al. Comparison of early invasive and conservative strategies in patients with unstable coronary syndromes treated with the glycoprotein IIb/IIIa inhibitor tirofiban. N Engl J Med 2001;344:1879–1887.

15. Rathore SS, Weinfurt KP, Gross CP, et al. Validity of a simple ST-elevation acute myocardial infarction risk index: are randomized trial prognostic estimates generalizable to elderly patients? Circulation 2003;107:811–816.

16. Patel MR, Roe MT. Pharmacological treatment of elderly patients with acute coronary syndromes without persistent ST segment elevation. Drugs Aging 2002;19: 633–646.

17. Cahalan MK, Hashimoto Y, Aizawa K, et al. Elderly, conscious patients have an accentuated hypotensive response to nitroglycerin. Anesthesiology 1992;77:646–655.

18. Yusuf S, Wittes J, Friedman L. Overview of results of randomized clinical trials in heart disease. II. Unstable angina, heart failure, primary prevention with aspirin, and risk factor modification. JAMA 1988;260:2259–2263.

19. Metoprolol in acute myocardial infarction (MIAMI). A randomised placebo-controlled international trial. The MIAMI Trial Research Group. Eur Heart J 1985;6: 199–226.

20. Randomised trial of intravenous atenolol among 16,027 cases of suspected acute myocardial infarction: ISIS-1. First International Study of Infarct Survival Collaborative Group. Lancet 1986;2:57–66.

21. Theroux P, Ouimet H, McCans J, et al. Aspirin, heparin, or both to treat acute unstable angina. N Engl J Med 1988;319:1105–1111.

22. Yüsuf S, Zhao F, Mehta SR, et al. Effects of clopidogrel in addition to aspirin in patients with acute coronary syndromes without ST-segment elevation. N Engl J Med 2001;345:494–502.

23. Mehta SR, Yusuf S, Peters RJ, et al. Effects of pretreatment with clopidogrel and aspirin followed by long-term therapy in patients undergoing percutaneous coronary intervention: the PCI-CURE study. Lancet 2001;358:527–533.

24. Steinhubl SR, Berger PB, Mann JT, 3rd, et al. Early and sustained dual oral antiplatelet therapy following percutaneous coronary intervention: a randomized controlled trial. JAMA 2002;288:2411–2420.

25. Boersma E, Harrington RA, Moliterno DJ, et al. Platelet glycoprotein IIb/IIIa inhibitors in acute coronary syndromes: a meta-analysis of all major randomised clinical trials. Lancet 2002;359:189–198.

26. Inhibition of platelet glycoprotein IIb/IIIa with eptifibatide in patients with acute coronary syndromes. The PURSUIT Trial Investigators. Platelet Glycoprotein IIb/IIIa in Unstable Angina: Receptor Suppression Using Integrilin Therapy. N Engl J Med 1998;339:436–443.

27. Hasdai D, Holmes DR Jr, Criger DA, et al. Age and outcome after acute coronary syndromes without persistent ST-segment elevation. Am Heart J 2000;139:858–866.

28. Inhibition of the platelet glycoprotein IIb/IIIa receptor with tirofiban in unstable angina and non-Q-wave myocardial infarction. Platelet Receptor Inhibition in Ischemic Syndrome Management in Patients Limited by Unstable Signs and Symptoms (PRISM-PLUS) Study Investigators. N Engl J Med 1998;338:1488–1497.

29. Novel dosing regimen of eptifibatide in planned coronary stent implantation (ESPRIT): a randomised, placebo-controlled trial. Lancet 2000;356:2037–2044.

30. Heeschen C, Hamm CW, Goldmann B, et al. Troponin concentrations for stratification of patients with acute coronary syndromes in relation to therapeutic efficacy of tirofiban. PRISM Study Investigators. Platelet Receptor Inhibition in Ischemic Syndrome Management. Lancet 1999;354:1757–7162.

31. Simoons ML. Effect of glycoprotein IIb/IIIa receptor blocker abciximab on outcome in patients with acute coronary syndromes without early coronary revascularisation: the GUSTO IV–ACS randomised trial. Lancet 2001;357:1915–1924.

32. Spinler SA, Evans CM. Update in unfractionated heparin, low-molecular-weight heparins, and heparinoids in the elderly (age >/= 65 years). J Thromb Thrombolysis 2000;9:117.

33. Campbell NR, Hull RD, Brant R, et al. Aging and heparin-related bleeding. Arch Intern Med 1996;156:857–860.

34. Weitz JI. Low-molecular-weight heparins. N Engl J Med 1997;337:688–698.

35. Oler A, Whooley MA, Oler J, et al. Adding heparin to aspirin reduces the incidence of myocardial infarction and death in patients with unstable angina. A meta-analysis. JAMA 1996;276:811–815.

36. Landefeld CS, Beyth RJ. Anticoagulant-related bleeding: clinical epidemiology, prediction, and prevention. Am J Med 1993;95:315–328.

37. Antman EM, Cohen M, Radley D, et al. Assessment of the treatment effect of enoxaparin for unstable angina/non-Q-wave myocardial infarction. TIMI 11B-ESSENCE meta-analysis. Circulation 1999;100:1602–1608.

38. Effects of tissue plasminogen activator and a comparison of early invasive and conservative strategies in unstable angina and non-Q-wave myocardial infarction. Results of the TIMI IIIB Trial. Thrombolysis in Myocardial Ischemia. Circulation 1994;89:1545–1556.

39. Boden WE, O'Rourke RA, Crawford MH, et al. Outcomes in patients with acute non-Q-wave myocardial infarction randomly assigned to an invasive as compared with a conservative management strategy. Veterans Affairs Non-Q-Wave Infarction Strategies in Hospital (VANQWISH) Trial Investigators. N Engl J Med 1998;338: 1785–1792.

40. Invasive compared with non-invasive treatment in unstable coronary-artery disease: FRISC II prospective randomised multicentre study. FRagmin and Fast Revascularisation during InStability in Coronary artery disease Investigators. Lancet 1999;354: 708–715.

41. Cannon CP, Weintraub WS, Demopoulos LA, et al. Invasive versus conservative strategies in unstable angina and non-Q-wave myocardial infarction following treatment with tirofiban: rationale and study design of the international TACTICS-TIMI 18 Trial. Treat Angina with Aggrastat and determine Cost of Therapy with an Invasive or Conservative Strategy. Thrombolysis In Myocardial Infarction. Am J Cardiol 1998;82:731–736.

42. Collinson J, Flather MD, Fox KA, et al. Clinical outcomes, risk stratification and practice patterns of unstable angina and myocardial infarction without ST elevation: Prospective Registry of Acute Ischaemic Syndromes in the UK (PRAIS-UK). Eur Heart J 2000;21:1450–1457.

43. Nasser TK, Fry ET, Annan K, et al. Comparison of six-month outcome of coronary artery stenting in patients <65, 65–75, and >75 years of age. Am J Cardiol 1997;80: 998–1001.

44. Weyrens FJ, Goldenberg I, Mooney JF, et al. Percutaneous transluminal coronary angioplasty in patients aged > or = 90 years. Am J Cardiol 1994;74:397–398.

45. Morrison DA, Bies RD, Sacks J. Coronary angioplasty for elderly patients with "high risk" unstable angina: short-term outcomes and long-term survival. J Am Coll Cardiol 1997;29:339–344.

46. Thompson RC, Holmes DR Jr, Gersh BJ, et al. Percutaneous transluminal coronary angioplasty in the elderly: early and long-term results. J Am Coll Cardiol 1991;17: 1245–1250.

47. Blackman DJ, Ferguson JD, Springings DC, et al. Revascularization for acute coronary syndromes in older people. Age Ageing 2003;32:129–135.

48. Trial of invasive versus medical therapy in elderly patients with chronic symptomatic coronary-artery disease (TIME): a randomised trial. Lancet 2001;358:951–957.

49. Bach RG, Cannon CP, DiBattiste PM, et al. Enhanced benefit of early invasive management of acute coronary syndromes in the elderly: results from TACTICS–TIMI 18. Circulation 2001;104:548.

50. Gibbons RJ, Abrams J, Chatterjee K, et al. ACC/AHA 2002 guideline update for the management of patients with chronic stable angina—summary article: a report of the American College of Cardiology/American Heart Association Task Force on practice guidelines (Committee on the Management of Patients With Chronic Stable Angina). J Am Coll Cardiol 2003;41:159–168.

51. Peterson ED, Jollis JG, Bebchuk JD, et al. Changes in mortality after myocardial revascularization in the elderly. The national Medicare experience. Ann Intern Med 1994;121:919–927.

52. Ivanov J, Weisel RD, David TE, et al. Fifteen-year trends in risk severity and operative mortality in elderly patients undergoing coronary artery bypass graft surgery. Circulation 1998;97:673–680.

52a. Grundy SM, Cleeman JI, Merz CNB, et al. Implications of recent clinical trials for the National Cholesterol Education Program Adult Treatment Panel III Guidelines. Circulation 2004;110:227–239.

53. Yusuf S, Sleight P, Pogue J, et al. Effects of an angiotensin-converting-enzyme inhibitor, ramipril, on cardiovascular events in high-risk patients. The Heart Outcomes Prevention Evaluation Study Investigators. N Engl J Med 2000;342:145–153.
54. Sacks FM, Pfeffer MA, Moye LA, et al. The effect of pravastatin on coronary events after myocardial infarction in patients with average cholesterol levels. Cholesterol and Recurrent Events Trial investigators. N Engl J Med 1996;335:1001–1009.
55. Cannon CP, Braunwald E, McCabe CH, et al. Intensive versus moderate lipid lowering with statins after acute coronary syndromes. N Engl J Med 2004;350:1495–1504.
56. Fried LP, Kronmal RA, Newman AB, et al. Risk factors for 5-year mortality in older adults: the Cardiovascular Health Study. JAMA 1998;279:585–592.
57. Hakim AA, Petrovitch H, Burchfiel CM, et al. Effects of walking on mortality among nonsmoking retired men. N Engl J Med 1998;338:94–99.
58. Pasquali SK, Alexander KP, Peterson ED. Cardiac rehabilitation in the elderly. Am Heart J 2001;142:748–755.

7

Percutaneous Coronary Intervention in the Elderly

Michael J. McWilliams, MD
and Eric J. Topol, MD

CONTENTS

INTRODUCTION
TREATMENT GOALS
PCI vs CABG
TRIALS OF PERCUTANEOUS CORONARY INTERVENTION
    IN THE ELDERLY
PCI FOR STABLE ANGINA
PCI FOR UNSTABLE ANGINA
ANTI-THROMBOTIC AND ANTIPLATELET THERAPY
    IN PCI
CONCLUSION
REFERENCES

INTRODUCTION

Cardiovascular disease (CVD) has been the number one cause of death each year in America since 1900, except for 1918, the year of the Spanish flu pandemic. As the population—particularly the baby-boomer generation—ages, this statistic is unlikely to change. The segment of the population that is older than age 80 is growing more rapidly and is living longer than age-matched populations from the late 19th century and from present-day Europe *(1)*. Those over 80 years old represent 3% of the current population and they are anticipated to increase threefold by the year 2050 *(2)*. This is expected to have a significant impact on public health resources as symptomatic coronary artery disease (CAD) is present

From: *Contemporary Cardiology: Cardiovascular Disease in the Elderly*
Edited by: G. Gerstenblith © Humana Press Inc., Totowa, NJ

in an estimated 30% of octogenarians with 50% expected to have CAD as their cause of death *(3,4)*. Given that elderly patients have greater risks associated with invasive therapies, questions persist regarding the safest and most efficacious treatments to manage CAD and alleviate anginal symptoms. Current indications for percutaneous coronary intervention (PCI) include stable angina, acute coronary syndromes (ACS), and myocardial infarctions (MIs). This chapter discusses issues pertaining to elective PCI in the aged patient population. The issues of safety, efficacy, and risk–benefit ratio are highlighted.

TREATMENT GOALS

CAD in elderly patients presents significant challenges not present in younger patients. Physicians must seriously deliberate the risks and benefits as well as patient expectations when treating this population. Patient age, life expectancy, and overall health are factors that may help guide physicians in their decision-making process. For example, a 65-year-old healthy patient with no physical impairment is expected to live an additional 13.6 years, whereas a healthy 85-year-old patient with no physical impairment is expected to live an additional 4.2 years *(5)*. The younger patient stands to lose substantial quality-of-life years from premature cardiac death or sustained symptomatic CAD, and, therefore, may appreciate a greater benefit from complete revascularization, with either PCI or coronary artery bypass grafting (CABG). In elderly patients, however, treatment goals may differ. A mortality benefit is unlikely to be achieved when the average life expectancy is already less than 5 years. Thus, it may be reasonable to pursue symptomatic improvement, minimization of complications, and shorter hospitalization as primary treatment objectives.

PCI VS CABG

An age-based approach to CAD treatment is particularly germane when considering a patient for PCI vs CABG. Although CABG in younger patients has relatively low morbidity and mortality, CABG in elderly patients poses substantial, life-altering risks including debilitating stroke, heart attack, long-term disability, and death. Any of these complications may affect a patient's ability to maintain autonomy or to care for a loved one. A complete discussion of risks, benefits, and alternatives should be presented to patients so they can weigh the risks of therapy with perceived values and therapeutic goals. Younger patients have a lower surgical risk and thus may be best served by complete revascularization. Conversely, older patients may benefit most from incremental symptomatic improvements and the lower risks associated with PCI.

Increased co-morbidities and arterial calcifications in elderly patients significantly increase the risks associated with CABG. O'Keefe et al. performed a retrospective, case–control study comparing coronary angioplasty and CABG in patients older than 70 years old *(6)*. In-hospital complication rates were greater for CABG and included mortality (9% vs 2%), serious in-hospital stroke (5% vs 0%), and Q-wave MI (6% vs 1%). The survival curves equilibrated after 1 year and showed no significant difference in the 5-year actuarial survival. Postoperative independence and quality of life were not reported, which may be important due to the significant difference in stroke (5% vs 0%) and the resultant loss of independence. Similar results were reached in the Department of Veterans Affairs Angina With Extremely Serious Operative Mortality (VA AWESOME) multicenter registry, which found that the 3-year survival rates for angioplasty vs bypass surgery were not significantly different (Fig. 1) *(7)*. More than 50% of patients in the VA AWESOME study were older than 70 years old, and interestingly, 68% of patients with anatomy suitable for either CABG or PCI, elected angioplasty instead of CABG when given the choice. Serruys et al. conducted the Comparison of Coronary-Artery Bypass Surgery and Stenting For The Treatment of Multivessel Disease (SOS trial). The SOS trial enrolled patients needing CABG or PCI in patients suitable for either therapy (Fig. 2) *(8)*. One major difference, however, is that the mean age in the SOS trial was 61 ± 10 years, notably younger than the O'Keefe et al. and the VA AWESOME registry. All three trials reported strikingly similar conclusions: there is no difference in actuarial survival between the two groups over 36-month follow-up and PCI is associated with increased unstable angina and need for repeat revascularization. Given the age-related co-morbidities and intrinsic limits on life expectancy, it is not surprising that survival benefits are not elucidated over the 3-year follow-up period. Deciding between a surgical and percutaneous approach to revascularization becomes a balance between acceptable risks and increased duration of hospitalization vs the increased potential for future unstable angina and repeat revascularization. These studies underscore the importance of communicating the procedural risks and benefits, and directly addressing age-related differences when selecting treatment options.

The risk of stroke with CABG increases dramatically with advancing age and occurs in 2.6% to 8.5% of elderly patients *(6,9–15)*. Roach et al. examined two categories of neurological injury following CABG: type I (focal injury, or stupor or coma at discharge) and type II (deterioration

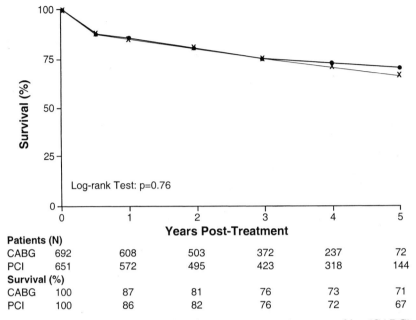

Fig. 1. Kaplan-Meier plots of survival for coronary artery bypass grafting (CABG) (●) vs percutaneous coronary interventions (PCI) (x) in physician-directed registry. (From ref. 7 with permission.)

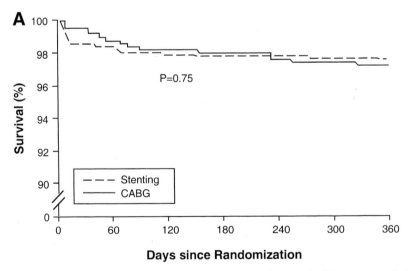

Fig. 2. Actuarial survival (**A**), Kaplan-Meier estimates of survival without myocardial infarction or cerebrovascular events (**B**), and Kaplan-Meier estimates of survival without cerebrovascular events, myocardial infarctions, or repeated revascularzation

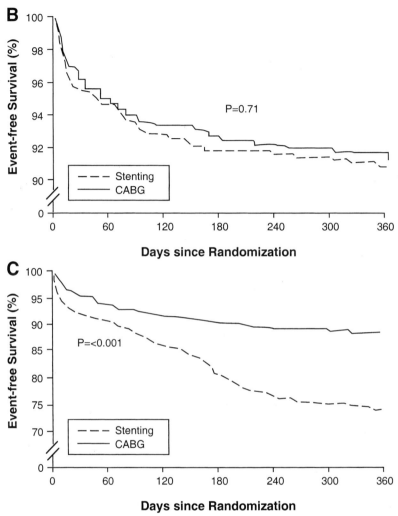

Fig. 2. *(Continued)* (**C**) among patients assigned to undergo stenting, as compared with those assigned to undergo coronary artery bypass grafting (CABG). There was a significant difference between the groups in survival without cerebrovascular events, myocardial infarctions, or repeat revascularization ($p < 0.001$ by the log-rank test). (From ref. *8*, with permission.)

in intellectual function, memory deficit, or seizure) *(9)*. Two major risk factors for type I and type II outcomes were age greater than 70 and prox-imal aortic calcification, which were found in more than 20% of patients over the age of 70. Age was the leading factor associated with both type I and II outcomes. The mortality associated with peri-operative stroke was 21% and was unchanged over the preceding decade. Perhaps more importantly, almost 50% of patients with type I outcomes required skilled nursing home or rehabilitation care upon discharge, compared to 30% with type II outcomes and 8% without obvious central nervous system injury.

Educating patients about treatments options is essential to ensire they are informed about the risks and benefits of revascularization, as well as realistic about their postprocedure quality of life. In essence, PCI is associated with fewer major adverse outcomes compared to CABG, but at the expense of more frequent episodes of unstable angina, Q-wave MIs, and revascularizations. The recovery time for PCI is measured in days, compared to longer hospitalizations and recovery time following CABG, especially if there is an adverse outcome.

TRIALS OF PERCUTANEOUS CORONARY INTERVENTION IN THE ELDERLY

Despite the higher prevalence of CAD in older patients, most randomized control trials (RCTs) fail to include a representative sample of elderly patients. To date, only a minority of patients enrolled in primary angioplasty studies are considered elderly; Lee et al. reported that only 2.8% of patients in recent primary angioplasty studies were age 75 or older (16). Older patients are still referred for PCI, as there is increasing data to support the safety and efficacy of its use. In the late 1980s and early 1990s, several small studies examined percutaneous transluminal coronary angioplasty (PTCA) in elderly patients (17–30). Although these reports demonstrated the safety of PCI in elderly patients, most were small, nonrandomized single-institution studies that were unable to draw strong conclusions regarding morbidity and mortality because of inadequate sample size. These smaller studies predate the stent era and modern antiplatelet therapies, and therefore, may not be applicable to contemporary practice.

From 1994 to 2001, several larger registry studies investigated PCI ± stenting in elderly patients. These studies clearly documented the increasing use of stents and decreasing use of other atheroablative procedures (7,14,31–32). In the VA AWESOME study, stent use increased from 26% in 1995 to 89% in 2001, and as stent use increased, the use of atherectomy devices and intra-aortic balloon counterpulsation decreased (7). This is corroborated by reports from The National Cardiovascular Network (NCN) that show increased stent use from 4% in 1994 to 66% in the last quarter of 1997 (31), and then to 78% in 1999 (33). They noted a similar decrease in atheroablative procedures, from 18% to 5% over the same time period *(14,31)*. From 1994 to 1997, Batchelor et al. used the NCN registry to demonstrate an 81% to 86% ($p = 0.009$) statistically significant improvement in procedural success and a nonstatistically significant decrease in the combined endpoint of death, MI, and cerebrovascular accident, from 6% to 3.8% ($p = 0.14$) *(31)*. Improved procedural success is likely related to improved operator skill, increased use of stents, and increased use of antiplatelet therapies, although antiplatelet therapy is not clearly documented. A trend suggests a possible mortality benefit with the addition of stenting, but did not reach statistical significance.

Although mortality is obviously an important endpoint, improving quality of life is an equal, if not more important, endpoint for aged patients. A study by Kahler et al. examined quality of life after angioplasty in octogenarians *(34)*. Not surprisingly, the angioplasty success rate for octogenarians was inferior to the younger group (88% vs 97%). Similar differences in success rates were observed in studies by Batchelor et al., 84% vs 89% ($p < 0.001$) *(31)* and DeGregorio et al., 90% vs 93% *(35)*. A study by Little et al., however, reported a statistically insignificant success rate favoring octogenarians over younger controls (89% vs 88%, $p = $NS) and demonstrated a higher clinical success rate in the octogenarian arm (93% vs 88%, $p = $NS).

These studies show that PCI is well tolerated and is associated with a high procedural and clinical success rate. More than 90% of patients reported satisfaction with their postprocedure quality of life and 88% stated they would undergo repeat PCI if needed *(36)*. Kahler et al. showed a quality-of-life improvement that was equivalent and, in some cases, greater for elderly patients compared to their younger cohort. Octogenarians are likely less active than the younger control group and may have a greater appreciation for any incremental symptomatic improvement that could help them maintain their autonomy.

PCI FOR STABLE ANGINA

There are several studies that address whether stenting with PCI improves outcomes in elderly patients with stable angina *(37–39)*. The Trial of Invasive Versus Medical Therapy in Elderly Patients With Chronic Symptomatic Coronary-Artery Disease (TIME) investigators performed a randomized, multicenter trial in patients aged 75 and older with angina, Canadian Cardiovascular Society class II or greater, and who were already treated with at least two anti-anginal medications. They examined major adverse cardiovascular events as well as changes in quality of life *(40)*. This intention-to-treat analysis randomized 305 patients to an invasive strategy (PCI or CABG) if indicated ($n = 155$) vs a noninvasive approach optimizing medical management alone ($n = 150$). Primary endpoints included quality of life at 6 months and the occurrence of major cardiac events including death, nonfatal MI, or hospital admission for ACS with or without the need for revascularization. Quality-of-life questionnaire data collection occurred at the time of enrollment and at 6 months follow-up. In the invasive arm, 79 patients underwent PTCA, 68 of whom received at least one stent, and 30 underwent CABG.

Fortunately, both invasive and noninvasive strategies demonstrated improved quality of life and decreased angina upon reassessment, but the improvement was greater following revascularization (Fig. 3). One-third of the medical management patients required revascularization secondary to refractory angina. Major adverse cardiac events were more frequent in the medical group (49%) vs invasive group (19%), with the majority of events being hospital admission for ACS with and without the need for revascularization. A nonsignificant excess mortality was associated with an invasive strategy, although half of these deaths occurred in patients unsuitable or unwilling to undergo revascularization. A similar increased mortality was shown *(42,43)* in previous studies, but these studies enrolled only patients with anatomy suitable for revascularization. Unfortunately, the symptomatic benefit observed with early revascularization at 6 months disappeared at 1-year follow-up, although the increased adverse cardiac events in the medical vs invasive group persisted at 1 year (64% vs 25.5%, $p < 0.001$) *(44)*. At 1-year, the TIME trial investigators concluded that elderly patients with refractory angina benefit from maximal medical therapy and then revascularization if angina persists.

PCI FOR UNSTABLE ANGINA

Morrison et al. addressed short- and long-term survival in "high-risk" elderly patients with unstable angina in a single-center, retrospective analysis *(46)*. They compared survival with PCI to CABG using predicted CABG short-term survival and US census long-term mortality rates. They observed PCI survival rates of 87% and predicted surgical survival rates of 85.5%. Of the 84% of patients who survived 6 months, subsequent yearly survival through 5 years was comparable to age-matched subjects in the US census. Quality of life and life free of anginal symptoms were not reported. Owing to the low number of patients followed, conclusions for the higher risk population, including patients with cardiogenic shock, intra-aortic balloon counterpulsation, and need for vasopressor agents could not be drawn.

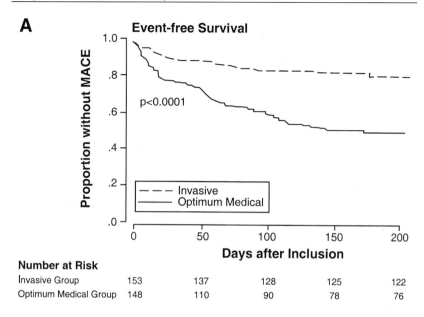

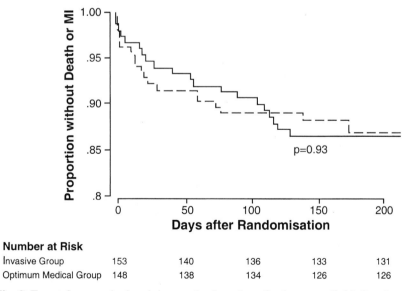

Fig. 3. Event-free survival and time to death and nonfatal myocardial infarction from the TIME trial. The invasive approach was associated with improved event-free survival but no difference in rates for time to death and nonfatal myocardial infarction. (From ref. *40*, with permission.)

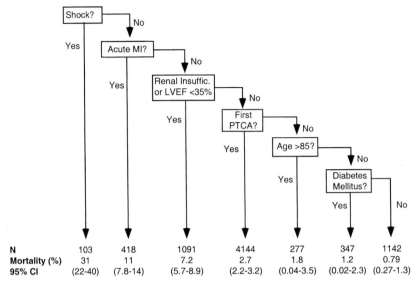

N	103	418	1091	4144	277	347	1142
Mortality (%)	31	11	7.2	2.7	1.8	1.2	0.79
95% CI	(22-40)	(7.8-14)	(5.7-8.9)	(2.2-3.2)	(0.04-3.5)	(0.02-2.3)	(0.27-1.3)

Fig. 4. Tree diagram illustrating the mortality for octogenarians stratified according to the independent predictors defined from the multivarable model. Patients are included into only one risk group considering the presence of each risk factor in descending order of predictive importance. The observed mortality and corresponding 95% confidence intervals are presented at the bottom. (From ref. *31*, with permission.)

Short-Term Outcomes

Several studies investigated potential risk factors associated with adverse outcomes and PCI. Not surprisingly, age is consistently a risk factor for procedural complications and has a curvilinear relationship with mortality *(31)*. Risk factors associated with increased mortality were shock (mortality 31%), acute MI (mortality 11%), renal insufficiency or left ventricular ejection fraction (EF) less than 35% (mortality 7.2%), first percutaneous coronary angioplasty (mortality 2.7%), age over 85 (mortality 1.8%), diabetes mellitus (mortality 1.2%), and no identifiable risk factors (mortality 0.79%) (Fig. 4) *(31)*. This algorithm presents a reasonable means of assessing pre-procedural risk of mortality with PCI. The reported mortality of 31% with shock is only about half the rate reported in the Should we Emergently Revascularize Occluded Coronaries for Cardiogenic Shock (SHOCK) trial and may underestimate the actual risk of death *(47)*.

Multivariate risk analysis by Gold et al. determined the following high-risk features for post-procedural mortality: left ventricular EF less than 40%, unstable angina at presentation, and incomplete revascularization at procedure termination *(6)*. A subsequent study using the NCN registry data collected from January 1998 to June 1999 created a scoring system to estimate the probability of in-patient mortality for octogenarians undergoing PCI. The scoring system uses the following variables: left ventricular end-diastolic pressure, EF, weight, and presence of acute MI, diabetes, emergent cases, and the absence of prior PCI. To determine mortality risk, points are allotted for each risk factor and then added together. The absolute point total reflects the cumulative mortality risk (Table 1).

A retrospective analysis in the pre-stent era by Malenka et al. examined 12,232 PTCA cases with 121 procedural and peri-procedural related deaths, and identified variables that increased the likelihood of death *(48)*. Factors associated with an increased mortality risk included advancing age (odds ratio [OR] 4.15 for age >80), female gender (OR 3.41), number of diseased coronary arteries, emergent cases, pre-procedural use of nitroglycerin, and use of an intra-aortic balloon pump. The modes of death for all ages were low-output failure (66.1%), ventricular arrhythmia (10.7%), stroke (4.1%), pre-existing renal failure (4.1%), bleeding (2.5%), ventricular rupture, respiratory failure, pulmonary embolism, and infection. The cause of death was procedure-related in 53.7% of cases, and when it was procedure-related, the patient was more likely female. It is unclear why procedure-related mortality is higher in elderly women.

Other complications occurring more frequently in octogenarians vs patients younger than 80 years old include a combined endpoint MI and cerebrovascular accident (4.9% vs 1.9%), Q-wave MI (1.9% vs 1.3%), cerebrovascular accident (0.58% vs 0.23%), renal failure (3.2% vs 1.0%), major blood loss defined as need for transfusion (9.9% vs 3.6%), and vascular complications (6.7% vs 3.3%) *(31)*. Although meticulousness is advised in all PCI cases, particular attention should be observed in patients with advanced age. Gaining arterial access with a single arterial puncture, using prehydration and careful manipulation of intra-aortic catheters may all decrease risk. When indicated, iso-osmolar nonionic contrast *(49)* and *N*-acetycysteine may decrease the risk of worsening renal insufficiency or acute renal failure *(50)*.

Long-Term Outcomes

Inherent difficulties exist in determining the long-term clinical benefit of PCI in elderly patients. Even in the acute setting, there is not evidence that angioplasty improves long-term survival. In fact, a retrospective analysis involving close to 100,000 MI patients older than 65 years by Thiemann et al. established that access to angioplasty or bypass surgery did not confer a survival advantage over hospitals without this technology, in agree-

170   Cardiovascular Disease in the Elderly

Table 1
Scoring System Estimating the Probability of In-Hospital Mortality
in Octogenarians Who Underwent Percutaneous Coronary Interventions

1. Find points for each predictive factor

LVEDP MmHg points	points	%	Points	kg	Points	Risk factor
5	8	10	60	40	71	Acute MI
		51				
10	17	20	51	50	47	No prior PCI
	34					
15	25	30	43	60	24	Emergent
		34				
20	33	40	34	70	11	Diabetes
		36				
25	42	50	26	80	9	
30	50	60	17	90	8	
35	58	70	9	100	6	
		80	0	110	5	
				120	3	
				130	2	

2. Add up points for all predictive factors
3. Look up risk corresponding to total points

Points	Probability of in-hospital mortality
8	0.1%
36	0.2%
65	0.4%
81	0.6%
93	0.8%
102	1%
131	2%
148	3%
160	4%
169	5%
200	10%
219	15%
233	20%
245	25%
255	30%
264	35%
273	40%
281	>45%

LVEDP, left ventricular end-diastolic pressure; MI, myocardial infarction; PCI, percutaneous coronary intervention. (From ref. *43*, with permission.)

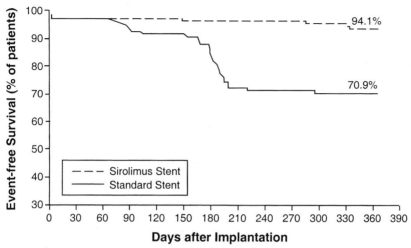

Fig. 5. Kaplan-Meier estimates of survival free of myocardial infarction and repeated revascularization among patients who received sirolimus-eluting stents and those who received bare metal stents. (From ref. 56, with permission.)

ment with the results of a previous studies *(51,52)*. Evidence suggests that although stenting does not improve survival more than angioplasty alone *(45)*, it may contribute to the increased procedural success rates *(31)*.

Abizaid et al. examined late outcomes with coronary stenting in three age groups: younger than 70 years old, 71 to 80 years old, and older than 80 years. Interestingly, at 1-year follow-up, they showed that cardiac events (death, MI, and need for revascularization) did not differ among the three groups *(53)*. There was no significant difference in revascularization among the three age groups, supporting the suggestion that instent restenosis (ISR) in elderly patients is similar to that in younger patients *(9,54,55)*. To the contrary, De Gregorio et al. suggested that angiographic ISR in elderly patients was significantly higher (47% vs 28%, $p = 0.0007$) than in younger patients *(35)*. Although they included a younger patient population (60.7 ± 10.4 years), Morice et al. showed significant survival free of MI and repeated revascularization over 3-year follow-up among patients receiving sirolimus-eluting stents compared to standard stents (Fig. 5) *(56)*. Similar results, if attained among elderly patients, may influence future decisions concerning CABG vs PCI and, therefore, potentially reduce morbidity and mortality associated with open heart surgery and repeat catheterizations. Further studies are necessary to determine whether aged patients are prone toward ISR and if chemical-coated stents influence the incidence of ACS or repeat revascularization.

ANTI-THROMBOTIC
AND ANTIPLATELET THERAPY IN PCI

The current 2002 American College of Cardiology/American Heart Association (ACC/AHA) Guidelines recommend three forms of anti-platelet and anti-thrombotic therapy for unstable angina or non-ST-segment elevation MI: aspirin, clopidogrel, and either unfractionated heparin or low-molecular-weight heparin. Even routine PCI in the non-acute setting, with or without stenting, requires antiplatelet therapy including aspirin, clopidogrel and often a glycoprotein (GP) IIb/IIIa inhibitor or direct thrombin inhibitor. Co-morbidities like gastrointestinal (GI) bleeds, malignancies, risk of trauma from falling, and hemorrhagic strokes create challenging risk–benefit decisions that complicate the routine administrations of these proven medications. Despite the high prevalence of coronary disease, there is a paucity of antiplatelet safety and efficacy trials in elderly patients; therefore, practitioners must use clinical judgment and risk–benefit assessments to determine which medications are most appropriate.

Most trials of GP IIb/IIIa inhibitors did not include the very old population. Sedeghi et al. followed 14,308 consecutive patients undergoing PCI between January 1998 and June 2001; 1392 were at least 80 years of age (9.7%) (57). Four hundred and fifty-nine (33% of the 1392 patients) received GP IIb/IIIa inhibitors: eptifibitide was used in 73% of cases, the remaining 27% of cases utilized abciximab. GP inhibitors were used more often in the following types of patients: male, MI less than 2 weeks prior, higher hematocrit (38.5 ± 5% vs 37.5 ± 5%), active ACS and triple-vessel CAD. Patients with a prior history of peptic ulcer disease and/or a history of peripheral vascular disease were less likely to receive GP IIb/IIIa inhibitors. Overall, the GP IIb/IIIa inhibitor patients were more likely to have access and nonaccess site-related bleeding, including GI bleeds, but did not have a significantly increased risk of transfusion (9.8% with GP IIb/IIIa inhibitor vs 8.6% without GP IIb/IIIa inhibitor, p = NS). On average, hospitalization was prolonged by 1 day with GP IIb/IIIa inhibitor use. No differences in retroperitoneal bleeds were noted and no intracranial hemorrhages were observed. Low-dose heparin and early sheath removal were encouraged to decrease risk of bleeding. In the accompanying editorial, Rogosta alludes to the clinical applicability of the study by Sedeghi et al. because it includes a real world patient population without the exclusion criteria of RCTs (58). There are no strict safety criteria to

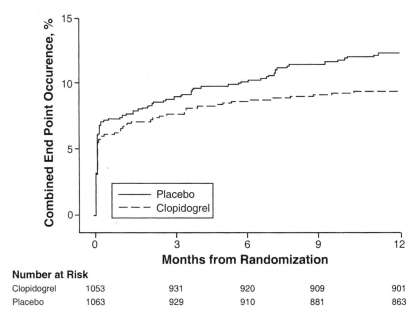

Fig. 6. CREDO trial results showing a decreased combined endpoint of death, MI, and stroke with clopidogrel vs placebo. (From ref. *60*, with permission).

define patients eligible for GP IIb/IIIa inhibitors; rather use is based on physician preference. Further studies to define higher risk features would help identify appropriate patient subgroups. The bivalirudin and provisional glycoprotein IIb/IIIa blockade compared with heparin and planned glycoprotein IIb/IIIa blockade during percutaneous intervention trial: REPLACE-2 randomized trial analyzed bivalirudin and provisional GP IIb/IIIa inhibitors compared to heparin and GP IIb/IIIa inhibition *(59)*. Unpublished data from the REPLACE-2 database confirm a uniform degree of bleeding reduction in all age groups, including the elderly, when bivalirudin and provisional GP IIb/IIIa inhibitors are used instead of heparin and GP IIb/IIIa inhibition. As expected, elderly patients are at greater risk for bleeding complications (Michael Lincoff, personal communication).

Clopidogrel loading 6 hours prior to PCI with short (1-month) and long-term (1-year) therapy was studied in the Clopidogrel for the Reduction of Events During Observation (CREDO) trial *(60)*. This randomized, double-blind, placebo-controlled trial enrolled 2116 patients scheduled to undergo elective PCI. At 1 year, a 26.9% relative risk reduction in death, MI, and stroke existed with clopidogrel compared to placebo (Fig. 6). There was a nonsignificant increased risk of bleeding of 8.8% with clopidogrel, compared to 6.7% with placebo (p = NS). Further studies are needed to demonstrate the safety of clopidogrel in the very-old population, as the in the mean age in the CREDO study was 61.5 years.

CONCLUSION

Although it does not extend life, PCI improves anginal symptoms and is associated with fewer major adverse events compared to CABG. PCI is, however, associated with more frequent repeat revascularization and hospitalizations for unstable angina. For elderly patients, where life is often measured by quality rather than quantity, PCI offers a relatively safe revascularization option that is proven to improve quality of life.

REFERENCES

1. Manton KG, Vaupel JW. Survival after the age of 80 in the United States, Sweden, France, England, and Japan. N Engl J Med 1995;333:1232–1235.
2. US Bureau of the Census. Sixty-five plus in America, P23-178RV; Population projections of the United States, by age, sex, race and Hispanic origin: 1993 to 2050. Washington, DC, US Bureau of the Census, 2003, pp. 23–178.
3. National Center for Health Statistics. Current Estimates from the National Interview Survey, 1989: Vital and Health Statistics Series 10. 2003. Washington, DC, US Government Printing Office;1990. No. 176.
4. O'Connor CM FGI. Aging and the heart. In: Topol EJ (ed.), Textbook of Cardiovascular Medicine. Lippincott-Raven, Philadelphia, 2003.
5. Manton KG, Land KC. Active life expectancy estimates for the U.S. elderly population: a multidimensional continuous-mixture model of functional change applied to completed cohorts, 1982–1996. Demography 2000;37:253–265.
6. O'Keefe JH Jr, Sutton MB, McCallister BD, et al. Coronary angioplasty versus bypass surgery in patients > 70 years old matched for ventricular function. J Am Coll Cardiol 1994;24:425–430.
7. Morrison DA, Sethi G, Sacks J, et al. Percutaneous coronary intervention versus coronary bypass graft surgery for patients with medically refractory myocardial ischemia and risk factors for adverse outcomes with bypass: The VA AWESOME multicenter registry: comparison with the randomized clinical trial. J Am Coll Cardiol 2002;39:266–273.
8. Serruys PW, Unger F, Sousa JE, et al. Comparison of coronary-artery bypass surgery and stenting for the treatment of multivessel disease. N Engl J Med 2001; 344:1117–1124.
9. Roach GW, Kanchuger M, Mangano CM, et al. Adverse cerebral outcomes after coronary bypass surgery. Multicenter Study of Perioperative Ischemia Research Group and the Ischemia Research and Education Foundation Investigators. N Engl J Med 1996;335:1857–1863.
10. Ko W, Krieger KH, Lazenby WD, et al. Isolated coronary artery bypass grafting in one hundred consecutive octogenarian patients. A multivariate analysis. J Thorac Cardiovasc Surg 1991;102:532–538.
11. Gold S, Wong WF, Schatz IJ, Blanchette PL. Invasive treatment for coronary artery disease in the elderly. Arch Intern Med 1991;151:1085–1088.

12. Faro RS, Golden MD, Javid H, et al. Coronary revascularization in septuagenarians. J Thorac Cardiovasc Surg 1983;86:616–620.
13. Dorros G, Lewin RF, Daley P, Assa J. Coronary artery bypass surgery in patients over age 70 years: report from the Milwaukee Cardiovascular Data Registry. Clin Cardiol 1987;10:377–382.
14. Alexander KP, Anstrom KJ, Muhlbaier LH, et al. Outcomes of cardiac surgery in patients > or = 80 years: results from the National Cardiovascular Network. J Am Coll Cardiol 2000;35:731–738.
15. Shimshak TM, McCallister BD. Coronary artery bypass surgery and percutaneous transluminal coronary angioplasty in the elderly patient with ischemic heart disease. In: Tresch DD, Aronow WS (eds.), Cardiovascular Disease in the Elderly. Marcel Dekker, New York, 1993, pp. 323–344.
16. Lee PY, Alexander KP, Hammill BG, Pasquali SK, Peterson ED. Representation of elderly persons and women in published randomized trials of acute coronary syndromes. JAMA 2001;286:708–713.
17. Forman DE, Berman AD, McCabe CH, Baim DS, Wei JY. PTCA in the elderly: the "young-old" versus the "old-old." J Am Geriatr Soc 1992;40:19–22.
18. Imburgia M, King TR, Soffer AD, Rich MW, Krone RJ, Salimi A. Early results and long-term outcome of percutaneous transluminal coronary angioplasty in patients age 75 years or older. Am J Cardiol 1989;63:1127–1129.
19. Jackman JD Jr, Navetta FI, Smith JE, et al. Percutaneous transluminal coronary angioplasty in octogenarians as an effective therapy for angina pectoris. Am J Cardiol 1991;68:116–119.
20. Jeroudi MO, Kleiman NS, Minor ST, et al. Percutaneous transluminal coronary angioplasty in octogenarians. Ann Intern Med 1990;113:423–428.
21. Kern MJ, Deligonul U, Galan K, et al. Percutaneous transluminal coronary angioplasty in octogenarians. Am J Cardiol 1988;61:457–458.
22. Maiello L, Colombo A, Gianrossi R, Thomas J, Finci L. Results of coronary angioplasty in patients aged 75 years and older. Chest 1992;102:375–379.
23. Peterson ED, Jollis JG, Bebchuk JD, et al. Changes in mortality after myocardial revascularization in the elderly. The national Medicare experience. Ann Intern Med 1994;121:919–927.
24. Rich JJ, Crispino CM, Saporito JJ, Domat I, Cooper WM. Percutaneous transluminal coronary angioplasty in patients 80 years of age and older. Am J Cardiol 1990;65:675–676.
25. Rizo-Patron C, Hamad N, Paulus R, Garcia J, Beard E. Percutaneous transluminal coronary angioplasty in octogenarians with unstable coronary syndromes. Am J Cardiol 1990;66:857–858.
26. Rozenman Y, Mosseri M, Lotan C, Hasin Y, Gotsman MS. Percutaneous Transluminal coronary angioplasty in octogenarians. Am J Geriatr Cardiol 1995;4:32–41.
27. Santana JO, Haft JI, LaMarche NS, Goldstein JE. Coronary angioplasty in patients eighty years of age or older. Am Heart J 1992;124:13–18.
28. Shapira I, Frimerman A, Rosenschein U, et al. Percutaneous transluminal coronary angioplasty in elderly patients. Cardiology 1994;85:88–93.
29. ten Berg JM, Bal ET, Gin TJ, et al. Initial and long-term results of percutaneous transluminal coronary angioplasty in patients 75 years of age and older. Cathet Cardiovasc Diagn 1992;26:165–170.
30. Thompson RC, Holmes DR Jr, Gersh BJ, Mock MB, Bailey KR. Percutaneous transluminal coronary angioplasty in the elderly: early and long-term results. J Am Coll Cardiol 1991;17:1245–1250.

31. Batchelor WB, Anstrom KJ, Muhlbaier LH, et al. Contemporary outcome trends in the elderly undergoing percutaneous coronary interventions: results in 7,472 octogenarians (National Cardiovascular Network Collaboration). J Am Coll Cardiol 2000; 36:723–730.

32. Lefevre T, Morice MC, Eltchaninoff H, et al. One-month results of coronary stenting in patients > or = 75 years of age. Am J Cardiol 1998;82:17–21.

33. Weintraub WS, Veledar E, Thompson T, Burnette J, Jurkovitz C, Mahoney E. Percutaneous coronary intervention outcomes in octogenarians during the stent era (National Cardiovascular Network). Am J Cardiol 2001;88:1407–1410, A6.

34. Kahler J, Lutke M, Weckmuller J, Koster R, Meinertz T, Hamm CW. Coronary angioplasty in octogenarians. Quality of life and costs. Eur Heart J 1999;20:1791–1798.

35. De Gregorio J, Kobayashi Y, Albiero R, et al. Coronary artery stenting in the elderly: short-term outcome and long-term angiographic and clinical follow-up. J Am Coll Cardiol 1998;32:577–583.

36. Little T, Milner MR, Lee K, Constantine J, Pichard AD, Lindsay J Jr. Late outcome and quality of life following percutaneous transluminal coronary angioplasty in octogenarians. Cathet Cardiovasc Diagn 1993;29:261–266.

37. Coronary angioplasty versus medical therapy for angina: the second Randomised Intervention Treatment of Angina (RITA-2) trial. RITA-2 trial participants. Lancet 1997;350:461–468.

38. Blumenthal RS, Cohn G, Schulman SP. Medical therapy versus coronary angioplasty in stable coronary artery disease: a critical review of the literature. J Am Coll Cardiol 2000;36:668–673.

39. Parisi AF, Folland ED, Hartigan P. A comparison of angioplasty with medical therapy in the treatment of single-vessel coronary artery disease. Veterans Affairs ACME Investigators. N Engl J Med 1992;326:10–16.

40. Trial of invasive versus medical therapy in elderly patients with chronic symptomatic coronary-artery disease (TIME): a randomised trial. Lancet 2001;358:951–957.

41. Rihal CS GBYS. Chronic coronary artery disease: coronary artery bypass surgery versus percutaneous transluminal coronary angioplasty versus medical therapy. In: Yusuf S, Cairns JA, Camm AJ, Fallen EL, Gersh JB (eds.), Evidence Based Cardiology. BMJ Books, London,1999, pp. 368–392.

42. Wallentin L, Lagerqvist B, Husted S, Kontny F, Stahle E, Swahn E. Outcome at 1 year after an invasive compared with a non-invasive strategy in unstable coronary-artery disease: the FRISC II invasive randomised trial. FRISC II Investigators. Fast Revascularisation during Instability in Coronary artery disease. Lancet 2000; 356:9–16.

43. Wennberg DE, Makenka DJ, Sengupta A, et al. Percutaneous transluminal coronary angioplasty in the elderly: epidemiology, clinical risk factors, and in-hospital outcomes. The Northern New England Cardiovascular Disease Study Group. Am Heart J 1999;137:639–645.

44. Pfisterer M, Buser P, Osswald S, et al. Outcome of elderly patients with chronic symptomatic coronary artery disease with an invasive vs optimized medical treatment strategy: one-year results of the randomized TIME trial. JAMA 2003;289:1117–1123.

45. Altmann DB, Racz M, Battleman DS, et al. Reduction in angioplasty complications after the introduction of coronary stents: results from a consecutive series of 2242 patients. Am Heart J 1996;132:503–507.

46. Morrison DA, Bies RD, Sacks J. Coronary angioplasty for elderly patients with "high risk" unstable angina: short-term outcomes and long-term survival. J Am Coll Cardiol 1997;29:339–344.

47. Hochman JS, Sleeper LA, Webb JG, et al. Early revascularization in acute myocardial infarction complicated by cardiogenic shock. SHOCK Investigators. Should We Emergently Revascularize Occluded Coronaries for Cardiogenic Shock. N Engl J Med 1999;341:625–634.

48. Malenka DJ, O'Rourke D, Miller MA, et al. Cause of in-hospital death in 12,232 consecutive patients undergoing percutaneous transluminal coronary angioplasty (The Northern New England Cardiovascular Disease Study Group). Am Heart J 1999;137:632–638.

49. Jakobsen JA. Renal experience with Visipaque. Eur Radiol 1996;6 Suppl 2:S16–S19.

50. Tepel M, van der GM, Schwarzfeld C, Laufer U, Liermann D, Zidek W. Prevention of radiographic-contrast-agent-induced reductions in renal function by acetylcysteine. N Engl J Med 2000;343:180–184.

51. Every NR, Parsons LS, Fihn SD, et al. Long-term outcome in acute myocardial infarction patients admitted to hospitals with and without on-site cardiac catheterization facilities. MITI Investigators. Myocardial Infarction Triage and Intervention. Circulation 1997;96:1770–1775.

52. Thiemann DR, Coresh J, Oetgen WJ, Powe NR. The association between hospital volume and survival after acute myocardial infarction in elderly patients. N Engl J Med 1999;340:1640–1648.

53. Abizaid AS, Mintz GS, Abizaid A, et al. Influence of patient age on acute and late clinical outcomes following Palmaz-Schatz coronary stent implantation. Am J Cardiol 2000;85:338–343.

54. Fishman RF, Kuntz RE, Carrozza JP Jr, et al. Acute and long-term results of coronary stents and atherectomy in women and the elderly. Coron Artery Dis 1995;6:159–168.

55. Lauer MS, Pashkow FJ, Snader CE, Harvey SA, Thomas JD, Marwick TH. Age and referral to coronary angiography after an abnormal treadmill thallium test. Am Heart J 1997;133:139–146.

56. Morice MC, Serruys PW, Sousa JE, et al. A randomized comparison of a sirolimus-eluting stent with a standard stent for coronary revascularization. N Engl J Med 2002;346:1773–1780.

57. Sadeghi HM, Grines CL, Chandra HR, et al. Percutaneous coronary interventions in octogenarians. glycoprotein IIb/IIIa receptor inhibitors' safety profile. J Am Coll Cardiol 2003;42:428–432.

58. Ragosta M. Percutaneous coronary intervention in octogenarians and the safety of glycoprotein IIb/IIIa inhibitors*. J Am Coll Cardiol 2003;42:433–436.

59. Lincoff AM, Bittl JA, Harrington RA, et al. Bivalirudin and provisional glycoprotein IIb/IIIa blockade compared with heparin and planned glycoprotein IIb/IIIa blockade during percutaneous coronary intervention: REPLACE-2 randomized trial. JAMA 2003;289:853–863.

60. Steinhubl SR, Berger PB, Mann JT, III, et al. Early and sustained dual oral antiplatelet therapy following percutaneous coronary intervention: a randomized controlled trial. JAMA 2002;288:2411–2420.

8   Cardiac Surgery in the Elderly

David D. Yuh, MD
and William A. Baumgartner, MD

CONTENTS

BACKGROUND

The elderly population is the most rapidly expanding sector of the US population, with an estimated 13 million citizens over the age of 75, including 1.6 million nonagenarians and 72,000 centenarians; these figures are expected to quadruple over the next half century *(1)*. Based on population studies, life expectancy at the age of 80 years is 8.5 years, and at the age of 85 and over, it is 6.3 years *(2)*. These striking demographics are, in large part, believed to be the result of improvements in the prevention and treatment of cardiovascular disease (CVD) in young and middle-aged adults, leading to improved survival and the delayed onset of disease until later years. Consequently, there has been a marked increase in the incidence and prevalence of cardiac disease in older adults *(3,4)*, making CVD the leading cause of morbidity and mortality in the elderly. Despite advances in medical therapies for CVDs, however, the morbidity and mortality of cardiac disease in older individuals remain high *(5–8)*. Hence, cardiac surgery, a well-established means of increasing survival and

From: *Contemporary Cardiology: Cardiovascular Disease in the Elderly*
Edited by: G. Gerstenblith © Humana Press Inc., Totowa, NJ

improving the quality of life in many patients under the age of 70 years, is becoming increasingly common in septuagenarians, octogenarians, and even nonagenarians *(9)*.

With respect to cardiac surgery, older patients generally present with lower functional reserve and more co-morbidities than do younger patients, which predispose them to complications and death. Consequently, with new emphasis being placed on procedural outcomes, many cardiologists and cardiac surgeons have become reluctant to offer elderly patients beneficial cardiac operations. Many cardiac surgeons shy away from geriatric patients based on advanced age alone. With the rise of percutaneous interventions, many cardiac surgeons are operating on older, sicker patients compared to their initial practices. This anticipated shift in patient demographics has prompted several cardiac groups to examine the consequences of cardiac surgery performed in the elderly.

Over the past decade, there has been a steadily increasing number of elderly patients with symptomatic coronary artery disease considered for coronary artery bypass grafting (CABG) surgery *(10)*. Indeed, CABG performed in octogenarians in the United States increased by 67% from 1987 to 1990 *(10–12)*. There are a significant number of published outcomes series of CABG performed in septuagenarians, octogenarians, and nonagenarians in recent years *(3,5,6,10,11,13–15)*. In general, however, most of these reports have reported quite varied morbidity and mortality rates reflecting comparatively small sample sizes and divergent experiences at single institutions (Table 1). For example, among octogenarians undergoing CABG surgery, reported mortality rates range from 8% to 24%, postoperative stroke rates from 2% to 9%, and postoperative renal failure rates from 2% to 13% *(16)*. Despite this variance in outcomes, most of these studies conclude that, in carefully selected older patients, cardiac operations can be performed with hospital mortality rates nearly comparable to those in younger populations, albeit at increased hospitalization costs owing to longer hospitalizations and higher intensities of illness. Identified predictors for in-hospital mortality include emergency operation *(8)*, operation complexity, and the presence of co-morbidities (e.g., renal failure, chronic obstructive pulmonary disease [COPD]) *(16)*.

EVALUATION OF THE ELDERLY PATIENT
FOR CARDIAC SURGERY

Operation Complexity

Alexander and colleagues examined outcomes in the elderly among several major cardiac operative classifications. As expected, CABG and

Table 1
Retrospective Reviews Reporting Postoperative Mortality
and Complications After Coronary Artery Bypass Grafting

	Year	n	Stroke	Renal insufficiency	In-hospital mortality
Mayo Clinic—Mullany	1977–1989	159	4%	—	10.7%
U Penn—Edmunds	1976–1987	41	—	—	24.0%[a]
Emory—Weintraub	1978–1989	154	5%	—	10.4%
St. Louis—Naumheim	1980–1989	71	—	—	13.0%
Duke—Glower	1983–1991	86	9%	5%	13.9%
NY/Cornell—Ko	1985–1989	100	3%	2%[b]	12.0%
Mt. Sinai—Williams	1989–1994	300	2%	13%	11.0%
Medicare—Peterson	1987–1990	24,461	—	—	11.5%
NY State—Hannan	1991–1992	1372	—	—	8.3%

[a]90-day postoperative mortality.
[b]Incidence of hemodialysis only.
From ref. 16.

181

CABG combined with valve surgery performed in octogenarians was associated with overall higher mortality and morbidity rates than observed in younger patients (Table 2). Among a subset of octogenarians without significant co-morbidity, Alexander's operative series revealed a 4.2% mortality with CABG only, 7% mortality with CABG with aortic valve replacement (AVR) and 18.2% mortality with CABG with mitral valve replacement (MVR). Comparing these results to the literature, it appears that the mortality rates for CABG only and combined CABG/AVR in these "ideal" octogenarians is comparable to outcomes in younger patients.

It is well established that the addition of valve replacement to CABG significantly increases operative mortality across all age groups. However, although AVR appears to increase mortality by the same amount across age categories, MVR adds increasingly to operative mortality risk with advancing age (Fig. 1). This observation may arise from the fact that patients with mitral valve disease often have significantly impaired left ventricular function that compounds the diminished physiological reserve in elderly patients. Furthermore, MVR usually requires more cardiopulmonary bypass time to complete than AVR; Kolh and associates noted that prolonged cardiopulmonary bypass increased in-hospital mortality in octogenarians (23).

These data suggest that adding complexity to a cardiac operation has a disproportionately high impact on mortality and morbidity rates in the elderly in comparison with younger patients. Consequently, it is generally wise to pragmatically balance these heightened risks vs the projected benefits of performing complex cardiac operations in the elderly.

An area that deserves mention in selecting the appropriate operation for a given elderly patient lies in valve prosthetic selection. In general, it is preferable to select a bioprosthetic valve (i.e., porcine or bovine pericardial) as opposed to a mechanical valve for most replacement procedures in the very elderly because these devices do not require long-term anticoagulation with coumadin. The potential for thrombotic and bleeding complications stemming from coumadin use in the elderly are heightened by increased rates of falling, pathological bone fracture, and inadequate anticoagulation dosing (e.g., confusion, forgetfulness). With improved design and tissue-fixation techniques, bioprosthetic durability and hemodynamics have improved significantly in recent years (17). With current mitral bioprostheses, structural valve deterioration resulting in valve failure averages 30% at 10 years and then accelerates with actuarial freedom from primary tissue failure ranging from 35% to 71% at 15 years (18). For stented aortic bioprostheses, large series indicate freedom from reoperation owing to structural valve deterioration is greater than 95% at 5 years, greater than 90% at 10 years, but less than 70% at 15 years (19).

Table 2
Outcomes of Cardiac Surgery by Age Category

All patients	CABG only		CABG/AVR		CABG/MVR	
	Age <80 $n = 60,161$	Age ≥80 $n = 4306$	Age <80 $n = 1690$	Age ≥80 $n = 345$	Age <80 $n = 1170$	Age ≥80 $n = 92$
In-hospital mortality	3.0%	8.1%[a]	7.9%	10.1%	12.2%	19.6%[a]
(95% CI)	(2.9–3.2)	(7.3–8.9)	(6.6–9.2)	(6.9–13.4)	(10.3–14.1)	(3.5–10.8)
All neurologic events (stroke, TIA, coma)	4.2%	10.2%[a]	9.1%	15.2%[a]	11.2%	22.5%[a]
Stroke only	1.8%	3.9%[a]	3.2%	4.9%	4.7%	8.8%
Renal failure	2.9%	6.9%	6.8%	12.1%[a]	11.4%	25.0%[a]
Perioperative MI	1.7%	2.5%	2.0%	3.0%	2.7%	1.5%
PLOS day[b]	6 (5,8)	7 (6,11)[a]	7 (5,10)	9 (6,15)[a]	9 (6,14)	11 (7,19)
Patients w/o comorbidity[b]	$n = 24,811$	$n = 1588$	$n = 571$	$n = 100$	$n = 196$	$n = 11$
(% of population)	(41.2%)	(36.9%)	(33.8%)	(29.0%)	(16.8%)	(12.0%)
In-hospital mortality	1.1%	4.2%[a]	4.0%	7.0%	7.1%	18.2%
(95% CI)	(1.0–1.3)	(3.2–5.2)	(2.4–5.7)	(1.9–12.1)	(3.5–10.8)	n/a

[a] $p < 0.05$ for comparison by age category.
[b] Subset of patients without significant comorbidity: EF < 35%, prior CABG, Hx CHF, COPD, vascular disease, renal insufficiency, MI within 21 days or emergency surgery (see Methods section); median and 25th and 75th quartiles.
AVR, aortic valve repair; CABG, coronary artery bypass grafting; MI, myocardial infarction; MVR, mitral valve repair or replacement; PLOS, postprocedural length of stay. (From ref. 16.)

183

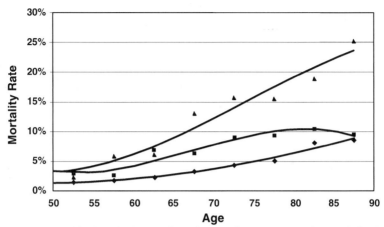

Fig. 1. Observed in-hospital mortality after cardiac surgery. Diamond, CABG; solid square, CABG/AVR; triangle, CABG/MVR; AVR, aortic valve replacement; CABG, coronary artery bypass grafting; MVR, mitral valve repair or replacement. (From ref. *16*.)

Valve-sparing techniques, including mitral valve repair (particularly in cases of marginal left ventricular function) and aortic valve-sparing techniques (e.g., Tirone-David, Ross procedures) represent alternatives to valve replacement therapies that also obviate the need for long-term anticoagulation. When considering valve-sparing procedures, it is important to realize that these operations often are more complex than standard valve replacement operations, imposing longer operative and cardiopulmonary bypass times with their attendant risks in elderly patients. Certainly, mechanical valve prosthetics should be considered in very healthy and vigorous elderly patients who would be most likely to outlive a bioprosthetic valve.

In the arena of coronary revascularization, "off-pump" techniques, in which CABG is performed on the beating heart without cardiopulmonary bypass support, have been postulated to be particularly beneficial in elderly patients. Indeed, the putative benefits of off-pump CABG continue to be debated in the form of conflicting study results. It is generally accepted that, compared to CABG performed with cardiopulmonary bypass, off-pump CABG confers less blood loss, fluid overload, early transient renal dysfunction, and myocardial enzyme leak. These advantages, however, have not consistently translated into improved clinical outcomes such as reduced hospitalization, wound complication rates, and postoperative pain. There is currently no compelling evidence that supports improved neurocognitive outcomes with off-pump CABG in any patient age group. Furthermore, there are several large, well-designed reviews suggesting that intermediate- to long-term graft patency, completeness of myocardial revascularization, and freedom from reintervention (i.e., angioplasty, reoperation) are compromised with the off-pump approach (20–22).

Nevertheless, off-pump techniques provide an excellent option for the cardiac surgeon in patients with high-grade ascending aortic atherosclerotic disease. Widely considered as the most substantial risk for embolic stroke, mechanical manipulation (i.e., clamping) of an atherosclerotic aorta can be avoided with the use of off-pump techniques and/or anastomotic stapling devices. Additionally, in elderly patients with poor left ventricular function, off-pump CABG precludes the global myocardial ischemia and "stunning" associated with cardioplegic arrest, potentially reducing the incidence for post-cardiotomy failure and mechanical ventricular assistance in this high-risk group.

Suitability for Operation

It is well demonstrated in the literature that judicious selection of cardiac surgical candidates among elderly patients is critical to maintaining acceptable outcomes. In general, predictors of poor operative outcomes in the elderly are similar to those in younger patients, however, their impact on operative mortality and morbidity tend to be much higher. Consequently, in relation to evaluating younger patients, these predictors should be considered more seriously in elderly candidates for cardiac surgery. Disregard of these considerations would result in an unacceptably high rate of morbidity and mortality in this population.

EMERGENCY OPERATION

Emergency operation is a strong positive predictor of increased in-hospital mortality when compared with a purely elective group Ko and associates reported mortality rates of 33.3% for emergent cases, 13.5% for urgent cases, and 2.8% for elective cases in octogenarians undergoing CABG (8) and identified emergency operation and decreased ejection fraction as two independent risk factors for mortality. Furthermore, these authors reported that morbidity rose strikingly, from 14% for elective CABG to 67% for emergency CABG in octogenarians. In a multivariate analysis of 182 octagenarians, Kolh and associates noted that urgent procedures significantly increased the risk for in-hospital mortality (23). Likewise, Alexander and associates demonstrated that preoperative shock, preoperative hemodynamic assist device, and emergency procedures were all predictive of in-hospital mortality after CABG in octogenarians *(16)*. Referring physicians should avoid feeling compelled to "at least give the patient a shot" under these dire circumstances because those patients who do manage to survive, and their families, are usually relegated to protracted hospitalizations only to be followed by institutional death or disability.

An illustrative example of prohibitively high surgical mortality is that of ascending aortic, or Stanford Type A, dissection repair in the very elderly. Neri and colleagues reviewed the outcomes of 24 consecutive octogenarians who underwent acute type A dissection repair from 1985 to 1999. The authors found that the overall hospital mortality was a staggering 83% *(24)*. Furthermore, none of the four surviving patients discharged from the hospital was capable of independent functioning and all eventually died after 6 months. In this circumstance, age in excess of 80 years was the most important independent patient risk factor associated with 30-day mortality and morbidity. Although these data do not conclusively suggest that this life-saving operation be denied octogenarians based on age alone, it represents an example of the heightened mortality associated with emergent cardiac surgery in the elderly.

SEVERE RESPIRATORY INSUFFICIENCY

Elderly patients suffering from severe COPD should be excluded from cardiac surgery. Protracted ventilatory dependence is common if the forced expiratory volume at 1 minute (FEV_1) is less than 65% of the vital capacity or if the FEV_1 is less than 1 L.

RENAL FAILURE

Preoperative renal failure should be considered a strong relative contraindication to cardiac surgery, primarily owing to the large fluid shifts and electrolyte alterations associated with cardiopulmonary bypass and high mortality rates. In a retrospective analysis, Engoren found that the survival rate among patients initiating dialysis postoperatively was 30% among octogenarians and 57% among septuagenarians *(10)*.

NEUROLOGICAL/PHYSICAL DISABILITY

Elderly patients who are physically disabled (e.g., nonambulatory) as a result of a history of strokes or other causes should not be considered for cardiac surgery as it is unlikely that the substantial physical and occupational rehabilitation requirements after cardiac surgery will be achieved. Most causes of physical disability in the very elderly are not cardiac related (e.g., arthritis, Alzheimer's disease, peripheral vascular disease [PVD]) and will not be ameliorated with cardiac surgery.

PERIOPERATIVE CONSIDERATIONS
Preoperative Evaluation

All patients considered for cardiac surgery undergo a preoperative evaluation to identify conditions that may preclude or alter the conduct of the operation and to provide an opportunity to optimize the conditions for a successful outcome. First and foremost, a detailed history and physical examination should be obtained from the patient, particularly the elderly, because their medical and surgical histories as well as medication regimens are quite often more complex than those for younger patients. Prior thoracic surgery (e.g., prior cardiac operation, lung or esophageal resection), peripheral vascular surgery, and saphenous vein stripping may have a direct impact on the planned cardiac operation. Prior mediastinal radiation may not only complicate the performance of a median sternotomy, but can adversely affect sternal wound healing and internal mam-mary graft patency. Medical conditions that increase morbidity and mortality in elderly cardiac surgical patients include COPD or restrictive pulmonary disease, diabetes, renal insufficiency, and PVD. If present, these conditions must be well characterized and treated optimally, if possible.

Second, a complete blood count, electrolyte panel, urinalysis, and coagulation profile should be obtained preoperatively to identify undiagnosed blood dyscrasias, electrolyte disturbances, renal insufficiency, active or chronic infections, and coagulopathy. Many of these conditions can be corrected or ameliorated preoperatively, effectively decreasing the risk of postoperative complications.

Third, a chest radiograph and 12-lead electrocardiogram should be obtained routinely to detect malignancy (i.e., new pulmonary nodule), aortic pathology (e.g., aneurysmal disease, heavy calcifications), arrhythmias, and nonviable myocardial territories.

Other optional preoperative tests include pulmonary function tests in the setting of significant pulmonary insufficiency, duplex venous ultrasonography in the setting of varicosities or suspect saphenous vein quality, dental examination to identify and treat caries in valve replacement candidates, and duplex carotid ultrasonography. In a retrospective analysis, Durand et al. identified age in excess of 65 years, carotid bruit, and history of cerebrovascular accident or transient ischemic attack as strong risk factors for hemodynamically significant carotid stenosis (i.e., $\geq 70\%$ luminal narrowing of the affected internal carotid artery) and perioperative stroke in CABG patients *(25)*. Because significant carotid stenosis has been identified as a risk factor for perioperative stroke in CABG patients *(26)*, concomitant or staged carotid endarterectomy and coronary bypass operations are often performed to reduce the incidence of perioperative stroke; the efficacy of this approach remains controversial.

Intraoperative Considerations

The conduct of cardiac operations in elderly patients is essentially identical to such procedures performed in younger patients. However, there are several considerations that are pertinent to older patients undergoing cardiac surgery. First, extra care should be afforded older patients during their positioning on the operating room table. Orthopedic and/or neurological injuries can occur owing to the less compliant cervicothoracic spine, hip, and extremity joints in elderly patients. Leg abduction to facilitate bladder catheter placement and saphenectomy, cervical extension during intubation, and arm abduction for intravascular line (e.g., radial arterial line, peripheral intravenous line) placement should be handled with this consideration.

The liberal use of transesophageal echocardiography should be encouraged in elderly patients to determine if the ascending thoracic aorta has high-grade atherosclerotic disease, which may predispose to perioperative stroke; simple palpation of the aorta by the surgeon is an extremely insensitive mode of inspection.

Higher cardiopulmonary bypass perfusion pressures are often used in elderly patients in an effort to improve end-organ perfusion during bypass. In a randomized trial, Gold and associates reported a significantly lower incidence of cardiac and neurological complications in CABG patients whose mean arterial pressure (MAP) was maintained between 80 and 100 mmHg on bypass as compared to those patients whose MAP was maintained from 50 to 60 mmHg *(27)*.

There is some evidence that relative anemia should be avoided in geriatric patients undergoing cardiac surgery. Floyd and colleagues report that anemia and advancing age are associated with increased cerebral blood flow after cardiac surgery and postulate that this hyperemia may play an important role in the higher incidence of perioperative stroke and cognitive dysfunction in elderly patients *(28)*. Furthermore, in a retrospective review, Wu et al. reported that avoiding anemia (hematocrit less than 30%) with blood transfusions is associated with a lower short-term mortality rate among elderly patients sustaining acute myocardial infarction *(29)*. Optimizing oxygen-carrying capacity by avoiding anemia in geriatric patients undergoing cardiac surgery may play a beneficial role.

Finally, cardiac surgery differs from other types of surgery due to the routine use of cardiopulmonary bypass. During bypass, blood is exposed to extracorporeal non-endothelial cell surfaces and continuously recirculated throughout the body. This contact with synthetic surfaces in the bypass circuit and a variety of tissues in the wound produces a massive humoral and cellular inflammatory cascade. This cascade, in turn produces thrombotic, vasoactive, and cytotoxic consequences affecting virtuallly every organ system. These consequences appear to be less well tolerated in elderly patients undergoing cardiac surgery and probably contributes substantially to the heightened morbidity and mortality associated with this age group. Consequently, particular attention should be paid to minimizing the duration of cardiopulmonary bypass when performing cardiac surgery on the elderly.

Postoperative Considerations

The postoperative care of elderly cardiac surgical patients is much like that afforded to younger patients. Special emphasis, however, is placed on early mobilization, physical and occupational therapy, and pulmonary toilet in order to reduce the heightened risks of bedsores, deep venous thrombosis/pulmonary embolism, and pneumonia in the older patient. Furthermore, the institution of environmental measures to reduce the high risk of "sundowning" or postoperative delirium in the hospitalized elderly patient is critical. These measures include quiet single rooms to facilitate normal sleep–wake cycles, signposts to time and location (e.g., clock, calendar, window), consistency in care staff, liberalized visitation by family and friends, correction of any pre-existing sensory impairments (e.g., hearing aids, eyeglasses), and the judicious use of opioid narcotics.

POSTOPERATIVE COMPLICATIONS

Although mortality rates in selected older patients appear to be acceptable, hospital morbidity remains a significant problem in elderly patients undergoing cardiac surgery. In a review of the literature on octogenarian patients, Bacchetta et al. reported postoperative morbidity ranging from at least 20% to 68%, and 30-day mortality from 6% to 29% (30). In their own series of nonagenarian surgical patients, these authors reported an overall morbidity rate of 67%, representing 28 of 42 patients suffering complications, including arrhythmias, respiratory (e.g., pneumonia, respiratory failure), infectious (e.g., wound, sepsis), and hemorrhage or emboli (e.g., postoperative bleeding, cerebrovascular accident). Although these complications occur in all patients undergoing cardiac surgery, several are particularly prevalent in the elderly population.

Delirium

Postoperative delirium and agitation is a neuropsychiatric complication of cardiac surgery associated with significantly increased morbidity (e.g., falls, infections, pressure sores), mortality, prolonged hospital stays and costs, and increased requirements for postdischarge institutionalization *(31)*. There is clear scientific evidence that geriatric patients experience a disproportionate incidence of delirium after cardiac surgery, however, owing to the variability in its presentation in this patient population, delirium is often overlooked, misdiagnosed, and mistreated. Several prospective and retrospective trials have attempted to better characterize postoperative delirium. Van der Mast and colleagues conducted a prospective study investigating the incidence of and preoperative predictors for delirium after cardiac surgery *(32)*. The investigators noted an incidence of postoperative delirium of 13.5%, which is in line with published incidences of 3% to 47% in prior studies. Age over 65 years and plasma albumin concentrations less than 40 g/L were strong predictors for delirium after cardiac surgery. Similar studies corroborate that risk factors include patient age, cerebral disease, and poor preoperative medical status *(33–35)*. Common precipitants of postoperative delirium include infection, hypoxia, myocardial ischemia, metabolic derangements, and anticholinergics. Taken together, these observations suggest that postoperative delirium in geriatric patients is multifactorial.

Outcome studies investigating the consequences of cardiac surgery in septuagenarians and octogenarians have concluded that cardiac surgery can be performed in the elderly with good hospital and late functional results, but at higher hospital costs and longer hospital stays than those for younger patients *(10)*. A significant cause of longer hospitalizations for geriatric cardiac patients lies in the propensity for transient postoperative neuropsychiatric dysfunction.

Unfortunately, delirium in the elderly and its treatment have not been well studied in the past owing to methodological hurdles, a lack of consensus about its definition, and a tacit acceptance that it is a natural manifestation of reduced physiological reserve in the geriatric set. Therefore, postoperative delirium in geriatric patients has been chronically underappreciated as an independent entity that requires thoughtful intervention beyond simply diagnosing it and searching in vain for an underlying cause. Clearly, there is a need for research aimed toward more effective treatment of delirium in geriatric patients sustained after cardiac surgery.

One therapeutic approach that we are investigating involves treating elderly patients suffering from postoperative delirium with scheduled regimens of neuroleptics and benzodiazepines. Neuroleptics are the cornerstone of pharmacological treatment for delirium as they ameliorate a range of symptoms, are effective both in patients with a hyperactive or hypoactive clinical profile and generally improve cognition *(36)*. Low-dose benzodiazepines can be useful adjuncts to neuroleptics in the treatment of delirium, particularly delirium associated with alcohol or sedative withdrawal. By maintaining a cyclical sleep-wake cycle with scheduled administration of these agents during acute states of delirium, we postulate that the total duration of delirium will be reduced compared to standard "prn" (as needed) administration of high-dose opioids, neuroleptics, and/or benzodiazepines.

Another experimental therapeutic approach is based on the premise that delirium occurring after cardiac surgery seems to result, at least in part, from serotoninergic receptor overstimulation. In a small study, Bayindir and colleagues demonstrated that ondansetron, a 5-HT$_3$ receptor antagonist, was safe and effective in reducing the severity of delirium in postcardiotomy patients (37).

Neurological Injury

Postoperative neurological complications increase with age. In a study examining the association of advanced age on neurological risk for CABG, Tuman and coauthors reported an incidence of postoperative neurological events to be 8.9% for patients 75 years of age and older, 3.6% for ages 65 to 74 years, and 0.9% for ages less than 65 years (38). Alexander and colleagues found that postoperative neurological events increase with advancing age in a parallel fashion to in-hospital mortality, with the steepest rise occurring after age 75 (Fig. 2) (16). Compared to younger patients, octogenarians experienced neurological complications twice as frequently. The rate of postoperative stroke in octogenarians after CABG was 3.9%, after combined CABG/AVR was 4.9%, and 8.8% after combined CABG/MVR. It is generally agreed that ascending aortic atherosclerotic disease is the most prominent source for embolic stroke in cardiac operations because manipulation of the ascending aorta (e.g., clamping) is required in most cases. The frequency and extent of ascending aortic disease increases with advancing age, resulting in higher stroke rates. Furthermore, the association of carotid and intracranial cerebrovascular disease with advancing age also contributes to the increase in perioperative neurological injury in the elderly. It is unclear precisely why valve replacement, when combined with CABG, increases the risk of postoperative stroke (39). However, the greater potential for generating embolic material with aortic and mitral valve debridement and introducing intracardiac air during valve replacement undoubtedly plays a role.

Renal Failure

Alexander and associates noted that, as with neurological injury, renal complications occurred twice as often in octogenarians as in younger patients. The rate of postoperative renal failure in octogenarians after

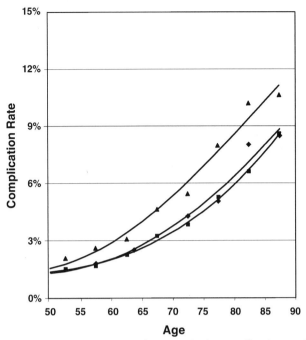

Fig. 2. In-hospital mortality, postoperative neurologic complications and postoperative renal failure after CABG by age. Diamond, mortality; square, renal failure; triangle, neurologic events. (From ref. *16*.)

CABG was 6.9%, 12.1% after combined CABG/AVR, and 25% after CABG/MVR.

Late Neurocognitive and Physical Functional Impairment

The literature yields very little meaningful data with respect to neurocognitive and physical functioning in the very elderly after undergoing cardiac surgery. Engoren and colleagues found that octogenarians as a group had lower levels of physical functioning and general health, but that both octogenarians and septuagenarians had similar and "acceptable" late functional outcomes postoperatively (Table 3) *(10)*. However, such outcome analyses to date have not determined what factors and patient characteristics correlate with good postoperative outcomes in the elderly. Most cardiac surgeons note, empirically, that a disproportionate number of their elderly patients are not discharged home as their younger counterparts, but rather to skilled nursing or rehabilitation facilities of varying acuity. What ultimately becomes of these patients is unclear. Certainly, further research in this area is needed and should be predi-

Table 3
Functional Outcomes of Septuagenarians
and Octogenarians After Undergoing Cardiac Surgery

Variables	Septuagenarians[a]	Octogenarians[a]
CVICU LOS, d	1 (1–3)	1 (1–3)
Postoperative LOS, d	6 (5–10)	6 (5–9)
Total LOS, d	8 (6–13)	9 (6–13)
Total costs, $	9383 (6321–16,992)[b]	12,624 (7836–22,124)[b]
Pre-operative	641 (410–1284)	743 (511–1710)
Anesthesia	279 (217–532)	356 (250–542)
Perfusion	1772 (1216–2540)	2224 (1461–2710)
Surgery	2299 (1773–3780)	3041 (1984–3787)
CVICU	816 (433–1867)	1154 (481–2858)
Postoperative room	655 (1094–2212)	761 (1492–2676)
Respiratory	67 (30–196)	146 (32–263)
Laboratory	217 (111–442)	258 (107–633)
Blood bank	102 (34–254)	91 (32–457)
ECC & vascular laboratory	29 (67–120)	31 (77–138)
Radiology	37 (11–134)	90 (26–426)
Pharmacy	592 (343–1226)	702 (450–1723)
Therapies	236 (106–439)	221 (139–523)
Supplies	70 (39–149)	95 (36–231)

[a]Values given as median (interquartile range). All p values are > 0.05 unless indicated.
LOS, length of stay.
[b]$p \leq 0.01$.
From ref. 10.

cated on identifying preoperative physiological metrics (e.g., "frailty") that can help determine operative risk (*see* next section).

FUTURE DIRECTIONS

Minimally Invasive Cardiac Surgery

The evolution and refinement of cardiac surgical techniques have recently focused on minimizing the trauma and physiological destabilization (e.g., cardiopulmonary bypass) traditionally associated with cardiac surgery. Minimally invasive techniques, including robot-assisted, endoscopic, and endovascular procedures, are examples of strong efforts made toward reducing the inherent morbidity of cardiovascular operations. Many surgeons believe that these new techniques may improve outcomes in elderly patients *(40)* by reducing postoperative pain, wound-healing complications, and sequelae of the systemic inflammatory response seen with extensive invasive operations. As such new surgical technologies become available for older patients with CVD, the decision criteria concerning eligibility for, and appropriateness of, these procedures for older patients need to be developed, which include a means of identifying high-risk older adults.

The Relationship Between Frailty and Cardiac Surgery

Recommendations regarding the appropriateness of cardiac surgical procedures are based on the results of clinical trials performed in younger patients with few co-morbidities. Thus, the validity of extrapolating from these results is limited for older patients with altered physiology, especially underlying vulnerability understood as "frailty," and various co-morbidities. The inherent heterogeneity of the aging process also complicates clinical decision making, in that it is difficult to differentiate physiological status from chronologic age (41). Clinically, it appears that there is a subset of frail older adults who tolerate cardiovascular procedures poorly, at least as they are currently performed (11,42). Their long-term cardiovascular outcomes also appear to be substantially adversely affected by their underlying frailty (15,43–45). Therefore, screening and interventions should consider parameters describing frailty, providing a basis for more appropriate, tailored approaches and treatments. More refined approaches to decision making regarding cardiac operations could, optimally, be based on knowing the specific aspects of frailty that most impact these outcomes (46,47). Developing such decision-making algorithms is predicated on defining and validating the concept of frailty, as it applies to these procedures.

Although it is generally accepted that frailty is prevalent in the elderly and confers high risk for mortality and morbidity, a standardized definition for frailty has heretofore been elusive. In its early use, the concept of frailty had been equated with disability, co-morbidity, or advanced old age (48–52). However, more recently, geriatricians have defined frailty as a distinct biological syndrome of decreased reserve and resistance to stressors, resulting from cumulative declines across multiple physiological systems, leading to increased susceptibility to adverse outcomes (48, 51,53). Bortz employs the notion of *symmorphosis* to suggest that frailty is a body-wide set of linked deteriorations including, but not confined to, the musculoskeletal, cardiovascular, metabolic, and immunological systems (54). There is growing agreement that characteristics of frailty include age-associated declines in lean body mass, strength, endurance, balance, walking performance, and low activity, and that multiple components must be present clinically to establish frailty. According to Fried et al., many of these components are related and can be unified into a hypothetical "cycle of frailty" associated with declining energetics and reserve (Fig. 3) *(55)*. Fried hypothesizes that this cycle is constructed on core elements that are commonly identified as clinical signs and symptoms of frailty and that a critical mass of phenotypic components in the cycle would, when present, identify the frailty syndrome. In a well-designed and presented study, Fried et al. developed a potential standardized definition for frailty in older adults based on this hypothetical construct (Table 4) *(55)*. The authors went on to validate this definition in community-dwelling older adults, establish an intermediate stage identifying those at high risk of frailty, and provide evidence that frailty is not synonymous with either co-morbidity or disability; rather co-morbidity is an etiological risk factor for, and disability is an outcome of, frailty. This definition provides a potential basis for clinical decision making: (a) identifying those older patients at high risk for morbidity or mortality after undergoing cardiac surgery and (b) identifying core physiologic deficiencies that could guide preoperative interventions to ameliorate or adjust for the condition of frailty, thereby improving patient outcomes.

Several studies have attempted to identify physiologic and metabolic markers of frailty (Table 5) *(56–58)* with an eye toward understanding the distinct pathological processes leading to frailty and to develop objective screening tests to identify frail patients. To date, there are no convincing studies that achieve this, however, there are several physiological and metabolic markers that display promising correlations with the state of frailty and appear to have a reasoned hypothetical basis for such linkage. Using the aforementioned definition of frailty, Newman and Fried identified a subset of frail patients in the Cardiovascular Health Study and demonstrated that, as they had hypothesized, frailty was associated with older age and a propensity toward clinical cardiovascular disease, particularly with congestive heart failure *(43)*.

In terms of metabolic markers of frailty, the most promising correlations appear to be related to inflammatory mechanisms. This is consistent with the notion that subclinical chronic disease processes, more prevalent in frail, older adults, are capable of triggering chronic inflammatory changes. Walston and Fried, using their operational definition of frailty, found that frail vs nonfrail individuals had increased serum levels of C-reactive protein, factor VIII, and D-dimer; these differences were independent of CVD *(56)*. Ershler and Keller demonstrated a relationship between elevated interleukin-6 levels and the development of disability and early mortality in healthy older adults *(58)*.

Other conditions associated with frailty include lower education and income, poorer health, and higher rates of co-morbid disease and disabil-

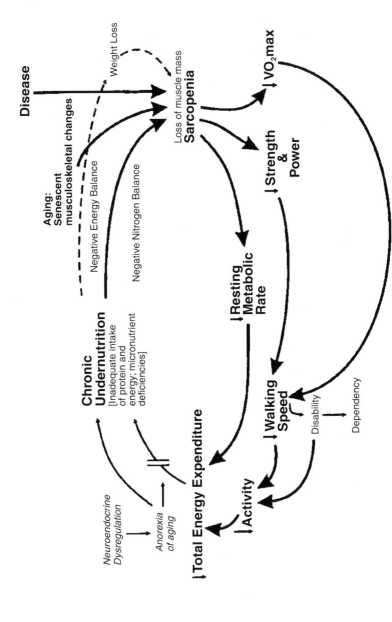

Fig. 3. Cycle of frailty hypothesized as consistent with demonstrated pairwise associations and clinical signs and symptoms of frailty. (From ref. 55.)

Table 4
Criteria Used to Define Frailty

- Weight loss: "In the last year, have you lost more than 10 pounds unintentionally (i.e., not due to dieting or exercise)?" If yes, then frail for weight loss criterion. At follow-up, weight loss was calculated as: (Weight in previous year – current measured weight/(weight in previous year) = K. If K ≥ 0.05 and the subject does not report that he/she was trying to lose weight (i.e., unintentional weight loss of at least 5% of previous year's body weight), then frail for weight loss = Yes.
- Exhaustion: Using the CES-D Depression Scale, the following two statements are read. (a) I felt that everything I did was an effort; (b) I could not get going. The question is asked "How often in the last week did you feel this way?" 0 = rarely or none of the time (<1 day), 1 = some or a little of the time (1–2 days), 2 = a moderate amount of the time (3–4 days), or 3 = most of the time. Subjects answering "2" or "3" to either of these questions are categorized as frail by the exhaustion criterion.
- Physical Activity: Based on the short version of the Minnesota Leisure Time Activity questionnaire, asking about walking, chores (moderately strenuous), mowing the lawn, raking, gardening, hiking, jogging, biking, exercise cycling, dancing, aerobics, bowling, golf, singles tennis, doubles tennis, racquetball, calisthenics, swimming. Kcals per week expended are calculated using standardized algorithm. This variable is stratified by gender. Men: Those with Kcals of physical activity per week <383 are frail. Women: Those with Kcals per week <270 are frail.
- Walk Time, stratified by gender and height (gender-specific cutoff a medium height).

Men	Cutoff for time to walk 15 feet criterion for frailty
Height ≤ 173 cm	≥7 seconds
Height > 173 cm	≥6 seconds
Women	
Height ≤ 159 cm	≥7 seconds
Height > 159 cm	≥6 seconds

- Grip Strength, stratified by gender and body mass index (BMI) quartiles:

Men	Cutoff for grip strength (Kg) criterion for frailty
BMI ≤ 24	<29
BMI 24.1–26	<30
BMI 26.1–28	<30
BMI > 28	<32
Women	
BMI ≤ 23	<17
BMI 23.1–26	<17.3
BMI 26.1–29	<18
BMI > 29	<21

From ref. 55.

Table 5
Biochemical Markers
of Inflammation Correlative with Frailty

C-reactive protein
Factor VIII
D-dimer
Interleukin-1B (IL-1B)
Interleukin-6 (IL-6)
Tumor necrosis factor-α (TNF-α)

ity. These include underlying diseases (e.g., malignancy, chronic disease, anemia, thyroid disease, diabetes mellitus), psychological impairment (e.g., depression, senile dementia), and lack of social or financial support. Thus, although frailty is associated with advanced age and increased physical disability, evidence suggests that neither old age nor disability alone accurately and predictively identify those older patients at highest risk of adverse outcomes after undergoing cardiac surgery.

SUMMARY

Clearly, the proportion of patients considered for cardiac surgery who are elderly will continue to increase. The very elderly present unique operative risk factors to the cardiac surgeon that require careful consideration and perioperative planning. Outcome reviews to date suggest that cardiac surgery can be performed in carefully selected elderly patients with acceptable results. Improved surgical techniques and accumulating clinical experience will undoubtedly maintain acceptable outcomes in these patients. However, cardiologists and cardiac surgeons should carefully evaluate these patients in order to provide the patient and their family members with realistic estimations of both the risk and expectations to be derived from surgery. Disregard of these considerations can only result in poor clinical outcomes, unanticipated anguish, and depriving the elderly patient the opportunity to live out his or her life with dignity. In time, well-designed clinical research will identify preoperative factors that will help assess operative risk and may facilitate interventions that can ameliorate these risks.

REFERENCES

1. U.S. Census Bureau. Population Projections Program. 2000, U.S. Census Bureau, Washington, D.C.
2. U.S. Census Bureau. Statistical abstract of the United States: 2000. U.S. Bureau of the Census, Washington, D.C., 2000, 85.

3. Roberts WC, Shirani J. Comparison of cardiac findings at necropsy in octogenarians, nonagenarians, and centenarians. Am J Cardiol 1998,82:627–631.

4. Foot DK, Lewis RP, Pearson TA, Bellu GA. Demography and cardiology, 1950–2050. J Am Coll Cardiol 2000; 35(4):1076–1081.

5. Craver JM, Puskas JD, Weintraub WW, et al. 601 octogenarians undergoing cardiac surgery: outcome and comparison with younger age groups. Ann Thorac Surg 1999; 67:1104–1110.

6. Tsai TP, Chaux A, Kass, M, et al. Aortocoronary bypass surgery in septuagenarians and octogenarians. J Cardiovasc Surg 1989;30:364–368.

7. Weintraub WS, Craver JM, Cohen C, et al. Influence of age on results of coronary artery surgery. Circulation 1991;84(Suppl 3):226–235.

8. Ko W, Krieger KH, Lazenby D, et al. Isolated coronary artery bypass grafting in one hundred consecutive octogenarian patients: a multivariate analysis. J Thorac Cardiovasc Surg 1991;102:532–538.

9. Kumar P, Zehr KJ, Chang A, et al. Quality of life in octogenarians after open heart surgery. Chest 1995;108:919–926.

10. Engoren M, Arslanian-Engoren C, Steckel D, et al. Cost, outcome, and functional status in octogenarians and septuagenarians after cardiac surgery. Chest 2002;122: 1309–1315.

11. Peterson ED, Cowper PA, Jollis JG. Outcomes of coronary artery bypass surgery in 24461 patients aged 80 years or older. Circulation 1995;92(Suppl II):II-85–II-95.

12. Peterson ED, Jollis JG, Bebchuk JD, et al. Changing mortality following myocardial revascularization in the elderly: the national Medicare experience. Ann Int Med 1994; 1212:919–927.

13. Smith KM, Lamy A, Arthur HM, et al. Outcomes and costs of coronary artery bypass grafting: comparison between octogenarians and septuagenarians at a tertiary care center. CMAJ 2001;165(6):759–764.

14. Mullaney CJ, Darling GE, Pluth JR, et al. Early and late results after isolated coronary artery bypass surgery in 159 patients aged 80 years and older. Circulation 1991;82 (Suppl IV):IV229–IV236.

15. Glower DD, Christopher TD, Milano CA. Performance status and outcome after coronary artery bypass grafting in persons 80 to 93 years. Am J Cardiol 1992;70: 567–571.

16. Alexander KP, Anstrom KJ, Muhlbaier LH, et al. Outcomes of cardiac surgery in patients age > 80 years: Results from the National Cardiovascular Network. J Am Coll Cardiol 2000;35:731–738.

17. Tseng EE, Lee CA, Cameron DE, et al. Aortic valve replacement in the elderly. Ann Surgery 1997;225(6):793–804.

18. Gudbjartsson T, Aranki S, Cohn LH. Mechanical/bioprosthetic mitral valve replacement In: Edmunds HL Jr (ed.), Cardiac Surgery in the Adult. McGraw-Hill, New York, 2003, pp. 951–986.

19. Desai ND, Christakis GT. Stented mechanical/bioprosthetic aortic valve replacement, In: Edmunds HL Jr (ed.), Cardiac Surgery in the Adult. McGraw-Hill, New York, 2003, pp. 825–855.

20. Khan NE, DeSouza A, Mister R, et al. A randomized comparison of off-pump and on-pump multivessel coronary artery bypass surgery. N Engl J Med 2004;350(1): 21–28.

21. Legare JF, Buth KJ, King S, et al. Coronary bypass surgery performed off pump does not result in lower in-hospital morbidity than coronary artery bypass grafting performed on pump. Circulation 2004;109(7):810–812.

22. Racz MJ, Hannan EL, Isom OW. A comparison of short- and long-term outcomes after off-pump and on-pump coronary artery bypass surgery with sternotomy. J Am Coll Cardiol 2004;43(4):557–564.
23. Kolh P, Kerzmann A, Lahaye L, et al. Cardiac surgery in octogenarians: perioperative outcome and long-term results. Eur Heart J 2001;22:1235–1243.
24. Neri E, Toscano T, Massetti, M, et al. Operation for acute type A aortic dissection in octogenarians: is it justified? J Thorac Cardiovasc Surg 2001;121:259–267.
25. Durand DJ, Perler BA, Roseborough GS, et al. Mandatory versus selective preoperative carotid screening: A retrospective analysis. Ann Thorac Surg 2004;77:TBD.
26. Naylor AR, Mehta Z, Rothwell PM, Bell PR, et al. Carotid artery disease and stroke during coronary artery bypass: a critical review of the literature. Eur J Vasc Endovasc Surg 2002;23(4):283–294.
27. Gold JP, Charlson ME, Williams-Russo P, et al. Improvement of outcomes after coronary artery bypass: a ramdomized trial comparing intraoperative high versus low mean arterial pressure. J Thorac Cardiovasc Surg 1995;110(5):1302–1311.
28. Floyd TF, McGarvey M, Ochroch EA, et al. Perioperative changes in cerebral blood flow after cardiac surgery: influence of anemia and aging. Ann Thorac Surg 2003;76 (6):2037–2042.
29. Wu WC, Rathore SS, Wang Y, et al. Blood transfusion in elderly patients with acute myocardial infarction. N Engl J Med 2001;345(17):1230–1236.
30. Bacchetta MD, Ko W, Girardi LN, et al. Outcomes of cardiac surgery in nonagenarians: a 10-year experience. Ann Thorac Surg 2002;75:1215–1220.
31. Van der Mast RC. Delirium after cardiac surgery. PhD Dissertation 1994.
32. Van der Mast RC, Van den Broek W, Fekkes, D, et al. Incidence of and preoperative predictors for delirium after cardiac surgery. J Psychosomatic Res 1998;46(5):479–483.
33. Rolfson DB, McElhaney JE, Rockwood K, et al. Incidence and risk factors for delirium and other adverse outcomes in older adults after coronary artery bypass graft surgery. Can J Cardiol 1999;15(7):771–776.
34. Bitondo Dyer C, Ashton CM, Teasdale TA. Postoperative delirium: a review of 80 primary data-collection studies. Arch Intern Med 1995;155:461–465.
35. Gokgoz L, Gunaydin S, Sinci V, et al. Psychiatric complications of cardiac surgery: postoperative delirium syndrome. Scand Cardiovasc J 1997;31:217–222.
36. Meagher DJ. Delirium: optimising management. BMJ 2001;322:144–149.
37. Bayindir O, Akpinar B, Can E, et al. The use of the 5-HT3-receptor antagonist ondansetron for the treatment of postcardiotomy delirium. J Cardiothorac Vasc Anesth 2000;14(3):288–292.
38. Taylor HL, Jacobs DR, Schuker B, et al. A questionnaire for the assessment of leisure-time physical activities. J Chronic Dis 1978;31:745–755.
39. Salazar JD, Wityk RJ, Grega MA, et al. Stroke after cardiac surgery: Short and long-term outcomes. Ann Thorac Surg 2001;72:1195–1202.
40. Plomondon ME, Cleveland JCJ, Ludwig ST, et al. Off-pump coronary artery bypass is associated with improved risk-adjusted outcomes. Ann Thorac Surg 2001;72:114–119.
41. Krumholz HM, Herrin J. Quality improvement studies: the need is there but so are the challenges. Am J Med 2000;109:501–503.
42. Gersh BJ, Kronmal RA, Frye RL. Coronary arteriography and coronary artery bypass surgery; morbidity and mortality in patients aged 65 years or older: a report from the Coronary Artery Surgery Study. Circulation 1983;67:483–491.
43. Newman AB, Gottdiener JS, McBurnie MA, et al. Associations of subclinical cardiovascular disease with frailty. J Gerontol A Biol Scie Med Sci 2001;56(3):M158–M166.

44. Fried LP, Kronmal RA, Newman AB, et al. Risk factors for 5-year mortality in older adults: the Cardiovascular Health Study. JAMA 1998;279(8):585–592.
45. Pendergast DR, Fisher NM, Calkins E. Cardiovascular, neuromuscular, and metabolic alterations with age leading to frailty. J Gerontol 1993;48:61–67.
46. Fried LP, Ettinger WH, Lind B, et al. Physical disability in older adults: a physiologic approach. Cardiovascular Health Study Research Group Clin Epidemiol 1994; 47(7):747–760.
47. Bild DE, Fitzpatrick A, Fried LP, et al. Age-related trends in cardiovascular morbidity and physical functioning in the elderly: the Cardiovascular Health Study. J Am Geriatr Soc 1993;41(10):1047–1056.
48. Fried LP, Walston J. Frailty and failure to thrive. In: Hazzard WR, Blass JP, Ettinger WHJ, Halter JB, Ouslander J (eds.), Principles of Geriatric Medicine and Gerontology. McGraw-Hill, New York, 1998, pp. 1387–1402.
49. Rockwood K, Stadnyk K, MacKnight C, et al. A brief clinical instrument to classify frailty in elderly people. Lancet 1999;353:205–206.
50. Winograd CH, Gerety MB, Chung M, et al. Screening for frailty: criteria and predictors of outcomes. J Am Geriatr Soc 1991;39:778–784.
51. Campbell AJ, Buchner DM. Unstable disability and the fluctuations of frailty. Age Aging 1997;26:315–318.
52. Winograd CH. Targeting strategies: an overview of criteria and outcomes. J Am Geriatr Soc 1991;39S:25S–35S.
53. Buchner DM, Wagner EH. Preventing frail health. Clin Geriatr Med 1992;8:1–17.
54. Bortz WM, II. A conceptual framework of frailty: a review. J Gerontol A Biol Sci Med Sci 2002;57(5):M283–M288.
55. Fried LP, Tangen CM, Walston J, et al. Frailty in older adults: evidence for a phenotype. J Gerontol A Biol Scie Med Sci 2001;56(3):M146–M156.
56. Walston J, McBurnie MA, Newman A, et al. Frailty and activation of the inflammation and coagulation systems with and without clinical comorbidities: results from the Cardiovascular Health Study. Arch Intern Med 2002;162(20):2333–2341.
57. Zieman SJ, Gerstenblith G, Lakatta EG, et al. Upregulation of the nitric oxide-cGMP pathway in aged myocardium: physiological response to L-arginine. Circ Res 2001;88:97–102.
58. Ershler WB Keller ET. Age-associated increased interleukin-6 gene expression, late-life diseases, and frailty. Ann Rev Med 2000;51:245–270.

9   Heart Failure in the Elderly

Michael W. Rich, MD

CONTENTS

EPIDEMIOLOGY AND SOCIETAL BURDEN
PATHOPHYSIOLOGY
CLINICAL FEATURES
MANAGEMENT
FUTURE DIRECTIONS
REFERENCES

EPIDEMIOLOGY AND SOCIETAL BURDEN

Heart failure (HF) affects approximately 5 million Americans, and more than 550,000 new cases are reported each year *(1,2)*. In addition, despite recent advances in the diagnosis and treatment of HF, as well as reductions in age-adjusted mortality rates from coronary heart disease and hypertensive cardiovascular disease (CVD) *(3,4)*, both the incidence and prevalence of HF are increasing, primarily owing to the aging of the population *(5)*. Indeed, HF is predominantly a disorder of the elderly, with prevalence rates increasing exponentially from less than 1% in the population under age 50 to about 10% in individuals over the age of 80 *(6)*. Consequently, more than 75% of hospitalizations for HF occur in persons 65 years of age or older *(7)*, the median age for all HF admissions is 75 years *(8)*, and HF is the leading indication for hospitalization in older adults *(2)*.

HF is also a major source of chronic disability and impaired quality of life in the elderly *(9)*, and it is a common factor contributing to institutionalization in a chronic care facility. Furthermore, HF is the most costly medical illness in the United States, with annual expenditures in excess of $40 billion, representing 5.4% of the total health care budget

From: *Contemporary Cardiology: Cardiovascular Disease in the Elderly*
Edited by: G. Gerstenblith © Humana Press Inc., Totowa, NJ

203

(10). HF also contributes to more than 250,000 deaths each year *(1,2)*, and 88% of these deaths are in persons over age 65 *(8)*.

These statistics emphasize the striking clinical and economic burden already imposed on our society by HF in older adults. Given the projected doubling in the number of Americans over 65 years of age in the next three decades, it may be anticipated that the magnitude of this burden will continue to rise, and that unless innovative strategies for the prevention and treatment of HF at elderly age are developed, HF in the elderly may develop into a true public health crisis. In this context, this chapter reviews the pathophysiology, clinical features, and management of HF in the elderly, and considers new approaches to prevention and treatment that may become available in the years ahead.

PATHOPHYSIOLOGY

Aging is associated with significant alterations in cardiovascular structure and function that diminish homeostatic reserve and predispose older individuals to the development of HF (Table 1) *(5,11,12)*. In general, cardiac output is determined by four factors—heart rate, preload, afterload, and contractile state—and age-related cardiovascular changes impact significantly on each of these parameters. Thus, diminished β-adrenergic responsiveness and degenerative changes in the sinoatrial node impair the heart rate response to stress; impaired myocardial relaxation and decreased compliance compromise ventricular filling and alter preload; increased vascular stiffness and a reduction in β_2-mediated systemic vasodilation serve to increase afterload; and reduced capacity of mitochondria to generate adenosine triphospate, in conjunction with diminished responsiveness to β_1-stimulation, lead to a decrease in contractile reserve. In the absence of CVD, these changes have minimal effect on resting cardiac performance; i.e., resting left ventricular systolic function and cardiac output are reasonably well preserved, even at very advanced age. However, a marked age-dependent reduction in cardiovascular reserve (Fig. 1) attenuates the heart's ability to respond to common stressors, such as ischemia, tachycardia (e.g., resulting from atrial fibrillation [AF]), systemic illness (e.g., infections), and physical exertion. As a result, clinical events that are generally well tolerated in younger individuals frequently precipitate HF in older persons.

An important feature that distinguishes HF in the elderly from HF in middle age is a striking increase in the proportion of cases that occur in the setting of normal or near-normal left ventricular systolic function *(13,14)*. As noted, aging is associated with impaired left ventricular filling owing to changes in myocardial relaxation and compliance. These

Table 1
Principal Effects of Aging on Cardiovascular Structure and Function

Increased vascular "stiffness," impedance to ejection, and pulse wave velocity

Impaired left ventricular early diastolic relaxation and mid- to late-diastolic compliance

Diminished responsiveness to neurohumoral stimuli, especially β_1 and β_2 adrenergic stimulation

Altered myocardial energy metabolism and reduced mitochondrial adenosine triphosphate-production capacity

Reduced number of sinus node pacemaker cells and impaired sinoatrial function

Endothelial dysfunction and vasomotor dysregulation

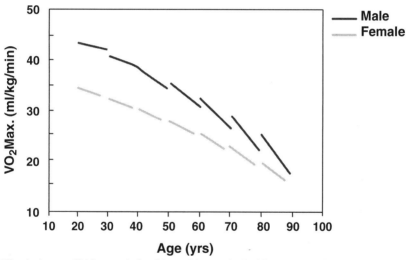

Fig. 1. Age and VO$_2$max in healthy subjects: the Baltimore Longitudinal Study on Aging. (From ref. *12a*.)

alterations lead to a shift in the left ventricular pressure–volume relationship, such that small increments in left ventricular volume result in greater increases in left ventricular diastolic pressure (Fig. 2) *(15)*. This increase in diastolic pressure further compromises left ventricular filling, and also leads to increases in left atrial, pulmonary venous, and pulmonary capillary pressures, thus predisposing to pulmonary congestion and HF. "Diastolic" HF, as it is often called, accounts for less than 10% of HF cases in persons under age 60, but more than 50% of cases after age 75 *(13,14,16)*. Diastolic HF is also more common in women

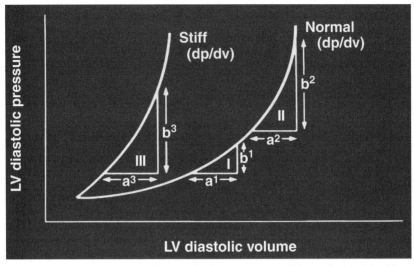

Fig. 2. Effect of age on the left ventricular pressure–volume relationship. Note that there is a shift to the left, such that small increases in left ventricular volume are associated with greater increases in left ventricular pressure compared to younger persons. (Adapted from ref. *15*, with permission.)

than in men, and accounts for nearly two-thirds of all HF cases among women over age 80 *(14)*.

CLINICAL FEATURES

Symptoms and Signs

Exertional dyspnea, orthopnea, lower extremity swelling, and impaired exercise tolerance are the cardinal symptoms of HF at both younger and older age. However, with increasing age, which is often accompanied by a progressively more sedentary lifestyle, exertional symptoms become less prominent *(17)*. Conversely, atypical symptoms, such as confusion, somnolence, irritability, fatigue, anorexia, or diminished activity level, become increasingly more common manifestations of HF, especially after age 80.

Physical signs of HF include elevated jugular venous pressure, hepato-jugular reflux, an S_3 gallop, pulmonary rales, and dependent edema. Each of these features occurs less commonly in older HF patients, in part because of the increasing prevalence of diastolic HF, in which signs of right HF are a late manifestation and a third heart sound is typically absent. On the other hand, behavioral changes and altered cognition, which may range from subtle abnormalities to overt delirium, frequently accompany HF at elderly age, particularly among institutionalized or hospitalized patients *(18)*.

Diagnosis

Accurate diagnosis of the HF syndrome at older age is confounded in part by the increasing prevalence of atypical symptoms and signs *(17)*. In addition, exertional symptoms may be attributable to noncardiac causes, such as pulmonary disease, anemia, depression, physical deconditioning, or aging itself. Likewise, peripheral edema may be the result of venous insufficiency, hepatic or renal disease, or medication side effects (e.g., calcium channel blockers), and pulmonary crepitus may be owing to atelectasis or chronic lung disease. Despite these limitations, careful clinical assessment for the presence of multiple symptoms and signs should lead to the correct diagnosis in most cases.

Chest radiography is indicated when HF is suspected, and it remains the most useful diagnostic test for determining the presence of pulmonary congestion. However, chronic lung disease or altered chest geometry (e.g., resulting from kyphosis) may confound interpretation of the chest radiograph in elderly individuals.

Recently, plasma B-type natriuretic peptide (BNP) levels were shown to be a valuable aid in distinguishing dyspnea owing to HF from that related to other causes, such as pulmonary disorders *(19)*. BNP levels tend to be elevated in both systolic and diastolic HF *(20,21)*, and they also correlate with response to therapy and prognosis *(22–24)*. However, BNP levels also increase with age in healthy individuals without HF, particularly women (Fig. 3), and, as a result, the specificity and predictive accuracy of BNP levels decline with age *(25)*. Nonetheless, in cases of diagnostic uncertainty, a low or normal BNP level effectively excludes acute HF, whereas a markedly elevated level provides strong evidence in support of the diagnosis.

Proper management of HF is critically dependent on establishing the pathophysiology of left ventricular dysfunction (i.e., systolic vs diastolic), determining the primary and any secondary etiologies (Table 2), and identifying potentially treatable precipitating or contributory factors (Table 3). Differentiating systolic from diastolic dysfunction requires an assessment of left ventricular contractility by echocardiography, radionuclide ventriculography, magnetic resonance imaging, or contrast angiography. Among these, echocardiography is the most widely used and clinically useful noninvasive test for evaluating systolic and diastolic function. In addition, echocardiography provides important information about left ventricular chamber size and wall thickness, atrial size, right ventricular function, the presence and severity of valvular lesions, and

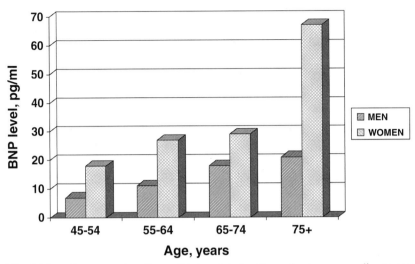

Fig. 3. Mean B-type natriuretic peptide levels in healthy volunteers according to age and gender. (Adapted from ref. *25*.)

pericardial disorders. For these reasons, echocardiography is recommended for all patients with newly diagnosed HF or unexplained disease progression *(26)*.

Other diagnostic studies that may be indicated in selected patients include an assessment of thyroid function (especially in the presence of AF), an exercise or pharmacological stress test to evaluate for the presence and severity of ischemia, and cardiac catheterization if revascularization or other corrective procedure (e.g., valve repair or replacement) is being contemplated.

Etiology and Precipitating Factors

Systemic hypertension and coronary heart disease account for 70 to 80% of HF cases at older age *(27,28)*. Hypertension is the most common etiology in older women, particularly those with preserved systolic function *(14,28)*. In older men, HF is more often attributable to coronary heart disease *(28)*. Other common etiologies include valvular heart disease (especially aortic stenosis and mitral regurgitation) and nonischemic cardiomyopathy (Table 2). Importantly, HF in the elderly is frequently multifactorial, and it is thus essential to identify all potentially treatable causes.

In addition to determining etiology, it is important to identify factors precipitating or contributing to HF exacerbations (Table 3). Noncompliance with medications and diet is the most common cause of recurrent

Table 2
Common Etiologies of Heart Failure in Older Adults

Coronary artery disease
  Acute myocardial infarction
  Chronic ischemic cardiomyopathy
Hypertensive heart disease
  Hypertensive hypertrophic cardiomyopathy
Valvular heart disease
  Aortic stenosis or insufficiency
  Mitral stenosis or insufficiency
  Prosthetic valve malfunction
  Infective endocarditis
Cardiomyopathy
  Dilated (nonischemic)
    Alcohol
    Chemotherapeutic agents
    Inflammatory myocarditis
    Idiopathic
  Hypertrophic
    Obstructive
    Nonobstructive
  Restrictive (especially amyloid)
Pericardial disease
  Constrictive pericarditis
High output syndromes
  Chronic anemia
  Thiamine deficiency
  Hyperthyroidism
  Arteriovenous shunting
Age-related diastolic dysfunction

HF exacerbations *(29,30)*, and patients should be closely questioned about their dietary and medication habits. Other common factors contributing to worsening symptoms include ischemia, volume overload as a result of excess fluid intake (self-inflicted or iatrogenic) *(31)*, tachyarrhythmias (especially AF or atrial flutter), intercurrent infections, anemia, thyroid disease, and various medications or toxins (e.g., alcohol).

Co-Morbidity

A hallmark of aging is the increasing prevalence of multiple co-morbid conditions, many of which impact directly or indirectly on the diagnosis, clinical course, treatment, and prognosis of HF in the elderly (Table 4) *(32)*. Discussion of individual co-morbidities is beyond the scope of

Table 3
Common Precipitants of Heart Failure in Older Adults

Myocardial ischemia or infarction
Uncontrolled hypertension
Dietary sodium excess
Medication noncompliance
Excess fluid intake
    Self-induced
    Iatrogenic
Arrhythmias
    Supraventricular, especially atrial fibrillation
    Ventricular
    Bradycardia, esp. sick sinus syndrome
Associated medical conditions
    Fever
    Infections, especially pneumonia or sepsis
    Hyperthyroidism or hypothyroidism
    Anemia
    Renal insufficiency
    Thiamine deficiency
    Pulmonary embolism
    Hypoxemia due to chronic lung disease
Drugs and medications
    Alcohol
    β-adrenergic blockers (including ophthalmolgicals)
    Calcium channel blockers
    Anti-arrhythmic agents
    Nonsteroidal anti-inflammatory drugs
    Glucocorticoids
    Mineralocorticoids
    Estrogen preparations
    Antihypertensive agents (e.g., clonidine, minoxodil)

this chapter, but it is important to recognize that HF in the elderly virtually never occurs in isolation; diagnosis and management must therefore be viewed in the context of the patient's other co-morbidities and competing risks.

MANAGEMENT

The principal goals of HF therapy are to relieve symptoms, maintain or enhance functional capacity and quality of life, preserve independence, and extend survival. Although it is often stated that quality of life is more important than quantity of life in the very elderly, this in fact is a

Table 4
Common Co-Morbidities in Older Patients

Condition	Implications
Renal dysfunction	Exacerbated by diuretics, ACE inhibitors
Anemia	Worsens symptoms and prognosis
Chronic lung disease	Contributes to uncertainty about diagnosis/volume status
Cognitive dysfunction	Interferes with dietary, medication, activity compliance
Depression, social isolation	Worsens prognosis, interferes with compliance
Postural hypotension, falls	Exacerbated by vasodilators, diuretics, β-blockers
Urinary incontinence	Aggravated by diuretics, ACE inhibitors (cough)
Sensory deprivation	Interferes with compliance
Nutritional disorders	Exacerbated by dietary restrictions
Polypharmacy	Compliance issues, drug interactions
Frailty	Exacerbated by hospitalization; increased fall risk

ACE, angiotensin-converting enzyme

matter of personal preference. Furthermore, because the elderly HF population is characterized by marked heterogeneity in terms of lifestyle, co-morbidity, and personal goals and perspectives, management of HF in the elderly must first and foremost be individualized to each patient's circumstances and needs.

The basic approach to HF management involves identification and treatment of the underlying etiology and contributing factors, implementation of an effective therapeutic regimen, and coordination of care through the use of a multidisciplinary team.

Etiology and Precipitating Factors

Although HF in the elderly is rarely "curable," proper treatment of the underlying etiology often improves symptoms and delays disease progression. Thus, hypertension should be treated aggressively (33), and coronary heart disease should be managed appropriately with medications and/or percutaneous or surgical revascularization. Similarly, therapy for diabetes and dyslipidemia should be optimized, smoking should be strongly discouraged, and a suitable level of regular physical activity should be prescribed. Alcohol intake should be limited to no more than two drinks per day in men and one drink per day in women, and alcohol use should be strictly proscribed in patients with suspected alcoholic cardiomyopathy.

Severe aortic stenosis is a common cause of HF in the elderly and can be effectively treated with aortic valve replacement *(34)*. Perioperative mortality rates are acceptable (less than 10%), and long-term results are excellent, even in octogenarians *(35)*. Severe mitral regurgitation may be amenable to surgical therapy (i.e., valve repair or replacement) in selected patients, but the operative results are somewhat less favorable than for aortic valve surgery *(36,37)*. Mitral valve replacement is also effective therapy for severe mitral stenosis; rarely, percutaneous mitral balloon valvuloplasty may be feasible in older patients *(38,39)*.

AF is a common precipitant of HF in elderly patients, especially in the setting of diastolic dysfunction. In patients with recent onset symptomatic AF, many clinicians recommend restoration and maintenance of sinus rhythm if feasible, although the long-term benefits of this approach have not been established *(40,41)*. In patients with chronic AF, the ventricular rate should be well controlled both at rest and during activity. Bradycardia is a less common primary cause of HF; when present, implantation of a permanent pacemaker provides definitive therapy (see section on devices). Anemia, thyroid disease, and other systemic illnesses should be identified and treated accordingly.

The importance of compliance with medications and dietary restrictions, including avoidance of excessive fluid intake, cannot be overemphasized. Nonsteroidal anti-inflammatory drugs are widely used by older individuals to treat arthritis and relieve chronic pain, but these agents promote sodium and water retention, interfere with the actions of angiotensin-converting enzyme (ACE) inhibitors and other antihypertensive agents, and may worsen renal function; their use should be avoided whenever possible *(42)*. Similarly, the use of other medications that may aggravate HF should be closely monitored.

Pharmacotherapy

The design of an effective therapeutic regimen is based in part on whether the patient has predominantly systolic or predominantly diastolic left ventricular dysfunction. Although these two abnormalities frequently coexist (indeed, virtually all individuals over age 70 have some degree of diastolic dysfunction), for purposes of this discussion patients with an ejection fraction (EF) less than 45% (i.e., moderate or severe left ventricular systolic dysfunction) will be considered as having systolic HF, whereas patients with an EF of 45% or more will be considered as having diastolic HF.

SYSTOLIC HEART FAILURE

In the past 20 years there has been considerable progress in the treatment of systolic HF. Although most studies have either excluded individuals over 75 to 80 years of age, or have enrolled too few elderly subjects to permit definitive conclusions, the available data indicate that older patients respond to standard therapies as well or better than younger patients. Therefore, current recommendations for drug treatment of systolic HF are similar in younger and older patients (26).

ACE Inhibitors. ACE inhibitors are the cornerstone of therapy for left ventricular systolic dysfunction, whether or not clinically overt HF is present (26), and there is strong evidence that ACE inhibitors are as effective in older as in younger patients, both in terms of reducing mortality and improving quality of life (43,44). On the other hand, older patients are more likely to have potential contraindications to ACE inhibitors (e.g., renal dysfunction, renal artery stenosis, orthostatic hypotension), and they may also be at increased risk for ACE inhibitor-related side effects, such as worsening renal function, electrolyte disturbances, and hypotension. Nonetheless, a trial of ACE inhibitors is indicated in virtually all older patients with documented left ventricular systolic dysfunction.

In most cases, ACE inhibitor therapy should be initiated at a low dose (e.g., 6.25–12.5 mg captopril three times a day [TID] or 2.5 mg enalapril 2.5 mg twice a day [BID]), and the dosage should be gradually titrated upward to the level shown to be effective in clinical trials (50 mg captopril TID, 10 mg enalapril BID, 20 mg lisinopril every day [qd], 10 mg ramipril qd) (43–47). Once a maintenance dose has been achieved, substituting a once-daily agent (e.g., lisinopril or ramipril) at equivalent dosage may facilitate compliance. Blood pressure, renal function, and serum potassium levels should be monitored closely during dose titration and periodically during maintenance therapy. In patients unable to tolerate standard ACE-inhibitor dosages because of side effects, dosage reduction is appropriate, as there is evidence that even very low doses of these agents (e.g., 2.5–5 mg lisinopril qd) provide some degree of benefit (48).

Angiotensin Receptor Blockers. Angiotensin receptor blockers (ARBs) have a more favorable side-effect profile than ACE inhibitors, but there is insufficient evidence to conclude that the effects of ARBs on major clinical outcomes (e.g., death, hospitalizations) are equivalent to those of ACE inhibitors (49–51). However, recent studies indicate that ARBs reduce mortality and hospitalizations in patients with systolic HF who are intolerant to ACE inhibitors owing to cough or other side effects (52,53). In addition, combining an ARB with an ACE inhibitor improves outcomes compared with an ACE inhibitor alone (54,55), although in one study triple therapy with an ACE inhibitor, β-blocker, and ARB was associated with increased mortality compared to treatment with only two of these classes of agents *(54)*. Based on available evidence, and pending the results of ongoing clinical trials, ACE inhibitors should still be considered first-line therapy for HF, but ARBs offer an excellent alternative for patients intolerant to ACE inhibitors, and as conjunctive therapy in patients with persistent symptoms despite conventional treatment.

Hydralazine and Isosorbide Dinitrate. The combination of 75 mg of hydralazine four times a day (QID) and 40 mg of isosorbide dinitrate QID was associated with decreased mortality in a small trial of HF patients less than 75 years of age *(56)*. Although ACE inhibitors are superior to hydralazine–nitrates in improving survival *(57)*, the combination provides an additional alternative for ACE inhibitor-intolerant patients. Side effects are common with both hydralazine and high-dose nitrates, and the QID dosing schedule is a particular disadvantage for older patients.

β-Blockers. β-Blockers, once widely viewed as contraindicated in patients with HF, have now been shown to improve left ventricular function and decrease mortality in a broad population of HF patients, including those with New York Heart Association (NYHA) class IV symptoms and patients up to 80 years of age *(58–61)*. As a result, β-blockers are now considered standard therapy for clinically stable patients without major contraindications *(26)*. Use of β-blockers in older patients may be limited by a higher prevalence of bradyarrhythmias and severe chronic lung disease, and older patients may also be more susceptible to the development of fatigue and impaired exercise tolerance during long-term β-blocker administration.

Carvedilol, metoprolol, and bisoprolol are all shown to improve outcomes in patients with systolic HF, and a recent study found that carvedilol (25 mg BID) was more effective than metoprolol (50 mg BID) in reducing mortality *(62)*. In most cases, β-blocker treatment should be initiated at low dosages in stable patients upon a background of ACE inhibitor and diuretic therapy. Recommended starting dosages are 3.125 mg of carvedilol twice a day, 6.25–12.5 mg of metoprolol twice a day, and a daily 1.25 mg dose of bisoprolol. The dose should be gradually increased at 2- to 4-week intervals to achieve maintenance dosages of carvedilol (25–50 mg BID), metoprolol (50–100 mg BID or sustained release metoprolol 100–200 mg qd), or bisoprolol (5–10 mg qd). Lower dosages and a slower titration protocol may be appropriate in patients over 75 years of age. Contraindications to β-blockade include marked sinus bradycardia (resting heart rate <45–50 beats per minute), PR interval longer than 0.24 seconds, heart block greater than first degree, systolic blood pressure less than 90–100 mmHg, active bronchospastic lung disease, and severe decompensated HF.

Digoxin. Digoxin improves symptoms and reduces hospitalizations in patients with symptomatic systolic HF treated with ACE inhibitors and diuretics, but has no effect on total or cardiovascular mortality *(63)*. Although these effects are similar in younger and older patients, including octogenarians *(64)*, a recent retrospective analysis has questioned the value of digoxin in women *(65)*. Nonetheless, digoxin remains a useful drug for the treatment of systolic HF in patients of all ages who have limiting symptoms despite standard therapy.

The volume of distribution and renal clearance of digoxin decline with age. In addition, recent data indicate that the optimal therapeutic concentration for digoxin is 0.5–0.8 ng/mL *(66)*; i.e., substantially lower than the traditional therapeutic range of 0.8–2.0 ng/mL. Moreover, higher concentrations of digoxin are associated with increased toxicity but no greater efficacy *(66,67)*. For most older patients with preserved renal function (estimated creatinine clearance ≥ 50 cc per minute), 0.125 mg of digoxin daily provides a therapeutic effect. Lower dosages should be used in patients with renal insufficiency. Although routine monitoring of serum digoxin levels is no longer recommended, it seems reasonable to measure the serum digoxin concentration 2 to 4 weeks after initiating therapy to ensure that the level does not exceed 0.8 ng/mL. In addition, a digoxin level should be obtained whenever digoxin toxicity is suspected.

Digoxin side effects include arrhythmias, heart block, gastrointestinal disturbances, and altered neurological function (e.g., visual disturbances). Although older patients are often thought to be at increased risk for digitalis toxicity, this was not confirmed in a recent analysis from the Digitalis Investigation Group trial *(64)*.

Diuretics. Diuretics are an essential component of therapy for most patients with HF, and are the most effective agents for relieving congestion and maintaining euvolemia. Some patients with mild HF can be effectively controlled with a thiazide diuretic, but the majority will require a loop diuretic such as furosemide or bumetanide. In patients with more severe HF or significant renal dysfunction (serum creatinine ≥ 2.0 mg/dL), the addition of 2.5–10 mg of metolazone daily may be necessary to achieve effective diuresis.

In general, diuretic dosages should be titrated to eliminate signs of pulmonary and systemic venous congestion. Common side effects include worsening renal function (often because of overdiuresis) and electrolyte disorders. To minimize these effects, renal function and serum electrolyte levels (sodium, potassium, magnesium) should be monitored closely during the initiation and titration phase of diuretic use, and periodically thereafter.

Aldosterone Antagonists. Spironolactone is a weak, potassium-sparing diuretic that acts by antagonizing aldosterone. Recently, the addition of 12.5–50 mg of spironolactone daily to standard HF therapy has been shown to reduce mortality in patients with NYHA class III–IV systolic HF, with similar benefits in older and younger patients *(68,69).* Eplerenone, a selective aldosterone antagonist, has also been shown to reduce mortality and sudden cardiac death in patients with left ventricular dysfunction following acute myocardial infarction (MI) *(70).* Spironolactone is contraindicated in patients with severe renal insufficiency or hyperkalemia, and up to 10% of patients develop painful gynecomastia. In addition, older patients receiving spironolactone in combination with an ACE inhibitor may be at increased risk for hyperkalemia, particularly in the presence of pre-existing renal insufficiency or diabetes, and at doses in excess of 25 mg per day *(71).*

Approach to Treatment. Figure 4 provides a suggested approach to the pharmacological treatment of systolic HF. All patients with left ventricular systolic dysfunction, whether asymptomatic or symptomatic, should receive an ACE inhibitor (or an ARB or alternative vasodilator if ACE inhibitors are contraindicated or not tolerated). Patients with stable symptoms and no contraindications should also receive a β-blocker, and diuretics should be administered in sufficient doses to maintain euvolemia. Digoxin and/or an ARB should be considered in patients who remain symptomatic despite the above regimen, and spironolactone should be used in patients with persistent NYHA class III–IV symptoms.

DIASTOLIC HEART FAILURE

Despite the fact that more than 50% of elderly HF patients have preserved left ventricular systolic function *(13,14),* until recently none of the major HF trials have specifically targeted this disorder. As a result, treatment of diastolic HF remains largely empiric. As with systolic HF, the underlying cardiac disorder and associated contributing conditions should be treated appropriately. In particular, hypertension and coronary heart disease should be managed aggressively. Diuretics should be used judiciously to relieve congestion while avoiding overdiuresis and pre-renal azotemia. Topical or oral nitrates may be beneficial in reducing pulmonary congestion and orthopnea. Based on the results of the Heart Outcomes Prevention Evaluation *(72),* an ACE inhibitor such as ramipril (2.5–10 mg daily) is appropriate for most older adults with vascular disease, but the value of ACE inhibitors in the treatment of diastolic HF *per*

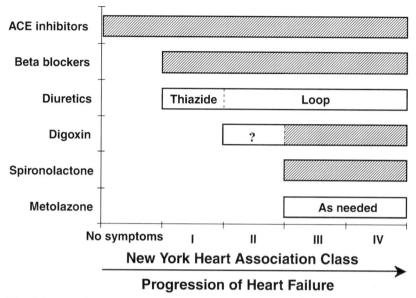

Fig. 4. Approach to treatment of systolic heart failure; see text for details. Shaded areas indicate therapies shown to be effective in prospective randomized clinical trials. ACE, angiotensin-converting enzyme.

se has not been established. Similarly, the role of ARBs in the management of diastolic HF is evolving. In the recently reported Candesartan in Heart failure: Assessment of Reduction in Mortality and morbidity (CHARM)-Preserved trial, the ARB candesartan reduced HF admissions by 16% but had no effect on mortality in patients with HF and a left ventricular EF greater than 40% *(73)*. Of note, the mean age of patients in CHARM-Preserved was 67 years, and 807 patients, comprising 27% of the total population, were at least 75 years of age.

β-Blockers are indicated in patients with coronary heart disease (especially prior MI), but the long-term effects of these agents in diastolic HF are unknown. Calcium channel blockers are effective antihypertensive agents in the elderly, and may provide symptomatic palliation in selected patients with diastolic HF *(74)*. Digoxin, in addition to its inotropic effect, also facilitates diastolic relaxation, and may improve symptoms and reduce hospitalizations in patients with HF and preserved systolic function *(63,64)*. In summary, the physician treating diastolic HF is presented with an array of therapeutic options, none of proven benefit, and therapy should be individualized and guided by prevalent co-morbidities and the observed response to specific therapeutic interventions.

Device Therapy

Although the majority of HF patients can be effectively managed with behavioral interventions and medications, implantable devices are playing an increasingly important role in the management of selected subgroups of the HF population.

CARDIAC PACEMAKERS

Aging is associated with a progressive decline in the number of functioning sinus nodal pacemaker cells, often leading to the "sick sinus syndrome," which is characterized by inappropriate sinus bradycardia, sinus pauses, and chronotropic incompetence (failure to adequately increase heart rate in response to increased demands) *(75)*. Because cardiac output is directly proportional to heart rate (cardiac output = heart rate × stroke volume), age-related bradyarrhythmias may contribute to HF symptoms and impaired exercise tolerance. Because there is no effective medical therapy for sick sinus syndrome, implantation of a pacemaker is appropriate in symptomatic patients. The use of β-blockers may also precipitate symptomatic bradyarrhythmias in elderly HF patients. Because β-blockers improve ventricular function and reduce mortality and hospitalizations in patients with systolic HF *(58–61)*, placement of a pacemaker is often preferable to discontinuation of β-blocker therapy.

CARDIAC RESYNCHRONIZATION THERAPY

Recently, a new role has evolved for pacemakers in treating selected patients with advanced HF. Approximately 30% of HF patients have left bundle branch block or other intraventricular conduction abnormality resulting in significant prolongation of the QRS interval (≥120 ms). In these patients, left ventricular contraction is often disynchronous and out of phase with right ventricular contraction. Biventricular pacing, with one lead pacing the right ventricle and a second lead pacing the left ventricle through retrograde insertion into the coronary sinus, can "resynchronize" ventricular contraction, thus improving EF and cardiac output *(76,77)*. The addition of atrial pacing may provide further benefit by optimizing the timing of atrial and ventricular contraction. The benefits of cardiac resynchronization therapy (CRT) in improving EF, reducing left ventricular cavity size, and enhancing exercise tolerance and quality of life have now been well documented in several randomized trials involving patients with advanced HF symptoms (NYHA class III–IV), reduced EFs, and prolonged QRS durations *(78–81)*. Although improved survival has not yet been proven *(80)*, CRT is a reasonable option for carefully selected older patients with advanced HF symptoms despite conventional therapies.

IMPLANTABLE CARDIOVERTER DEFIBRILLATORS

Approximately 40%–50% of all deaths in patients with HF are attributable to ventricular tachycardia (VT) and ventricular fibrillation (VF). Implantable cardioverter defibrillators (ICDs) have the capacity to recognize VT and VF, and to restore normal rhythm either by pacing techniques (in the case of VT) or by delivering an intracardiac electrical shock (refractory VT or VF). Moreover, ICDs have been shown to significantly improve survival in certain high-risk subgroups of the HF population, including those with resuscitated cardiac arrest, symptomatic sustained VT, and ischemic or nonischemic cardiomyopathy with EF less than 30%–35% *(82–84a)*. Importantly, the survival benefit of ICDs is greatest in patients over 70 years of age with EFs less than 35% and NYHA class III or IV HF symptoms *(85)*.

In the United States, more than half of ICDs are implanted in patients 65 years of age or older. However, despite the established benefits of ICDs in appropriately selected patients, the clinical role of ICDs in elderly HF patients remains a subject of debate *(86–88)*. These devices are expensive, with a total cost of approximately $40,000–$50,000 per device, although a $10,000 "generic" version has recently gained approval. In addition, the societal cost burden is likely to increase substantially as the indications for these devices continue to expand. There are also ethical questions, such as how and when to turn off the device in the terminal stages of HF, or in cases where another life-threatening illness (e.g., stroke or cancer) develops. In part because of these reasons, many older patients may elect to forego ICD implantation, even though survival may be enhanced. Although additional study is needed, it is clear that the use of ICDs must be individualized, but that older age should not constitute the sole grounds for withholding ICD therapy.

Multidisciplinary Care

The presence of multiple co-morbid conditions, polypharmacy, dietary concerns, and a host of psychosocial and financial issues frequently complicate the management of HF in older patients. Moreover, these factors often contribute to poor outcomes in older adults, including frequent hospitalizations *(30,89)*. To address these issues, and to provide comprehensive yet individualized care for older HF patients, a coordinated multidisciplinary approach is recommended. Several recent studies have documented the efficacy of multidisciplinary HF disease management programs in reducing hospitalizations and improving quality of life in older patients, and these interventions have also been reported to lower overall medical costs *(90–92)*.

Elements of an effective HF disease management program include patient and caregiver education, enhancement of self-management skills, optimization of pharmacotherapy (including consideration of polypharmacy issues), and close follow-up. The structure of a HF disease management team is similar to that of a multidisciplinary geriatric assessment team, and typically includes a nurse coordinator or case manager, dietitian, social worker, clinical pharmacist, home health representative, primary care physician, and cardiology consultant. Specific goals of disease management are to improve patient compliance with medications, diet, and exercise recommendations by enhancing education and self-management skills; provide close follow-up and improved health care access through telephone contacts, home health visits, and nurse or physician office visits; and optimize the medication regimen by promoting physician adherence to recommended HF treatment guidelines (26), simplifying and consolidating the regimen when feasible, eliminating unnecessary medications, and minimizing the risks for drug–drug and drug–disease interactions.

Exercise

Both HF and normal aging are associated with reduced exercise capacity, in part because of sarcopenia (loss of muscle mass) and alterations in skeletal muscle blood flow and metabolism. Regular physical activity improves exercise performance in healthy older adults, as well as in those with HF, and regular exercise is now recommended for most older HF patients (26,93–97). Although supervised exercise programs have been associated with the greatest improvements in exercise performance, such programs are not feasible for most older patients owing to lack of availability, travel concerns, and cost constraints. Therefore, most older HF patients should be encouraged to engage in a self-monitored home exercise program that includes stretching and resistance exercises and aerobic activities. Stretching increases or maintains muscle flexibility and reduces the risk of injury. A daily stretching routine lasting 15 to 30 minutes and involving all major muscle groups is recommended. Resistance training increases muscle mass and strength and reduces the risk of falls and frailty (98). Older adults initiating a strength-training program should use light weights and perform two to three sets of 8 to 12 repetitions for each of 8 to 12 exercises approximately two to three times per week; as with stretching, all major muscle groups should be included in the strength-training program.

Aerobic exercise leads to improved physical performance and quality of life, and may increase the likelihood that older adults will remain independent in activities of daily living (94–97). For most older adults, walking is the most suitable form of aerobic exercise, but stationary cycling and swimming are appropriate alternatives. Older adults embarking on an exercise program should be advised to begin at a comfortable pace and exercise for a comfortable period of time. For HF patients, this may be as little as a few minutes of walking at a slow pace, but patients should not be discouraged by the fact that they are starting at a low level; indeed, data show that the greatest improvements occur in patients with the lowest baseline activity levels. Patients should exercise at least 4 to 5 days per week, gradually increasing the duration of exercise (but not the intensity) until it is possible to exercise comfortably and continuously for 20 to 30 minutes. Once this level of exercise capacity has been achieved, patients may consider further increasing the duration of exercise (e.g., up to 45 minutes) or gradually increasing the intensity. In either case, older HF patients should not exercise strenuously or to exhaustion. Additionally, patients should be instructed to stop exercising and contact their physician if they develop chest pain, undue shortness of breath, dizziness or syncope, or any other symptom that may indicate clinical instability. Finally, contraindications to exercise in elderly HF patients include decompensated HF, unstable coronary disease or arrhythmias, neurological or muscular disorders that preclude participation in an exercise program, or any other condition that would render exercise unsafe.

End of Life

The overall 5-year survival rate for older patients with established HF is less than 50% (i.e., the prognosis is worse than for most forms of cancer [99–101]). Clinical features portending a less favorable outcome include older age, more severe symptoms and functional impairment, lower left ventricular EF, underlying coronary heart disease, and impaired renal function (102). Older patients with advanced HF, as evidenced by NYHA class III–IV symptoms, have a 1-year mortality rate of 25% to 50%; for these patients, HF can properly be considered a terminal illness. In addition, all HF patients are at risk for sudden arrhythmic death, which may occur during periods of apparent clinical stability. For these reasons, it is appropriate to address end-of-life issues early in the course of HF, and to reconsider these issues periodically as the disease progresses or when changes in clinical status occur.

Although discussing end-of-life issues is often challenging for health care providers, as well as patients and families, specific measures should be undertaken to plan for and facilitate end-of-life care (103). These include the development of an advance directive and appointment of durable power of attorney. The advance directive should be as explicit as possible in defining circumstances under which the patient does not want to

Table 5
Effect of Antihypertensive Therapy on Incident Heart Failure in Older Adults

Trial	N	Age range (years)	Reduction in HF
EWPHE (107)	840	>60	22%
Coope (108)	884	60–79	32%
STOP-HTN (109)	1627	70–84	51%
SHEP (110)	4736	≥60	55%
Syst-Eur (111)	4695	≥60	36%
STONE (112)	1632	60–79	68%

HF, heart failure; EWPHE, European Working Party on Hypertension in the Elderly; SHEP, Systolic Hypertension in the Elderly Program; STONE, Shanghai Trial of Nifedipine in the Elderly; STOP-HTN, Swedish Trial in Old Patients with Hypertension; Syst-Eur, Systolic Hypertension in Europe Trial.

be hospitalized, intubated, subjected to other life-sustaining interventions (e.g., a feeding tube), or resuscitated. Because patients often change their minds about these issues as clinical circumstances evolve (104), it is important to maintain open communication throughout the disease process.

End-stage HF is frequently accompanied by considerable discomfort and anxiety, and data from the SUPPORT study indicate that most patients and families express concerns about the quality of end-of-life care (105, 106). A cardinal principal of end-of-life care is to provide adequate relief of pain and suffering through the judicious use of conventional therapies in conjunction with narcotics (e.g., morphine), sedatives (e.g., benzodiazepines), and other comfort measures. Equally important is the provision of emotional support for the patient and family, assisted by nurses, members of the clergy, social service representatives, and other qualified health care professionals.

FUTURE DIRECTIONS

In light of the high prevalence and poor prognosis associated with HF in the elderly, it is evident that more effective means for the prevention and treatment of this disorder are needed. At present, the most effective preventive strategies involve aggressive treatment of established risk factors for the development of HF (i.e., hypertension and coronary heart disease). Several studies have shown that even modest reductions in blood pressure are associated with substantial reductions in incident HF among elderly hypertensive patients (Table 5) (107–112). Likewise, treatment of elevated cholesterol levels with an hydroxymethylglutaryl-coen-

Table 6
New Approaches to the Treatment of Chronic Heart Failure

Pharmacological agents
Neutral endopeptidase inhibitors
Endothelin receptor antagonists
Cytokine inhibitors
Calcium sensitizers
Therapeutic angiogenesis and anti-angiogenesis
Inhibition of apoptosis
Gene therapy and pharmacogenomics
Hereditary disorders (e.g., cardiomyopathies, dyslipidemias)
Modulation of signaling pathways
Targeted therapy based on specific genetic profile
Biventricular pacing
Implantable assist devices
Cell transplantation and growth factor therapy
Xenotransplantation
Prevention of cardiovascular aging

zyme A reductase inhibitor ("statin") has been shown to decrease incident HF following an acute coronary event (113). Similarly, it is likely that smoking cessation, weight control in obese patients, and aggressive control of diabetes will all lead to a reduction in HF. Finally, thrombolysis and coronary angioplasty reduce infarct size and the subsequent risk for HF in patients with acute MI, and the more widespread application of reperfusion therapies in elderly patients with acute MI should be strongly encouraged.

Asymptomatic left ventricular systolic dysfunction is associated with a high rate of progression to clinical HF, and ACE inhibitors have been shown to reduce the incidence of HF in these patients (45,114). Therefore, documented systolic dysfunction mandates ACE inhibitor therapy even in the absence of symptoms. Although routine screening for left ventricular dysfunction is not justified at the present time, screening echocardiography may be worthwhile in high-risk older patients, such as those with known coronary heart disease or multiple coronary risk factors (115).

In addition to existing therapies, several new treatments for HF, both pharmacological and technological, are currently under active investigation (Table 6). Although it is difficult to project which of these new therapies will ultimately come into widespread clinical use, it is likely that the management of HF will undergo substantial evolution over the course of the next several decades; indeed, we may be on the threshold of radical changes in the paradigm of HF prevention and therapy.

Finally, current treatment of HF in the elderly is characterized by marked underutilization of proven therapies *(116)*, insufficient evidence to guide treatment in major patient subgroups (e.g., octogenarians and beyond, nursing home residents, patients with advanced co-morbidities, and individuals with diastolic HF), and inattention to critically important psychobehavioral issues (e.g., compliance, personal preferences, and end-of-life care). Thus, there is a need for additional research aimed at developing more effective strategies for the prevention and treatment of acute and chronic HF in older adults.

REFERENCES

1. American Heart Association. Heart disease and stroke statistics—2003 update. Dallas, TX: American Heart Association, 2002. http://www.americanheart.org
2. National Heart, Lung, and Blood Institute. Congestive heart failure in the United States: a new epidemic. National Heart, Lung, and Blood Institute Data Fact Sheet, 1996. http://www.nhlbi.nih.gov/health/public/heart/other/HF_abs.htm.
3. Centers for Disease Control and Prevention. Trends in ischemic heart disease mortality—United States, 1980–1988. MMWR 1992;41:548–549; 555–556.
4. Centers for Disease Control and Prevention. Cerebrovascular disease mortality and Medicare hospitalization—United States, 1980–1990. MMWR 1992;41:477–480.
5. Rich MW. Epidemiology, pathophysiology, and etiology of congestive heart failure in older adults. J Am Geriatr Soc 1997;45:968–974.
6. Kannel WB, Belanger AJ. Epidemiology of heart failure. Am Heart J 1991;121: 951–957.
7. Hall MJ, Frances CJ. 2001 National Hospital Discharge Survey. Advance data from vital and health statistics; no. 332. Hyattsville, MD: National Center for Health Statistics, 2003.
8. Popovic JR. 1999 National Hospital Discharge Survey: Annual summary with detailed diagnosis and procedure data. National Center for Health Statistics. Vital Health Stat 2001;13(151).
9. Hobbs FDR, Kenkre JE, Roalfe AK, Davis RC, Hare R, Davies MK. Impact of heart failure and left ventricular systolic dysfunction on quality of life. A cross-sectional study comparing common chronic cardiac and medical disorders and a representative adult population. Eur Heart J 2002;23:1867–1876.
10. O'Connell JB. The economic burden of heart failure. Clin Cardiol 2000;23(Suppl III):III-6–III-10.
11. Wei JY. Age and the cardiovascular system. N Engl J Med 1992;327:1735–1739.
12. Lakatta EG. Cardiovascular aging in health. Clin Geriatr Med 2000;16:419–443.
12a. Fleg JL, Bos AG, Brant LH, O'Connor FC. Longitudinal decline of aerobic capacity accelerates with age. Circulation 2000;102(Suppl II):II-602.
13. Vasan RS, Larson MG, Benjamin EJ, Evans JC, Reiss CK, Levy D. Congestive heart failure in subjects with normal versus reduced left ventricular ejection fraction: prevalence and mortality in a population-based cohort. J Am Coll Cardiol 1999; 33:1948–1955.
14. Kitzman DW, Gardin JM, Gottdiener JS, et al. Importance of heart failure with preserved systolic function in patients ≥ 65 years of age. CHS Research Group. Cardiovascular Health Study. Am J Cardiol 2001;87:413–419.

15. Gaasch WH, Levine HJ, Quinones MA, Alexander JK. Left ventricular compliance: Mechanisms and clinical implications. Am J Cardiol 1976;38:645–653.
16. Wong WF, Gold S, Fukuyama O, Blanchette PL. Diastolic dysfunction in elderly patients with congestive heart failure. Am J Cardiol 1989;63:1526–1528.
17. Tresch DD. Clinical manifestations, diagnostic assessment, and etiology of heart failure in elderly patients. Clin Geriatr Med 2000;16:445–456.
18. Rockwood K. Acute confusion in elderly medical patients. J Am Geriatr Soc 1989; 37:150–154.
19. Maisel AS, Krishnaswamy P, Nowak RM, et al. Rapid measurement of B-type natriuretic peptide in the emergency diagnosis of heart failure. N Engl J Med 2002; 347:161–167.
20. Krishnaswamy P, Lubien E, Clopton P, et al. Utility of B-natriuretic peptide levels in identifying patients with left ventricular systolic or diastolic dysfunction. Am J Med 2001;111:274–279.
21. Lubien E, DeMaria A, Krishnaswamy P, et al. Utility of B-natriuretic peptide in detecting diastolic dysfunction: comparison with Doppler velocity recordings. Circulation 2002;105:595–601.
22. Kazanegra R, Cheng V, Garcia A, et al. A rapid test for B-type natriuretic peptide correlates with falling wedge pressures in patients treated for decompensated heart failure: a pilot study. J Card Fail 2001;7:21–29.
23. Anand IS, Fisher LD, Chiang YT, et al. Changes in brain natriuretic peptide and norepinephrine over time and mortality and morbidity in the Valsartan Heart Failure Trial (Val-HeFT). Circulation 2003;107:1278–1283.
24. de Lemos JA, McGuire DK, Drazner MH. B-type natriuretic peptide in cardiovascular disease. Lancet 2003;362:316–322.
25. Redfield MM, Rodeheffer RJ, Jacobsen SJ, Mahoney DW, Bailey KR, Burnett JC Jr. Plasma brain natriuretic peptide concentration: impact of age and gender. J Am Coll Cardiol 2002;40:976–982.
26. Hunt SA, Baker DW, Chin MH, et al. ACC/AHA guidelines for the evaluation and management of chronic heart failure in the adult. J Am Coll Cardiol 2001;38: 2101–2113.
27. Gottdiener JS, Arnold AM, Aurigemma GP, et al. Predictors of congestive heart failure in the elderly: the Cardiovascular Health Study. J Am Coll Cardiol 2000;35: 1628–1637.
28. Levy D, Larson MG, Vasan RS, Kannel WB, Ho KK. The progression from hypertension to congestive heart failure. JAMA 1996;275:1557–1562.
29. Ghali JK, Kadakia S, Cooper R, Ferlinz J. Precipitating factors leading to decompensation of heart failure: traits among urban blacks. Arch Intern Med 1988;148: 2013–2016.
30. Vinson JM, Rich MW, Shah AS, Sperry JC. Early readmission of elderly patients with congestive heart failure. J Am Geriatr Soc 1990;38:1290–1295.
31. Rich MW, Freedland KE, Shah AS, Vinson JM, Kuru T, Sperry JC. Iatrogenic congestive heart failure in older adults: Clinical course and prognosis. J Am Geriatr Soc 1996;44:638–643.
32. Rich MW, Kitzman DW. Heart failure in octogenarians: a fundamentally different disease. Am J Geriatr Cardiol 2000;9(Suppl):97–104.
33. Chobanian AV, Bakris GL, Black HR, et al. The Seventh Report of the Joint National Committee on Prevention, Detection, Evaluation, and Treatment of High Blood Pressure: the JNC 7 report. JAMA 2003;289:2560–2572.
34. Slaughter MS, Ward HB. Surgical management of heart failure. Clin Geriatr Med 2000;16:567–592.

35. Geholt A, Mullany CJ, Ilstrup D, et al. Aortic valve replacement in patients aged eighty years and older: early and long-term results. J Thorac Cardiovasc Surg 1996; 111:1026–1036.
36. Bolling SF, Deeb GM, Bach DS. Mitral valve reconstruction in elderly, ischemic patients. Chest 1996;109:35–40.
37. Marzo K, Prigent FM, Steingart RM. Interventional therapy in heart failure management. Clin Geriatr Med 2000;16:549–566.
38. Shapiro LM, Hassanein H, Crowley JJ. Mitral balloon valvuloplasty in patients > 70 years of age with severe mitral stenosis. Am J Cardiol 1995;75:633–636.
39. Sutaria N, Elder AT, Shaw TR. Long term outcome of percutaneous mitral balloon valvotomy in patients age 70 and over. Heart 2000;83:433–438.
40. Wyse DG, Waldo AL, DiMarco JP, et al. A comparison of rate control and rhythm control in patients with atrial fibrillation. N Engl J Med 2002;347:1825–1833.
41. Van Gelder IC, Hagens VE, Bosker HA, et al. A comparison of rate control and rhythm control in patients with recurrent persistent atrial fibrillation. N Engl J Med 2002;347:1834–1840.
42. Page J, Henry D. Consumption of NSAIDs and the development of congestive heart failure in elderly patients. An underrecognized public health problem. Arch Intern Med 2000;160:777–784.
43. Garg R, Yusuf S, for the Collaborative Group on ACE Inhibitor Trials. Overview of randomized trials of angiotensin-converting enzyme inhibitors on mortality and morbidity in patients with heart failure. JAMA 1995;273:1450–1456.
44. Flather MD, Yusuf S, Kober L, et al. Long-term ACE-inhibitor therapy in patients with heart failure or left-ventricular dysfunction: a systematic overview of data from individual patients. Lancet 2000;355:1575–1581.
45. Pfeffer MA, Braunwald E, Moyé LA, et al. Effect of captopril on mortality and morbidity in patients with left ventricular dysfunction after myocardial infarction. N Engl J Med 1992;327:669–677.
46. The SOLVD Investigators. Effect of enalapril on survival in patients with reduced left ventricular ejection fractions and congestive heart failure. N Engl J Med 1991; 325:293–302.
47. The Acute Infarction Ramipril Efficacy (AIRE) Study Investigators. Effect of ramipril on mortality and morbidity of survivors of acute myocardial infarction with clinical evidence of heart failure. Lancet 1993;342:821–828.
48. Packer M, Poole-Wilson PA, Armstrong PW, et al. Comparative effects of low and high doses of the angiotensin-converting enzyme inhibitor, lisinopril, on morbidity and mortality in chronic heart failure. Circulation 1999;100:2312–2318.
49. Pitt B, Segal R, Martinez FA, et al. Randomised trial of losartan versus captopril in patients over 65 with heart failure (Evaluation of Losartan in the Elderly Study, ELITE). Lancet 1997;349:747–752.
50. Pitt B, Poole-Wilson PA, Segal R, et al. Effect of losartan compared with captopril on mortality in patients with symptomatic heart failure: randomized trial—the Losartan Heart Failure Survival Study ELITE II. Lancet 2000;355:1582–1587.
51. Dickstein K, Kjekshus J for the OPTIMAAL Steering Committee of the OPTIMAAL Study Group. Effects of losartan and captopril on mortality and morbidity in high-risk patients after acute myocardial infarction: the OPTIMAAL randomized trial. Optimal Trial in Myocardial Infarction with Angiotensin II Antagonist Losartan. Lancet 2002;360:752–760.
52. Maggioni AP, Anand I, Gottlieb SO, et al. Effects of valsartan on morbidity and mortality in patients with heart failure not receiving angiotensin-converting enzyme inhibitors. J Am Coll Cardiol 2002;40:1414–1421.

53. Granger CB, McMurray JJV, Yusuf S, et al. Effects of candesartan in patients with chronic heart failure and reduced left-ventricular systolic function intolerant to angiotensin-converting-enzyme inhibitors: the CHARM-Alternative trial. Lancet 2003; 362:772–776.

54. Cohn JN, Tognoni G and the Valsartan Heart Failure Trial Investigators. A randomized trial of the angiotensin-receptor blocker valsartan in chronic heart failure. N Engl J Med 2001;345:1667–1675.

55. McMurray JJV, Ostergren J, Swedberg K, et al. Effects of candesartan in patients with chronic heart failure and reduced left-ventricular systolic function taking angiotensin-converting-enzyme inhibitors: the CHARM-Added trial. Lancet 2003;362: 767–771.

56. Cohn JN, Archibald DG, Ziesche S, et al. Effect of vasodilator therapy on mortality in chronic congestive heart failure. Results of a Veterans Administration Cooperative Study. N Engl J Med 1986;314:1547–1552.

57. Cohn JN, Johnson G, Ziesche S, et al. A comparison of enalapril with hydralazine-isosorbide dinitrate in the treatment of chronic congestive heart failure. N Engl J Med 1991;325:303–310.

58. Packer M, Bristow MR, Cohn JN, et al. The effect of carvedilol on morbidity and mortality in patients with chronic heart failure. N Engl J Med 1996;334:1349–1355.

59. CIBIS-II Investigators and Committees. The Cardiac Insufficiency Bisoprolol Study II (CIBIS II): a randomized trial. Lancet 1999;353:9–13.

60. Effect of metoprolol CR/XL in chronic heart failure: Metoprolol CR/XL Randomised Intervention Trial in Congestive Heart Failure (MERIT-HF). Lancet 1999; 353:2001–2007.

61. Packer M, Coats AJS, Fowler MB, et al. Effect of carvedilol on survival in severe chronic heart failure. N Engl J Med 2001;344:1651–1658.

62. Poole-Wilson PA, Swedberg K, Cleland JGF, et al. Comparison of carvedilol and metoprolol on clinical outcomes in patients with chronic heart failure in the Carvedilol Or Metoprolol European Trial (COMET): randomised controlled trial. Lancet 2003;362:7–13.

63. The Digitalis Investigation Group. The effect of digoxin on mortality and morbidity in patients with heart failure. N Engl J Med 1997;336:525–533.

64. Rich MW, McSherry F, Williford WO, Yusuf S, for the Digitalis Investigation Group. Effect of age on mortality, hospitalizations, and response to digoxin in patients with heart failure: The DIG Study. J Am Coll Cardiol 2001;38:806–813.

65. Rathore SS, Wang Y, Krumholz HM. Sex-based differences in the effect of digoxin for the treatment of heart failure. N Engl J Med 2002;347:1403–1411.

66. Rathore SS, Curtis JP, Wang Y, Bristow MR, Krumholz HM. Association of serum digoxin concentration and outcomes in patients with heart failure. JAMA 2003;289: 871–878.

67. Slatton ML, Irani WN, Hall SA, et al. Does digoxin provide additional hemodynamic and autonomic rhythm? J Am Coll Cardiol 1997;29:1206–1213.

68. Pitt B, Zannad F, Remme WJ, et al. The effect of spironolactone on morbidity and mortality in patients with severe heart failure. Randomized Aldactone Evaluation Study Investigators. N Engl J Med 1999;341:709–717.

69. Pitt B, Perez A, for the Randomized Aldactone Study Investigators. Spironolactone in patients with heart failure. N Engl J Med 2000;342:133–134.

70. Pitt B, Remme W, Zannad F, et al. Eplerenone, a selective aldosterone blocker, in patients with left ventricular dysfunction after myocardial infarction. N Engl J Med 2003;348:1309–1321.

71. Wrenger E, Muller R, Moesenthin M, Welte T, Frolich JC, Neumann KH. Interaction of spironolactone with ACE inhibitors or angiotensin receptor blockers: analysis of 44 cases. BMJ 2003;327:147–149.
72. Yusuf S, Sleight P, Pogue J, Bosch J, Davies R, Dagenais G. Effects of an angiotensin-converting-enzyme inhibitor, ramipril, on cardiovascular events in high-risk patients. The Heart Outcomes Prevention Evaluation Study Investigators. N Engl J Med 2000;342:145–153.
73. Yusuf S, Pfeffer MA, Swedberg K, et al. Effects of candesartan in patients with chronic heart failure and preserved left-ventricular ejection fraction: the CHARM-Preserved trial. Lancet 2003;362:777–781.
74. Setaro JF, Zaret BL, Schulman DS, Black HR, Soufer R. Usefulness of verapamil for congestive heart failure associated with abnormal left ventricular diastolic filling and normal left ventricular systolic performance. Am J Cardiol 1990;66: 981–986.
75. Adan V, Crown LA. Diagnosis and treatment of sick sinus syndrome. Am Fam Phys 2003;67:1725–1732.
76. Kerwin WF, Botvinick EH, O'Connell JW, et al. Ventricular contraction abnormalities in dilated cardiomyopathy: effect of biventricular pacing to correct interventricular dyssynchrony. J Am Coll Cardiol 2000;35:1221–1227.
77. Bakker P, Meijburg H, de Bries J, et al. Biventricular pacing in end-stage heart failure improves functional capacity and left ventricular function. J Interv Cardiac Electrophysiol 2000;4:395–404.
78. Abraham WT, Fisher WG, Smith AL, et al. for the MIRACLE Study Group. Cardiac resynchronization in chronic heart failure. N Engl J Med 2002;346:1845–1853.
79. Linde C, Leclercq C, Rex S, et al. Long-term benefits of biventricular pacing in congestive heart failure: results from the Multisite STimulation in Cardiomyopathy (MUSTIC) Study. J Am Coll Cardiol 2002;40:111–118.
80. Bradley DJ, Bradley EA, Braughman KL, et al. Cardiac resynchronization and death from progressive heart failure: a meta-analysis of randomized controlled trials. JAMA 2003;289:730–740.
81. Young JB, Abraham WT, Smith AL, et al. Combined cardiac resynchronization and implantable cardioversion defibrillation in advanced chronic heart failure: the MIRACLE ICD Trial. JAMA 2003;289:2685–2694.
82. Moss AJ, Zareba W, Hall WJ, et al. Prophylactic implantation of a defibrillator in patients with myocardial infarction and reduced ejection fraction. N Engl J Med 2002;346:877–883.
83. Moss AJ, Hall WJ, Cannom DS, et al. Improved survival with an implanted defibrillator in patients with coronary disease at high risk for ventricular arrhythmia. Multicenter Automatic Defibrillator Implantation Trial Investigators. N Engl J Med 1996;335:1933–1940.
84. Ezekowitz JA, Armstrong PW, McAlister FA. Implantable cardioverter defibrillators in primary and secondary prevention: a systematic review of randomized, controlled trials. Ann Intern Med 2003;138:445–452.
84a. Bardy GH, Lee KL, Mark DB, et al. Amiodarone or an implantable cardioverter-defibrillator for congestive heart failure. N Engl J Med 2005;352:225–237.
85. Sheldon R, Connolly S, Krahn A, Roberts R, Gent M, Gardner M. Identification of patients most likely to benefit from implantable cardioverter-defibrillator therapy: the Canadian Implantable Defibrillator Study. Circulation 2000;101:1660–1664.
86. Camm AJ, Nisam S. The utilization of the implantable defibrillator—a European enigma. Eur Heart J 2000;21:1998–2004.

87. Exner DV, Klein GJ, Prystowsky EN. Primary prevention of sudden death with implantable defibrillator therapy in patients with cardiac disease: Can we afford to do it? (Can we afford not to?) Circulation 2001;104:1564–1570.

88. Weiss JP, Saynina O, McDonald KM, McClellan MB, Hlatky MA. Effectiveness and cost-effectiveness of implantable cardioverter defibrillators in the treatment of ventricular arrhythmias among Medicare beneficiaries. Am J Med 2002;112: 519–527.

89. Krumholz HM, Butler J, Miller J, et al. Prognostic importance of emotional support for elderly patients hospitalized with heart failure. Circulation 1998;97:958–964.

90. Rich MW. Heart failure disease management: A critical review. J Cardiac Failure 1999;5:64–75.

91. McAlister FA, Lawson FM, Teo KK, Armstrong PW. A systematic review of randomized trials of disease management programs in heart failure. Am J Med 2001; 110:378–384.

92. Rich MW, Nease RF. Cost-effectiveness analysis in clinical practice: the case of heart failure. Arch Intern Med 1999;159:1690–1700.

93. Pina IL, Apstein CS, Balady GJ, et al. Exercise and heart failure: A statement from the American Heart Association Committee on exercise, rehabilitation, and prevention. Circulation 2003;107:1210–1225.

94. McKelvie RS, Teo KK, Roberts R, et al. Effects of exercise training in patients with heart failure: the Exercise Rehabilitation Trial (EXERT). Am Heart J 2002; 144:23–30.

95. Hambrecht R, Gielen S, Linke A, et al. Effects of exercise training on left ventricular function and peripheral resistance in patients with chronic heart failure: A randomized trial. JAMA 2000;283:3095–3101.

96. Belardinelli R, Georgiou D, Cianci G, Purcaro A. Randomized controlled trial of long-term moderate exercise training in chronic heart failure: effects on functional capacity, quality of life, and clinical outcome. Circulation 1999;99:1173–1182.

97. Keteyian SJ, Levine AB, Brawner CA, et al. Exercise training in patients with heart failure: A randomized, controlled trial. Ann Intern Med 1996;124:1051–1057.

98. Hare DL, Ryan TM, Selig SE, Pellizzer AM, Wrigley TV, Krum H. Resistance exercise training increases muscle strength, endurance, and blood flow in patients with chronic heart failure. Am J Cardiol 1999;83:1674–1677.

99. Croft JB, Giles WH, Pollard RA, Keenan NL, Casper ML, Anda RF. Heart failure survival among older adults in the United States: a poor prognosis for an emerging epidemic in the Medicare population. Arch Intern Med 1999;159:505–510.

100. MacIntyre K, Capewell S, Stewart S, et al. Evidence of improving prognosis in heart failure. Trends in case fatality in 66,547 patients hospitalized between 1986 and 1995. Circulation 2000;102:1126–1131.

101. Stewart S, MacIntyre K, Hole DJ, et al. More "malignant" than cancer? Five-year survival following a first admission for heart failure. Eur J Heart Failure 2001;3: 315–322.

102. Krumholz HM, Chen YT, Vaccarino V, et al. Correlates and impact on outcomes of worsening renal function in patients ≥ 65 years of age with heart failure. Am J Cardiol 2000;85:1110–1113.

103. Freisinger GC, Butler J. End-of-life care for elderly patients with heart failure. Clin Geriatr Med 2000;16:663–675.

104. Krumholz HM, Phillips RS, Hamel MB, et al. Resuscitation preferences among patients with severe congestive heart failure: results from the SUPPORT project.

Study to Understand Prognoses and Preferences for Outcomes and Risks of Treatments. Circulation 1998;98:648–655.

105. Levenson JW, McCarthy EP, Lynn J, Davis RB, Phillips RS. The last six months of life for patients with congestive heart failure. J Am Geriatr Soc 2000;48:S101–S109.

106. Baker R, Hyg MS, Wu AW, et al. Family satisfaction with end-of-life care in seriously ill hospitalized adults. J Am Geriatr Soc 2000;48:S61–S69.

107. Amery A, Birkenhager W, Brixko P, et al. Mortality and morbidity results from the European Working Party on High Blood Pressure in the Elderly Trial. Lancet 1985; I:1349–1354.

108. Coope J, Warrender TS. Randomised trial of treatment of hypertension in elderly patients in primary care. BMJ 1986;293:1145–1151.

109. Dahlof B, Lindholm LH, Hannson L, Schersten B, Ekbom T, Wester PO. Morbidity and mortality in the Swedish Trial in Old Patients with Hypertension (STOP-Hypertension). Lancet 1991;338:1281–1285.

110. The Systolic Hypertension in the Elderly Program (SHEP) Cooperative Research Group. Prevention of stroke by antihypertensive drug treatment in older persons with isolated systolic hypertension: final results of SHEP. JAMA 1991;265:3255–3264.

111. Staessen JA, Fagard R, Thijs L, et al. Randomised double-blind comparison of placebo and active treatment for older patients with isolated systolic hypertension. The Systolic Hypertension in Europe (Syst-Eur) Trial Investigators. Lancet 1997; 350:757–764.

112. Gong L, Zhang W, Zhu Y, et al. Shanghai Trial of Nifedipine in the Elderly (STONE). J Hypertens 1996;14:1237–1245.

113. Kjekshus J, Pedersen TR, Olsson AG, Faergeman O, Pyorala K. The effects of simvastatin on the incidence of heart failure in patients with coronary heart disease. J Card Failure 1997;3:249–254.

114. The SOLVD Investigators. Effect of enalapril on mortality and the development of heart failure in asymptomatic patients with reduced left ventricular ejection fractions. N Engl J Med 1992;327:685–691.

115. McMurray JV, McDonagh TA, Davie AP, Cleland JG, Francis CM, Morrison C. Should we screen for asymptomatic left ventricular dysfunction to prevent heart failure? Eur Heart J 1998;19:842–846.

116. Krumholz HM, Wang Y, Parent EM, Mockalis J, Petrillo M, Radford MJ. Quality of care for elderly patients hospitalized with heart failure. Arch Intern Med 1997; 157:2242–2247.

10   Valvular Heart Disease in the Elderly

Milind Y. Desai, MD
and Gary Gerstenblith, MD

CONTENTS

INTRODUCTION
DISEASES OF THE AORTIC VALVE
DISEASES OF THE MITRAL VALVE
CONCLUSION
REFERENCES

INTRODUCTION

Valvular disease continues to be an important cause of morbidity and mortality across the globe with an increasing number of elderly patients affected by "degenerative" valvular diseases on top of a background incidence of unrecognized rheumatic and infective endocarditis (1–3). Although there are no recent population-based data regarding the prevalence of valvular heart disease in the elderly, several studies have provided relevant information (4,5) (Table 1). Aortic stenosis and ischemic mitral regurgitation are the most common valvular disorders in the elderly.

The diagnosis and management of valvular disease in the elderly have been influenced by the dramatic increase in the life expectancy and the number of geriatric patients in the last half of the 20th century. In the United States, for instance, it is estimated that the number of octogenarians was around 7.4 million in the early 1990s (3% of the population) with a life expectancy of 6.9 years in men and 8.7 years in women. The number exceeded 10 million by the year 2000 and constituted 4.3% of the population (6). As the human life span increases and health care

From: Contemporary Cardiology: Cardiovascular Disease in the Elderly
Edited by: G. Gerstenblith © Humana Press Inc., Totowa, NJ

Table 1
Prevalence of Significant Valvular Heart Disease in the Elderly

Valvular abnormality	60–69 years	>70 years
Aortic stenosis	—	5%
Aortic regurgitation	3.7%	2.2%
Mitral regurgitation	2.3%	5.5%
Tricuspid regurgitation	0.9%	3.6%

Adapted from refs. *4* and *5.*

quality improves, more people are reaching an advanced age to present with cardiac disorders that might be treated uneventfully in younger patients. However, in the elderly, there is an important balance between enhanced initial risks and eventual benefits, which are often reduced in the geriatric population. This can lead to difficult medical, as well as ethical and economic decisions. Although there is a substantial variation between chronological and physiological ages, the capacity of elderly patients to withstand a major insult like cardiac surgery is usually reduced because of associated co-morbidities, diminished functional reserve of vital organs, and reduced adaptation capacities *(6)*. It is estimated that the prevalence of co-morbidities in octogenarians with valvular heart disease is as follows: 40%–60% coronary artery disease (CAD), 15%–25% obstructive lung disease, 5%–10% renal insufficiency, 2%–10% peripheral vascular disease, 20%–50% hypertension, 10%–20% diabetes mellitus (DM), and 5%–25% cerebrovascular disease *(6)*. In addition, transesophageal echocardiography (TEE) has demonstrated that 20% of patients older than 70 years have complex atherosclerosis in the ascending aorta and the transverse arch *(7)*, which significantly increases the risk of embolization during cardiac surgical procedures. Finally, impaired cerebral perfusion is another factor that should be considered in the geriatric age group. Potential contributors include non-pulsatile bypass flow, altered cerebral autoregulation, and atherosclerosis, all of which lead to delayed awakening, agitation, and incomplete return of cognitive function, the effects of which can be devastating. It is estimated that 15% to 20% of elderly patients have focal or diffuse neurological deficits after cardiac surgery *(6)*. Fortunately, major advances in cardiac surgery have improved the outcomes of surgical treatment in elderly patients who in the past might not have been operative candidates. Also, studies have shown that among surgical survivors, function and quality of life are similar to those in a general population of age-matched subjects *(8–10)*. Hence, the classic thought that valve surgery should be considered only for elderly patients in excellent general health is being challenged as higher success rates are being obtained in elderly patients with non-serious co-morbidities *(11)*. This chapter will provide a detailed outline of the diagnosis and management of commonly encountered valvular problems in the geriatric age group.

DISEASES OF THE AORTIC VALVE
Aortic Stenosis
ETIOLOGY, RISK FACTORS, AND PATHOPHYSIOLOGY

Calcific aortic stenosis is the most common valvular abnormality in the geriatric age group and accounts for 82% of cases in patients over 65 years *(12)* and 90% of aortic valve replacements in patients over 75 years *(13)*. In the Helsinki Aging Study, the prevalence of at least moderate aortic stenosis in patients aged 75 to 86 years was 5% and that of critical aortic stenosis was 6% at 86 years of age *(5)*. Recent studies demonstrate a similarity in risk-factor profile for atherosclerosis and calcific aortic stenosis. The Cardiovascular Health Study demonstrated that the risk factors for the development of calcific aortic stensosis were age, with a twofold increased risk with every decade; male gender, also a twofold increased risk; current smoking, 35% increased risk; hypertension, 20% increased risk; and elevated low-density lipoprotein and lipoprotein (a) levels *(14)*.

The pathophysiological hallmark of calcific aortic stenosis is gradually progressive obstruction to left ventricular emptying, leading to an adaptive hypertrophic response, to generate greater systolic pressure. The multiple pathophysiological sequelae of aortic stenosis are schematically demonstrated in Fig. 1.

CLINICAL FEATURES

Aortic stenosis is characterized by a long latent period during which patients are asymptomatic and, often, the diagnosis is incidentally made at the time of a routine physical examination. However, advanced aortic stenosis is associated with dyspnea/congestive heart failure (CHF), angina pectoris, and syncope. Dyspnea on exertion can be the result of a combination of systolic and diastolic dysfunction with overt heart failure and in the setting of significant left ventricular dysfunction is a late and terminal finding. Association of atrial fibrillation (AF) is unusual with isolated aortic stenosis, but can occur in association with heart failure, and its occurrence can trigger significant debilitation. Syncope can occur for various reasons: hypotension owing to exercise-induced vasodilatation in the setting of a fixed obstruction, a tachy- or bradyarrhythmia, and/or an abnormal baroreceptor response. Effort-related angina can be the result

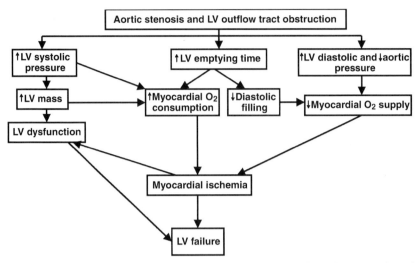

Fig. 1. Schematic representation of the various pathophysiological sequelae of aortic stenosis.

of concomitant CAD (in about 50% of the cases) and/or to other mechanisms as demonstrated in Fig. 1. Increased cardiac mass can lead to increased myocardial oxygen demand, reduced coronary flow reserve, reduced coronary perfusion time and pressure, and compression of intramyocardial arteries *(15)*. Once these symptoms develop, the prognosis is grim without surgical intervention. It is reported that the time from symptom onset to death is 2 years with heart failure, 3 years with syncope, and 5 years with angina *(16)*. Another common finding in patients with calcific aortic stenosis is gastrointestinal bleeding, commonly owing to angiodysplasia (Heyde's syndrome) *(17)*. The risk of bleeding is thought to be caused by an acquired von Willebrand syndrome owing to disruption of von Willebrand multimers during passage through the narrowed valve *(18)*. There is a linear relationship between the severity of the von Willebrand factor abnormality and the mean aortic gradient *(18)*. Infective endocarditis is a rare sequelae of calcific aortic stenosis and isolated reports describe systemic embolic events associated with calcific aortic stenosis. However, in a cohort study comparing 515 patients with calcific aortic stenosis, 300 with a calcified nonstenotic aortic valve and 562 controls, there were no significant differences in stroke rates *(19)*.

Physical examination is often useful in determining the severity of aortic stenosis and it has been demonstrated that the delay of carotid upstroke, timing, and intensity of the murmur and absence of the aortic component of second heart sound correlate with aortic stenosis severity *(20)*. The arterial pulse is characteristically described as *parvus et tardus* i.e., weak and slow rising, best appreciated in the carotid artery and associated with a thrill. Age-associated increased central vascular stiffness, however, may result in a normal pressure rise in the setting of significant stenosis. The apical impulse is sustained and usually not displaced until late in the course of the disease when left ventricular dilatation occurs. Upon auscultation, S1 is usually normal, the aortic component of S2 is diminished and at times absent. S2 can be paradoxically split when stenosis is severe or ventricular dysfunction develops. An S4 gallop might also be present. A harsh systolic murmur heard best at the base of the heart with radiation to the carotids is characteristic. The murmur peaks early in mild stenosis and moves later with advancing degrees of stenosis. When the murmur radiates to the apex, it might have a musical quality and mimic that of mitral regurgitation (Gallivardin phenomenon). An associated diastolic aortic regurgitation murmur is common in older patients with calcified rigid aortic valves.

DIAGNOSIS

Although physical examination is important in the diagnosis of aortic stenosis, there is a significant role of diagnostic modalities in ascertaining the severity of the disease and the feasibility of a surgical operation. The electrocardiogram (EKG) may demonstrate left ventricular hypertrophy (LVH). AF is uncommon early in the course of the disease and its presence often indicates concomitant mitral valve disease. The chest radiograph is usually normal in early cases, but might show changes of LVH and valvular calcification in later stages. Echocardiography is a very reliable modality in assessing the severity of the disease (Fig. 2). In degenerative aortic stenosis, it usually demonstrates thickened calcific valves with a reduced excursion and a significantly reduced aortic orifice. In later stages, there is evidence of concentric LVH. Doppler examination usually allows estimation of aortic gradients (both peak and mean) and calculation of aortic valve area by the continuity equation. Aortic valve area can also be calculated by planimetry during TEE. Table 2 details the criteria for determining the severity of aortic stenosis. The American College of Cardiologists (ACC)/American Heart Association (AHA) guidelines detailing the role of echocardiography in aortic stenosis are listed in Table 3 *(11)*.

The importance of cardiac catheterization for assessment of the severity of aortic stenosis has lessened in the last few years but still remains an important modality in cases where noninvasive techniques are inadequate. It can be used to assess the peak and mean valve gradients and to

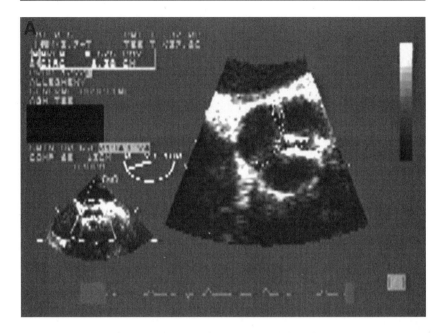

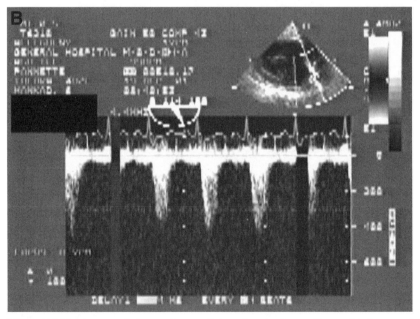

Fig. 2. (**A**) Planimetered short axis two-dimensional echocardiographic image of the aortic valve demonstrating severe calcific aortic stenosis. (**B**) A continuous-wave Doppler image in the same patient with the sample volume in the left ventricular outflow tract demonstrating significantly elevated gradient consistent with severe aortic stenosis.

Table 2
Criteria for Determining the Severity of Aortic and Mitral Stenosis

Aortic stenosis severity	Mean gradient (mmHg)	Valve area (cm²)
Mild	<25	>1.5
Moderate	25–50	1.0–1.5
Severe	>50	<1.0
Critica	>80	<0.7
Mitral stenosis severity	Mean gradient (mmHg)	Valve area (cm²)
Mild	<5.0	>1.5
Moderate	5.0–10.0	1.0–1.5
Severe	>10.0	<1.0

calculate the valve area using the Gorlin formula, which is useful in low cardiac output states *(21)*. Coronary angiography is often performed to assess whether concomitant bypass surgery is also indicated.

MANAGEMENT

Medical management, except for endocarditis prophylaxis, has a minimal role in the management of aortic stenosis. Aortic valve replacement, along with coronary revascularization, which is commonly indicated in elderly patients, remains the mainstay of treatment for symptomatic severe aortic stenosis, and accounts for 60% to 70% of the valve surgery cases *(22,23)*. The indications for surgery are similar to those for younger patients, angina, dyspnea, and syncope, and most surgeons will consider valve replacement for moderate stenosis in patients undergoing coronary revascularization. This is based on the knowledge that valve replacement increases the risk only slightly, but the progression of aortic stenosis can be very rapid in the elderly, and can quickly negate the benefits of coronary revascularization.

A controversial but important issue in aortic valve disease is the choice of a bioprosthesis or a mechanical valve. The major concerns with mechanical prostheses include thromboembolism and complications of chronic anticoagulation *(24)*. Bioprosthetic valves, however, degenerate more quickly and are less durable. The older the patient, the less of an issue the shorter functional lifetime of the bioprosthetic valve becomes. On the other hand, mechanical valves have smaller transvalvular gradients than bioprostheses and provide better hemodynamics, especially in

Table 3
Current Guidelines
for Echocardiography in Various Valvular Diseases

Aortic stenosis indication	*Class*
1. Diagnosis and assessment of severity of aortic stenosis	I
2. Assessment of left ventricular size and function	I
3. Re-evaluation of patient with known aortic stenosis and changing clinical scenario	I
4. Re-evaluation of asymptomatic patients with severe aortic stenosis	I
5. Re-evaluation of asymptomatic patients with mild to moderate aortic stenosis and left ventricular dysfunction or hypertrophy	IIa
6. Routine re-evaluation of asymptomatic patients with mild aortic stenosis and normal ventricular size and function	III

Aortic regurgitation indication	*Class*
1. Confirmation of the presence and severity of aortic regurgitation	I
2. Diagnosis of chronic aortic regurgitation in patients with equivocal findings	I
3. Assessment of the etiology of regurgitation	I
4. Assessment of left ventricular dimensions and function	I
5. Semi-quantitative estimate of severity of regurgitation	I
6. Re-evaluation of patients with mild, moderate or severe regurgitation and changing clinical scenario	I
7. Yearly evaluation of asymptomatic patients and stable physical examination and normal ventricular dimensions	III

Mitral stenosis indications for transthoracic echocardiography	*Class*
1. Diagnosis of stenosis, hemodynamic severity, and assessment of right ventricular size and function	I
2. Assessment of valve morphology to determine suitability for percutaneous mitral balloon valvuloplasty	I
3. Diagnosis and assessment of concomitant valvular lesions	I
4. Re-evaluation of patient with known mitral stenosis and changing clinical scenario	I
5. Assessment of hemodynamic response of mean gradient and pulmonary artery pressure by exercise echocardiography in patients with discrepant findings	IIa
6. Re-evaluation of asymptomatic patients with moderate to severe mitral stenosis to assess pulmonary artery pressure	IIb
7. Routine re-evaluation of asymptomatic patient with stable clinical findings	III

Table 3 (Continued)

Indications for transesophageal echocardiography	Class
1. Assessment for the presence of left atrial thrombus prior to cardioversion or percutaneous balloon valvuloplasty	IIa
2. Routine evaluation of mitral valve when transthoracic images are satisfactory	III

Mitral regurgitation indications for transthoracic echocardiography	Class
1. For baseline evaluation to quantify severity of regurgitation and left ventricular function	I
2. To delineate the mechanism of regurgitation	I
3. To follow left ventricular function in asymptomatic severe regurgitation	I
4. To re-evaluate after a change in symptoms	I
5. Baseline evaluation following mitral valve repair or replacement	I
6. Routine follow-up of mild regurgitation with normal dimensions and systolic function	III

Indications for transesophageal echocardiography	Class
1. Intraoperatively to establish the anatomic basis of regurgitation and to guide repair	I
2. Evaluation of patients when transthoracic images are suboptimal	I
3. Routine follow-up of patients with native valve regurgitation	III

Adapted from ref. *11*.

patients with a small annulus (<21 mm) *(25)*. A small annulus is an issue in some patients, particularly elderly females, as it leads to the selection of a smaller prosthesis leading to a residual transprosthetic gradient and hence, patient–prosthesis mismatch, which may be associated with poorer hemodynamics, less functional improvement, and higher in-hospital mortality *(26,27)*. In practice, most surgeons accept the higher residual gradient of a bioprosthesis or choose to enlarge the aortic annulus or to use the new stentless biological valve, which offers the largest opening surface and the smallest transvalvular gradient *(28)*. Thus, the vast majority of aortic valve surgeries in the elderly involve bioprosthesis, 88% in one report *(29)*, as early mortality and actuarial survival are similar with the two types of valves.

Factors affecting postoperative mortality include age, with a 14% mortality in one report for those over 80 years *(8)*, poor preoperative status, left ventricular dysfunction *(22)*, valvular calcification, and concurrent coronary artery bypass grafting (CABG) or other cardiac surgery. Post-operative mortality rates are reported in the range of 5% to 10% for iso-lated aortic valve surgery *(23,30)*, but increase to as high as 15% to 20% with concurrent coronary revascularization or other cardiac procedures *(25)*. However, octogenarians who survive the perioperative period often do well *(8,25,29)*. The 30-day cardiac and all-cause mortalities were 4% and 6.6%, respectively, whereas the actuarial survival at 1, 5, and 8 years was 89%, 69%, and 46%, respectively *(29)*.

Percutaneous balloon aortic valvuloplasty has a very limited role in the elderly because the aortic valve is usually severely calcified without com-missural fusion, making it unsuitable for dilatation. The procedure is also associated with a high incidence of residual or recurrent stenosis and serious complications including death, stroke, and aortic rupture *(31)*. Hence, it is now rarely performed. Possible reasons for its use would be to transiently improve hemodynamics prior to non-ardiac surgery and, as part of an assessment of the improvement a patient would experience with aortic valve surgery. It is not an alternative to valve replacement when the patient is a candidate for surgery. More recently, a percutaneous aortic valve stent, composed of three pericardial leaflets inserted within a balloon-expandable stainless steel stent, has been developed and its feasibility has been demonstrated in humans *(32)*. A recent study employ-ing this technique, demonstrated hemodynamic, clinical and echocar-diographic improvement in five out of six patients with end-stage calcific aortic stenosis, not considered to be surgical candidates *(33)*. Thus, it has the potential of becoming an important therapeutic option for patients not amenable to surgical valve replacement.

Aortic Sclerosis

Aortic sclerosis is defined as focal areas of thickening and echoge-nicity on the aortic valve without commissural fusion or increase in aor-tic valvular velocities (velocities <2–2.5 m/s) on echocardiography *(1)* (Fig. 3). It can be detected in up to 29% of those over age 65 and in 48% of those over age 85 *(1,5)*. Its significance stems from the findings that it can progress to aortic stenosis and it is a marker for increased cardio-vascular risk. Studies have demonstrated that the early lesion of aortic valve sclerosis involves an active process demonstrating the following findings resembling atherosclerosis *(34–38)*. Focal areas of accumula-tion of apolipoproteins B, (a) and E, areas of lipid accumulation in con-junction with macrophage and T lymphocyte infiltration and evidence of early valve calcification, including expression of osteopontin and other proteins. Echocardiographically detected aortic sclerosis progressed to

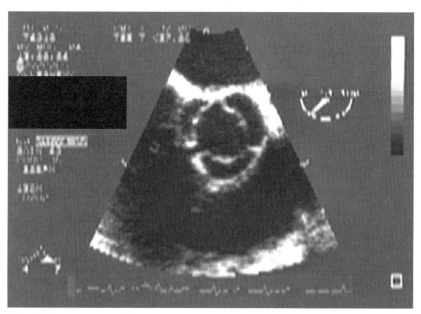

Fig. 3. Short axis two-dimensional echocardiographic image of the aortic valve demonstrating leaflet calcification, but with normal valvular excursion, consistent with aortic sclerosis.

aortic stenosis in 16% patients within 7 years (mild to moderate in 84% and severe in 16%) (39). In the 29% of patients with aortic sclerosis in the Cardiovascular Health Study, the all-cause and cardiovascular mortality, after a mean follow up of 5 years, were 22% and 10%, respectively and the relative risks of cardiovascular death and of myocardial infarction in those with aortic sclerosis without coronary disease at baseline were 1.5 and 1.4, respectively as compared to those participants with normal valves (1). Similarly, in another study of 1980 patients, baseline aortic valve sclerosis was independently associated with new cardiac events at 4 years with a risk ratio of 1.8 (40). Aortic sclerosis does not lead to left ventricular obstruction and hence in itself, is not an indication for surgery. However, because it is a risk factor for coronary heart disease and because it can progress to significant aortic stenosis, it has important implications for patient management. There are no controlled trials to confirm whether aggressive control of blood pressure or other cardiac risk factors reduce the progression of aortic valve sclerosis. Small observational studies suggest that statins slow the increase in valve leaflet calcification in aortic sclerosis (41,42). However, in the absence of a prospective randomized trial of

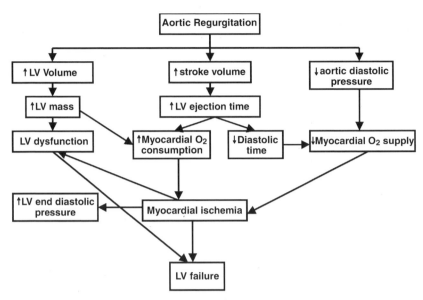

Fig. 4. Schematic representation of the various pathophysiological sequelae of aortic regurgitation.

treatment for aortic sclerosis, a prudent approach would be to stringently control cardiac risk factors including hypercholesterolemia.

Aortic Regurgitation

ETIOLOGY AND PATHOPHYSIOLOGY

Inadequate closure of the aortic valve leaflets, because of either damage to the valve leaflets or dilatation of the ascending aorta and the aortic root, leads to aortic regurgitation. In the elderly, the most common etiologies include hypertension-related dilatation of the ascending aorta, calcific aortic stenosis, and occasionally, primary aortic disease or a bicuspid aortic valve. Endocarditis or aortic dissection account for the vast majority of the acute cases. The prevalence of aortic regurgitation has been reported to be 13% in the Framingham Heart study *(4)* and 29% in the Helsinki Aging study *(5)*. The main pathophysiological phenomenon that occurs with aortic regurgitation is left ventricular volume overload. In the acute setting, there is inadequate time for compensatory ventricular dilatation leading to an inability to increase total stroke volume, and thus a decline in effective forward stroke volume and cardiac output culminating in cardiogenic shock and pulmonary edema. The multiple pathophysiological sequelae of chronic aortic regurgitation are schematically demonstrated in Fig. 4.

CLINICAL FEATURES

Patients with chronic aortic regurgitation can remain asymptomatic for decades and occasionally complain of an uncomfortable awareness of the heart beat, atypical chest pain induced by a mechanical interaction between the heart and the chest wall, and palpitations. Eventually, symptoms of left-sided CHF occur. Angina is uncommon with isolated aortic regurgitation, and its presence suggests either underlying CAD or subendocardial ischemia.

Physical findings in aortic regurgitation result from increased stroke volume leading to an abrupt distension of the peripheral arteries, whereas regurgitation back into the left ventricle leads to quick collapse of the arteries. This results in a wide pulse pressure and a "water-hammer" or Corrigan's pulse, best appreciated by palpation of the radial or brachial arteries (exaggerated by raising the arm) or the carotid pulses. Other commonly identified findings related to a hyperdynamic pulse include deMusset's sign (head bob occurring with each heart beat), Traube's sign (pistol shot pulse heard over the femoral arteries), Duroziez's sign (diastolic bruit heard when the femoral artery is partially compressed), Quincke's pulses (capillary pulsations in the fingertips or lips), and Mueller's sign (systolic pulsations of the uvula). However, none of these signs are specific for aortic regurgitation. Auscultatory sounds include a soft S1, variable S2, and an S3, the latter associated with left ventricular dilatation and dysfunction. A high-pitched, blowing decrescendo diastolic murmur begins immediately after A2 and may be soft, often appreciated only when the patient is sitting up, leaning forward, and holding his or her breath in expiration. The timing varies with severity of the disease process: blowing and occurring in early diastole in the presence of mild disease, and a rougher quality and holodiastolic in the setting of severe disease. The murmur may shorten as left ventricular diastolic pressure rises in the setting of severe decompensation. The murmur is classically heard best along the left sternal border, at the third and fourth intercostal space when due to valvular disease or at the right sternal border and apex when due to aortic root disease. Another diastolic murmur, the Austin Flint murmur, is a mid- to late-diastolic rumble heard at the apex and is the result of antegrade turbulent diastolic blood flow from the left atrium competing with the retrograde regurgitant flow from the aorta. The murmur can be distinguished from that of mitral stenosis by the absence of both a loud S1 and an opening snap of the mitral valve. A systolic ejection murmur, owing to increased forward aortic flow is often present.

In cases of acute aortic regurgitation, there is evidence of hypotension, hemodynamic collapse, tachycardia, cyanosis, and pulmonary edema.

The pulse pressure is usually normal or only slightly widened and peripheral signs are not as impressive. The early diastolic murmur is lower pitched and shorter and an Austin flint murmur, if present, is brief.

DIAGNOSIS

EKG evidence of LVH is associated with advanced regurgitation. In addition, repolarization abnormalities on the resting or exercise EKG also correlate with left ventricular size and function. The absence of these EKG abnormalities is associated with a normal left ventricular systolic dimension and a resting ejection fraction (EF) of more than 45%. In contrast, 83% of patients with resting or exercise ST-segment abnormalities had an enlarged left ventricle (>55 mm) or a reduced EF of less than 45% (43). On chest radiography, there is evidence of cardiomegaly owing to the dilatation of the left ventricle, and the ascending aorta and often the aortic arch or knob are typically markedly dilated. Echocardiography is extremely useful in determining whether the etiology of the aortic regurgitation is valvular and/or aortic, as well as to determine the hemodynamic effects, including the severity/amount of the regurgitant flow and ventricular dimensions (Figs. 5 and 6). Occasionally, a high-frequency, diastolic fluttering of the anterior leaflet of the mitral valve might be seen. The ACC/AHA recommendations for the use of echocardiography in aortic regurgitation are listed in Table 3. The role of cardiac catheterization in the diagnosis of aortic regurgitation has diminished significantly with the advent of echocardiography.

MANAGEMENT

Management of aortic regurgitation is dependent on the acuity of the process. In acute cases owing to endocarditis, early initiation of antibiotics following blood cultures is essential, and emergency replacement of the aortic root with a valve homograft (with coronary artery re-implantation) is a consideration in endocarditis not responsive to antibiotics. However, because of potential associated excessive mortality for the elderly, debridement of the annulus and valve replacement may be a better alternative (6). In cases of aortic dissection and associated regurgitation in the elderly, resection of the dissected aorta should be limited to the ascending aorta and hypothermic circulatory arrest should be avoided, if possible, particularly if the aortic arch is at a low risk for rupture (6). In chronic cases, medical therapy using vasodilators (hydralazine, nifedipine, and angiotensin-converting enzyme inhibitors) has been utilized to help reduce the degree of regurgitation (44,45), along with routine use of endocarditis prophylaxis. Valve replacement surgery for pure aortic regurgitation represents approximately 3%–5% of valve surgeries in the elderly (22).

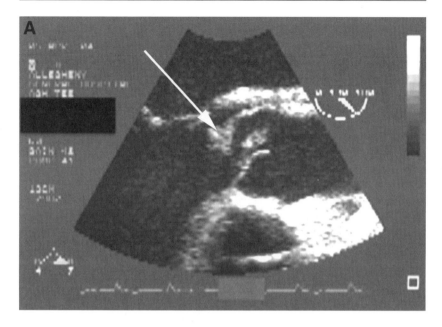

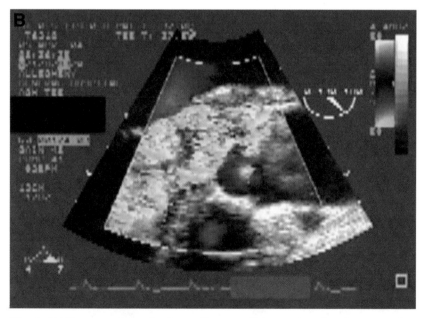

Fig. 5. (A) Transesophageal echocardiogram of the aortic valve demonstrating large echo densities (arrow) on both the leaflets, consistent with endocarditis. (B) Color Doppler image in the same view of the same patient demonstrating severe eccentric aortic regurgitation.

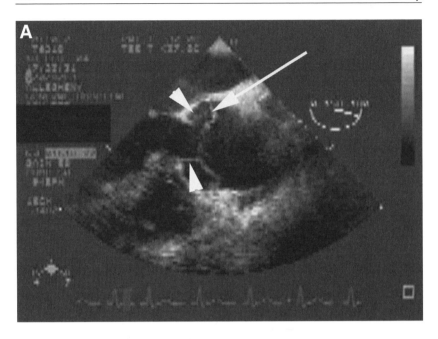

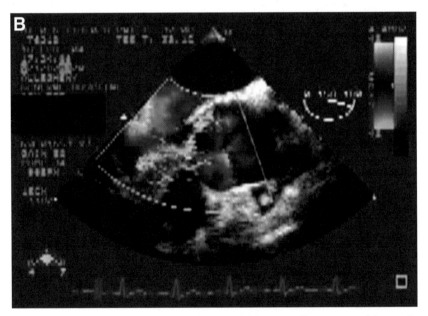

Fig. 6. (A) Transesophageal echocardiogram of the ascending aorta and the aortic valve (arrow heads) demonstrating an intimal flap (arrow), consistent with type A aortic dissection. (B) Color Doppler image in the same view of the same patient demonstrating eccentric aortic regurgitation.

In elderly patients, especially those over 80 years, surgery is generally recommended when symptoms are present. However, mild symptoms and mild heart failure should alert the physician to consider surgery. Because of a high incidence of concomitant significant CAD (approximately 33%), it might be necessary to combine CABG with aortic valve surgery. The following risk factors increase the operative mortality and morbidity: increased age, ventricular dysfunction, extensive CAD, infective endocarditis, DM, and chronic renal or pulmonary disease. Survival is approximately 80% at 5 years and 60% to 70% at 10 years postsurgery in a low-risk cohort *(46)*. The type of valve to be used is generally determined by age and the patient's ability to undergo chronic anticoagulation. Mechanical valves are less prone to deterioration than are bioprosthetic valves, particularly in the aortic position. But the incidence of systemic thromboembolism is 1%–2% per year even with adequate anticoagulation *(47)*.

Although aortic valve replacement is usually the treatment of choice for acute or chronic aortic regurgitation, aortic valve repair is sometimes possible in aortic regurgitation owing to endocarditis, and valve-sparing operations are a major consideration in patients with aortic dissection. However, if conservative surgery in these patients is not possible or questionable, standard valve replacement should be performed.

DISEASES OF THE MITRAL VALVE
Rheumatic Mitral Valve Disease

Rheumatic mitral valve disease usually manifests in young adults, but various autopsy studies have demonstrated a 2.5%–5% incidence of rheumatic mitral valve involvement in older patients. In contrast to younger patients who have thin leaflets and commissural fusion, commissural and leaflet calcification is more common in older patients *(48)*. About two-thirds of elderly patients with rheumatic mitral disease have regurgitation and a combination of regurgitation and stenosis is fairly common, along with approximately a 75% prevalence of pulmonary hypertension. This pattern is particularly common in women *(49)*. Older patients may also exhibit any of the sequelae of rheumatic disease, including AF, heart failure, and thromboembolism, a particularly common problem, and infective endocarditis, which is common in the setting of combined mitral stenosis and regurgitation.

Mitral Stenosis
ETIOLOGY AND PATHOPHYSIOLOGY

Valvular mitral stenosis continues to affect young people, and rheumatic fever remains the leading cause of mitral stenosis in all age groups

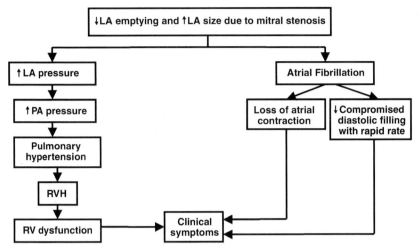

Fig. 7. Schematic representation of the various pathophysiological sequelae of mitral stenosis.

(50). However, mitral valvular obstruction due to protuberant mitral annular calcification (MAC) is increasingly being recognized in the elderly. In a series of 100 patients at least 62 years of age with MAC, 6% had mitral obstruction *(51).* The process is accelerated by the presence of systemic hypertension, DM, and genetic abnormalities of the fibrous skeleton, such as Marfan syndrome *(52).* Also, conditions associated with chronically increased left ventricular systolic pressures (such as LVH, hypertrophic cardiomyopathy, aortic stenosis, and systemic hypertension) either enhance stress on the mitral valve and apparatus, and/or promote abnormal valve motion; these effects accelerate the degenerative process, leading to calcium deposition *(53).* The primary pathophysiological mechanism in mitral stenosis is progressive impediment to left atrial emptying. The multiple pathophysiological sequelae related to mitral stenosis are schematically demonstrated in Fig. 7.

CLINICAL FEATURES

Progressive dyspnea is a very common finding and occurs with any condition that causes an increase in blood flow across the narrowed mitral valve or reduces the time for such blood flow to occur (e.g., exertion, emotional stress, fever, and AF). Fatigue, orthopnea, and pulmonary edema occur with progressive disease but can also be precipitated by rapid AF. Other symptoms include hemoptysis, those related to systemic or pulmonary thromboembolism, infective endocarditis, vocal hoarseness, and progressive right-sided heart failure.

On physical examination, it is common, particularly in older females, to find typical mitral facies of purple-pinkish patches on the cheeks. In older patients with a calcific mitral valve, S1 is soft and with the development of pulmonary hypertension, P2 is accentuated. An opening snap (OS) of the mitral valve may be present with mild to moderate mitral stenosis. As the mitral stenosis progresses and left atrial pressure increases, the OS moves closer to A2. Thus, the shorter the A2-OS interval, the more severe the mitral stenosis. The classic murmur is a low-pitched diastolic rumble, heard best at the apex. In mild stenosis, the murmur is heard late in diastole. With severe stenosis, the diastolic murmur becomes holodiastolic with a presystolic accentuation, particularly when the patient is in sinus rhythm. The diastolic murmur may be inaudible or absent when mitral stenosis is very severe, owing to the very slow and reduced flow across the mitral valve. This is the case with many older patients. Pulmonary hypertension may be associated with pulmonary insufficiency, termed a Graham Steell murmur, and with tricuspid regurgitation, which results in a holosystolic murmur best heard along the right sternal border and which increases with inspiration.

DIAGNOSIS

The electrocardiogram may show left atrial enlargement (classically known as "P-mitrale"), AF, and right ventricular hypertrophy. Chest radiography might reveal elevation of the left bronchus related to left atrial enlargement, mitral valve calcification (Fig. 8), cephalization of pulmonary blood flow to upper lobes and Kerley B lines indicating interstitial fluid accumulation. Echocardiography is very useful in diagnosing mitral stenosis and can accurately determine doming of the mitral leaflets, degree of calcification, left atrial size, and mitral valve gradient/area. Dobutamine or exercise echocardiography is also useful in evaluating patients with symptoms that are out of proportion to the calculated resting valve area *(54)*. Table 2 details the criteria for determining the severity of mitral stenosis. The ACC/AHA recommendations for the use of echocardiography in mitral stenosis are listed in Table 3. The widespread availability of echocardiography has led to a very limited role for left ventricular angiography in mitral stenosis. Angiography can determine movement of the mitral valve and the presence of mitral regurgitation, and may give some additional information about the subvalvular apparatus.

MANAGEMENT

Medical management of mitral stenosis is similar in young and elderly patients, and includes endocarditis prophylaxis, appropriate antibiotic coverage for infective endocarditis, rate control, and anticoagulation in

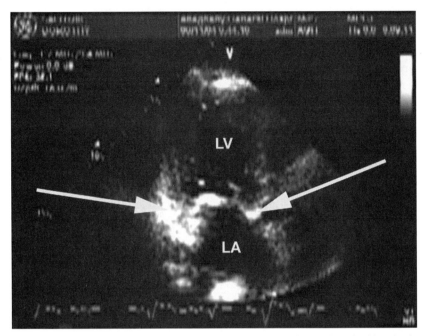

Fig. 8. Transthoracic two-dimensional echocardiograpic image in apical long axis view demonstrating severe mitral annular calcification (arrows). LA, left atrium; LV, left ventricle.

AF. Preferred surgical treatment is usually valve repair (commisurotomy) and is generally reserved for symptomatic patients. From a technical standpoint, valve repair is usually not feasible in elderly patients because of calcification, rigidity and retraction of valvular components. An alternative is percutaneous balloon commisurotomy (with a favorable valve morphology) in high-risk patients, which has a procedural mortality of 5% and an immediate significant hemodynamic improvement in 50% of patients *(55)*. It is not indicated in patients with mitral obstruction caused by mitral annular calcification. Surgery has a mortality of as high as 20%, but was required in about 50% of patients within 3 years of valvuloplasty, owing to restenosis. Mitral valvuloplasty is considered only a temporary, palliative measure in the elderly as its hemodynamic benefits dissipate quickly *(6)*.

Mitral Regurgitation

ETIOLOGY AND PATHOPHYSIOLOGY

Mitral regurgitation is a very common valvular abnormality in the elderly, with a reported prevalence of mild regurgitation in 19% of indi-

viduals older than 60 years in a Framingham echocardiography study
(4). There are several important causes of significant mitral regurgitation *(50)*. One category is mitral regurgitation owing to intrinsic disease
of the mitral leaflets or subvalvular apparatus. These include mitral
valve prolapse; flail mitral leaflet owing to trauma or infective endocarditis; ruptured chordae tendineaee that may be spontaneous, traumatic,
or the result of infective endocarditis; rheumatic fever or progressive
mitral annular calcification. A second category is ischemic mitral regurgitation owing to reversible ischemia or to papillary muscle infarction,
with or without rupture. A third category is nonischemic mitral regurgitation resulting from annular dilatation induced by left ventricular enlargement of any cause. A less common etiology is prosthetic valve dysfunction
owing to deterioration of tissue leaflets, ring or strut fracture, perival-
vular leak from ruptured sutures, infective endocarditis, and/or deterioration of the disc or ball of the prosthetic. In elderly patients, the most
common causes of mitral regurgitation are prolapse and ischemic heart
disease *(56)*.

From a pathophysiological standpoint, the hallmark of mitral regurgitation is excessive volume overload leading to various left ventricular compensatory changes over a protracted period of time, arbitrarily
divided as acute stage, chronic compensated stage and chronic decompensated stage. The pathophysiological sequelae of mitral regurgitation
are demonstrated in Fig. 9.

CLINICAL FEATURES

Acute mitral regurgitation usually presents as a dramatic event with
the sudden onset and rapid progression of pulmonary edema, hypotension, and signs and symptoms of cardiogenic shock. Examination reveals
evidence of poor tissue perfusion, thready pulse, and neck vein distension.
The murmur of acute mitral regurgitation may be early or midsystolic,
or holosystolic and is often soft, low-pitched and decrescendo, ending
before A2.

The majority of patients with chronic mitral regurgitation remain asymptomatic unless the left ventricle fails. The most common symptoms
include weakness, fatigue, and exercise intolerance. Further advancement
of the disease leads to symptomatic CHF with pulmonary congestion and
edema. Other symptoms such as thromboembolism, hemoptysis, and
right-sided CHF do occur, but are less common than with mitral stenosis,
whereas infective endocarditis is more common.

On examination, there is leftward displacement of the apical impulse,
diminished S1, accentuated P2 with pulmonary hypertension, and an S3
with worsening left ventricular function. The murmur of mitral regurgi-

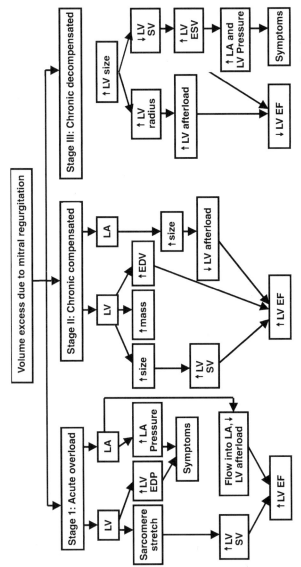

Fig. 9. Schematic representation of the various pathophysiological sequelae of mitral regurgitation.

252

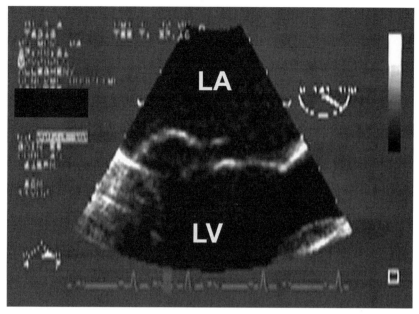

Fig. 10. Transesophageal echocardiographic image demonstrating a flail posterior mitral leaflet. LA, left atrium; LV, left ventricle.

tation is systolic but its characteristics depend on the etiology and component of the mitral apparatus that is diseased. In most cases, the murmur is blowing, high-pitched, holosystolic and is best heard over the apex, radiating to the axilla and when very loud may radiate to the back. However, when the posterior leaflet is involved the murmur may radiate to the base and when the anterior leaflet is involved (owing to prolapse or chordal rupture), the murmur radiates to the back, and may be heard on the top of the head. A midsystolic click may be heard with mitral valve prolapse.

DIAGNOSIS

In chronic cases, the electrocardiogram reveals evidence of left atrial enlargement and in later stages, left and right ventricular hypertrophy. Chest radiography reveals cardiomegaly and might reveal mitral annular calcification. Echocardiography, especially TEE, is usually helpful in establishing the etiology and hemodynamic consequences of mitral regurgitation (Fig. 10). The ACC/AHA recommendations for the use of echocardiography in mitral regurgitation are listed in Table 3. Similar to other valvular disorders, there is currently a very limited role for left ventricular angiography in mitral regurgitation.

MANAGEMENT

Nonsurgical treatment for acute, hemodynamically significant mitral regurgitation includes left ventricular unloading agents, including intra-aortic balloon pump placement but the patient should undergo urgent or emergent surgery. Vasodilator therapy may reduce diastolic filling pressures and the degree of mitral regurgitation and these efforts may stabilize the patients before surgery (57). Chronic mitral regurgitation is the second most common reason for valve surgery in the elderly, representing 30% to 35% of cases (23). Unlike younger individuals in whom surgery is often recommended even when they are asymptomatic, in patients over age 80, it is preferred to proceed with surgery when symptoms are present. Also, important issues to remember include the observations that regurgitation in those with ischemic cardiomyopathy often regresses with myocardial revascularization, whereas extensive valvular calcification makes both valve repair and replacement more difficult. It is vital to distinguish between mitral regurgitation owing to intrinsic valve disease, and that which is caused by ischemia, particularly in the elderly, because the latter will improve with revascularization and increased myocardial perfusion. Intraoperative echocardiography may help in making a decision regarding valve replacement or repair: mild and moderate regurgitation after induction of anesthesia is usually left alone, whereas severe regurgitation should be corrected.

Mitral valve repair, if feasible, is the surgical treatment of choice for mitral regurgitation as it preserves all components of the valve, avoids the use of a prosthesis with its attendant complications, and is associated with lower rates of morbidity and mortality than mitral valve replacement. In one study of primary isolated mitral valve repair degenerative mitral valve disease, the in-hospital mortality was 0.3% (58). In another study, the long-term survival after an 8-year post-repair follow up was 91% (59). It can often be achieved by use of applicable and reliable techniques. Resection of the part of the leaflets and remodeling the annulus with a ring are usually successful, in experienced hands. Mitral valve replacement can be performed with preservation of the subvalvular apparatus in myxomatous cases, but might not work in cases of ischemic regurgitation. Preservation of the subvalvular apparatus avoids unfavorable remodeling of the left ventricle.

The choice of the prosthesis is also controversial. Some surgeons prefer a bioprosthesis to avoid anticoagulation, but the implantation is more technically challenging. As a result, many surgeons prefer mechanical prosthesis, particularly in the presence if AF An additional consideration is that the stented commissures of a bioprosthesis tend to protrude into the left ventricular outflow tract, leading to subaortic obstruction (6).

Another issue is that of mitral annular calcification, which could extend to the epicardium of the atrioventricular groove. Extensive decalcification can lead to nonrepairable atrioventricular disconnection or ruptured left ventricle, whereas incomplete decalcification can lead to paraprosthetic leaks caused by maladaptation of the prosthesis ring to the annulus *(6)*.

Outcomes after surgery in elderly patients vary with age and disease severity and are better after mitral valve repair than replacement. Mitral valve repair produces good results in elderly patients. The in-hospital mortality of patients over 70 years age was 6.5% with valve repair alone, 13.2% when annuloplasty was combined with another reparative procedure, and 17% when combined with CABG *(60)*. For patients who undergo isolated mitral valve replacement with a bioprosthetic or mechanical valve, the 30-day mortality is reported to be 10.4% *(61)* and actuarial survival at 1, 3, and 5 years to be 79%, 64%, and 41%; the values were the same with both types of valves. Elderly patients with combined CABG and mitral valve replacement had a higher in-hospital mortality of 19.6% *(62)*.

Recent promising reports of experimental percutaneous mitral valve annuloplasty have generated significant interest and the field is evolving rapidly *(63,64)*. Percutaneous annuloplasty exploits the anatomic relationship of the coronary sinus to the mitral valve. A clip is placed in the mid portion of the tips of the two cusps, turning the orifice into a figure of eight. Animal studies have demonstrated its feasibility and a significant improvement in the degree of mitral regurgitation; however long-term safety and efficacy of this technique are not yet demonstrated.

CONCLUSION

Valvular disease in the elderly continues to be an important cause of morbidity and mortality, with degenerative aortic stenosis and mitral regurgitation accounting for the majority of the cases. Because of major advances in medications and surgical techniques, it is now possible to offer a myriad of treatment options to elderly patients unlike in the past when many were considered ineligible for any kind of intervention. Also encouraging are the findings that if the patient survives surgery, they often do so without a significant deterioration in the level of function and quality of life. Improved percutaneous techniques will allow a new therapeutic strategy, which is likely to have a major impact on the treatment of valvular diseases in the elderly.

ACKNOWLEDGMENTS

The authors would like to thank Sunil Mankad MD, of Allegheny General Hospital, Pittsburgh, PA for providing the echocardiographic images for this chapter.

REFERENCES

1. Otto CM, Lind BK, Kitzman DW, Gersh BJ, Siscovick DS. Association of aortic-valve sclerosis with cardiovascular mortality and morbidity in the elderly. N Engl J Med 1999;341(3):142–147.
2. Schneider EL, Guralnik JM. The aging of America. Impact on health care costs. JAMA 1990;263(17):2335–2340.
3. Passik CS, Ackermann DM, Pluth JR, Edwards WD. Temporal changes in the causes of aortic stenosis: a surgical pathologic study of 646 cases. Mayo Clin Proc 1987; 62(2):119–123.
4. Singh JP, Evans JC, Levy D, et al. Prevalence and clinical determinants of mitral, tricuspid, and aortic regurgitation (the Framingham Heart Study). Am J Cardiol 1999;83(6):897–902.
5. Lindroos M, Kupari M, Heikkila J, Tilvis R. Prevalence of aortic valve abnormalities in the elderly: an echocardiographic study of a random population sample. J Am Coll Cardiol 1993;21(5):1220–1225.
6. Pretre R, Turina MI. Cardiac valve surgery in the octogenarian. Heart 2000;83(1): 116–121.
7. Katz ES, Tunick PA, Rusinek H, Ribakove G, Spencer FC, Kronzon I. Protruding aortic atheromas predict stroke in elderly patients undergoing cardiopulmonary bypass: experience with intraoperative transesophageal echocardiography. J Am Coll Cardiol 1992;20(1):70–77.
8. Olsson M, Granstrom L, Lindblom D, Rosenqvist M, Ryden L. Aortic valve replacement in octogenarians with aortic stenosis: a case–control study. J Am Coll Cardiol 1992;20(7):1512–1516.
9. Olsson M, Janfjall H, Orth-Gomer K, Unden A, Rosenqvist M. Quality of life in octogenarians after valve replacement due to aortic stenosis. A prospective comparison with younger patients. Eur Heart J 1996;17(4):583–589.
10. Shapira OM, Kelleher RM, Zelingher J, et al. Prognosis and quality of life after valve surgery in patients older than 75 years. Chest 1997;112(4):885–894.
11. Bonow RO, Carabello B, de Leon AC Jr, et al. Guidelines for the management of patients with valvular heart disease: executive summary. A report of the American College of Cardiology/American Heart Association Task Force on Practice Guidelines (Committee on Management of Patients with Valvular Heart Disease). Circulation 1998;98(18):1949–1984.
12. Iung B, Baron G, Butchart EG, et al. A prospective survey of patients with valvular heart disease in Europe: The Euro Heart Survey on Valvular Heart Disease. Eur Heart J 2003;24(13):1231–1243.
13. Dare AJ, Veinot JP, Edwards WD, Tazelaar HD, Schaff HV. New observations on the etiology of aortic valve disease: a surgical pathologic study of 236 cases from 1990. Hum Pathol 1993;24(12):1330–1338.
14. Stewart BF, Siscovick D, Lind BK, et al. Clinical factors associated with calcific aortic valve disease. Cardiovascular Health Study. J Am Coll Cardiol 1997;29(3): 630–634.
15. Julius BK, Spillmann M, Vassalli G, Villari B, Eberli FR, Hess OM. Angina pectoris in patients with aortic stenosis and normal coronary arteries. Mechanisms and pathophysiological concepts. Circulation 1997;95(4):892–898.
16. Ross J Jr, Braunwald E. Aortic stenosis. Circulation 1968;38(1 Suppl):61–67.
17. King RM, Pluth JR, Giuliani ER. The association of unexplained gastrointestinal bleeding with calcific aortic stenosis. Ann Thorac Surg 1987;44(5):514–516.

18. Vincentelli A, Susen S, Le Tourneau T, et al. Acquired von Willebrand syndrome in aortic stenosis. N Engl J Med 2003;349(4):343–349.
19. Boon A, Lodder J, Cheriex E, Kessels F. Risk of stroke in a cohort of 815 patients with calcification of the aortic valve with or without stenosis. Stroke 1996;27(5): 847–851.
20. Munt B, Legget ME, Kraft CD, Miyake-Hull CY, Fujioka M, Otto CM. Physical examination in valvular aortic stenosis: correlation with stenosis severity and prediction of clinical outcome. Am Heart J 1999;137(2):298–306.
21. Gorlin R, Gorlin SG. Hydraulic formula for calculation of the area of the stenotic mitral valve, other cardiac valves, and central circulatory shunts. I. Am Heart J 1951; 41(1):1–29.
22. Akins CW, Daggett WM, Vlahakes GJ, et al. Cardiac operations in patients 80 years old and older. Ann Thorac Surg 1997;64(3):606–614.
23. Freeman WK, Schaff HV, O'Brien PC, Orszulak TA, Naessens JM, Tajik AJ. Cardiac surgery in the octogenarian: perioperative outcome and clinical follow-up. J Am Coll Cardiol 1991;18(1):29–35.
24. Kvidal P, Bergstrom R, Malm T, Stahle E. Long-term follow-up of morbidity and mortality after aortic valve replacement with a mechanical valve prosthesis. Eur Heart J 2000;21(13):1099–1111.
25. Elayda MA, Hall RJ, Reul RM, et al. Aortic valve replacement in patients 80 years and older. Operative risks and long-term results. Circulation 1993;88(5 Pt 2):II11–II16.
26. Arom KV, Goldenberg IF, Emery RW. Long-term clinical outcome with small size Standard St Jude Medical valves implanted in the aortic position. J Heart Valve Dis 1994;3(5):531–536.
27. Pibarot P, Dumesnil JG, Lemieux M, Cartier P, Metras J, Durand LG. Impact of prosthesis–patient mismatch on hemodynamic and symptomatic status, morbidity and mortality after aortic valve replacement with a bioprosthetic heart valve. J Heart Valve Dis 1998;7(2):211–218.
28. David TE. Aortic valve replacement with stentless porcine bioprostheses. J Card Surg 1998;13(5):344–351.
29. Asimakopoulos G, Edwards MB, Taylor KM. Aortic valve replacement in patients 80 years of age and older: survival and cause of death based on 1100 cases: collective results from the UK Heart Valve Registry. Circulation 1997;96(10):3403–3408.
30. Gehlot A, Mullany CJ, Ilstrup D, et al. Aortic valve replacement in patients aged eighty years and older: early and long-term results. J Thorac Cardiovasc Surg 1996; 111(5):1026–1036.
31. Bernard Y, Etievent J, Mourand JL, et al. Long-term results of percutaneous aortic valvuloplasty compared with aortic valve replacement in patients more than 75 years old. J Am Coll Cardiol 1992;20(4):796–801.
32. Cribier A, Eltchaninoff H, Bash A, et al. Percutaneous transcatheter implantation of an aortic valve prosthesis for calcific aortic stenosis: first human case description. Circulation 2002;106(24):3006–3008.
33. Cribier A, Eltchaninoff H, Tron C, et al. Early experience with percutaneous transcatheter implantation of heart valve prosthesis for the treatment of end-stage inoperable patients with calcific aortic stenosis. J Am Coll Cardiol 2004;43(4):698–703.
34. Otto CM, Kuusisto J, Reichenbach DD, Gown AM, O'Brien KD. Characterization of the early lesion of 'degenerative' valvular aortic stenosis. Histological and immunohistochemical studies. Circulation 1994;90(2):844–853.
35. O'Brien KD, Kuusisto J, Reichenbach DD, et al. Osteopontin is expressed in human aortic valvular lesions. Circulation 1995;92(8):2163–2168.

36. O'Brien KD, Reichenbach DD, Marcovina SM, Kuusisto J, Alpers CE, Otto CM. Apolipoproteins B, (a), and E accumulate in the morphologically early lesion of 'degenerative' valvular aortic stenosis. Arterioscler Thromb Vasc Biol 1996;16(4): 523–532.

37. Olsson M, Rosenqvist M, Nilsson J. Expression of HLA-DR antigen and smooth muscle cell differentiation markers by valvular fibroblasts in degenerative aortic stenosis. J Am Coll Cardiol 1994;24(7):1664–1671.

38. Olsson M, Dalsgaard CJ, Haegerstrand A, Rosenqvist M, Ryden L, Nilsson J. Accumulation of T lymphocytes and expression of interleukin-2 receptors in non-rheumatic stenotic aortic valves. J Am Coll Cardiol 1994;23(5):1162–1170.

39. Cosmi JE, Kort S, Tunick PA, et al. The risk of the development of aortic stenosis in patients with "benign" aortic valve thickening. Arch Intern Med 2002;162(20): 2345–2347.

40. Aronow WS, Ahn C, Shirani J, Kronzon I. Comparison of frequency of new coronary events in older subjects with and without valvular aortic sclerosis. Am J Cardiol 1999;83(4):599–600, A598.

41. Shavelle DM, Takasu J, Budoff MJ, Mao S, Zhao XQ, O'Brien KD. HMG CoA reductase inhibitor (statin) and aortic valve calcium. Lancet 2002;359(9312): 1125–1126.

42. Pohle K, Maffert R, Ropers D, et al. Progression of aortic valve calcification: association with coronary atherosclerosis and cardiovascular risk factors. Circulation 2001;104(16):1927–1932.

43. Chen J, Okin PM, Roman MJ, et al. Combined rest and exercise electrocardiographic repolarization findings in relation to structural and functional abnormalities in asymptomatic aortic regurgitation. Am Heart J 1996;132(2 Pt 1):343–347.

44. Scognamiglio R, Rahimtoola SH, Fasoli G, Nistri S, Dalla Volta S. Nifedipine in asymptomatic patients with severe aortic regurgitation and normal left ventricular function. N Engl J Med 1994;331(11):689–694.

45. Cohn LH, Birjiniuk V. Therapy of acute aortic regurgitation. Cardiol Clin 1991;9(2): 339–352.

46. Cosgrove DM, Lytle BW, Taylor PC, et al. The Carpentier–Edwards pericardial aortic valve. Ten-year results. J Thorac Cardiovasc Surg 1995;110(3):651–662.

47. Segal BL. Valvular heart disease, Part 1. Diagnosis and surgical management of aortic valve disease in older adults. Geriatrics 2003;58(9):31–35.

48. Limas CJ. Mitral stenosis in the elderly. Geriatrics 1971;26(11):75–79.

49. Waller BF, Howard J, Fess S. Pathology of mitral valve stenosis and pure mitral regurgitation—Part I. Clin Cardiol 1994;17(6):330–336.

50. Olson LJ, Subramanian R, Ackermann DM, Orszulak TA, Edwards WD. Surgical pathology of the mitral valve: a study of 712 cases spanning 21 years. Mayo Clin Proc 1987;62(1):22–34.

51. Aronow WS, Kronzon I. Correlation of prevalence and severity of mitral regurgitation and mitral stenosis determined by Doppler echocardiography with physical signs of mitral regurgitation and mitral stenosis in 100 patients aged 62 to 100 years with mitral anular calcium. Am J Cardiol 1987;60(14):1189–1190.

52. Merjanian R, Budoff M, Adler S, Berman N, Mehrotra R. Coronary artery, aortic wall, and valvular calcification in nondialyzed individuals with type 2 diabetes and renal disease. Kidney Int 2003;64(1):263–271.

53. Fulkerson PK, Beaver BM, Auseon JC, Graber HL. Calcification of the mitral annulus: etiology, clinical associations, complications and therapy. Am J Med 1979; 66(6):967–977.

54. Cheitlin MD. Stress echocardiography in mitral stenosis: when is it useful? J Am Coll Cardiol 2004;43(3):402–404.

55. Iung B, Cormier B, Farah B, et al. Percutaneous mitral commissurotomy in the elderly. Eur Heart J 1995;16(8):1092–1099.
56. Lee EM, Porter JN, Shapiro LM, Wells FC. Mitral valve surgery in the elderly. J Heart Valve Dis 1997;6(1):22–31.
57. Carabello BA, Crawford FA Jr. Valvular heart disease. N Engl J Med 1997;337(1): 32–41.
58. Gillinov AM, Cosgrove DM, Blackstone EH, et al. Durability of mitral valve repair for degenerative disease. J Thorac Cardiovasc Surg 1998;116(5):734–743.
59. Flameng W, Herijgers P, Bogaerts K. Recurrence of mitral valve regurgitation after mitral valve repair in degenerative valve disease. Circulation 2003;107(12):1609–1613.
60. Grossi EA, Zakow PK, Sussman M, et al. Late results of mitral valve reconstruction in the elderly. Ann Thorac Surg 2000;70(4):1224–1226.
61. Asimakopoulos G, Edwards MB, Brannan J, Taylor KM. Survival and cause of death after mitral valve replacement in patients aged 80 years and over: collective results from the UK heart valve registry. Eur J Cardiothorac Surg 1997;11(5):922–928.
62. Alexander KP, Anstrom KJ, Muhlbaier LH, et al. Outcomes of cardiac surgery in patients > or = 80 years: results from the National Cardiovascular Network. J Am Coll Cardiol 2000;35(3):731–738.
63. Block PC. Percutaneous mitral valve repair for mitral regurgitation. J Interv Cardiol 2003;16(1):93–96.
64. Liddicoat JR, Mac Neill BD, Gillinov AM, et al. Percutaneous mitral valve repair: a feasibility study in an ovine model of acute ischemic mitral regurgitation. Catheter Cardiovasc Interv 2003;60(3):410–416.

11 Arrhythmia Management in the Elderly

Jonathan P. Piccini, MD
and Hugh Calkins, MD

CONTENTS

INTRODUCTION

Arrhythmias cause significant mortality and impair quality of life in the elderly. The prevalences of cardiac arrhythmias and disorders of impulse formation and conduction, increase with age *(1,2)*. As the US population ages and as cardiovascular care for coronary disease and heart failure improves, the prevalence and burden of electrophysiological disorders will continue to rise. In fact, among Medicare beneficiaries, hospitalization rates for many common arrhythmias, including atrial fibrillation (AF), sinoatrial node (SAN) dysfunction, atrial flutter, and ventricular fibrillation (VF), continue to outpace elderly population growth *(3)*.

From: *Contemporary Cardiology: Cardiovascular Disease in the Elderly*
Edited by: G. Gerstenblith © Humana Press Inc., Totowa, NJ

These disorders almost always require the involvement of cardiovascu-lar specialists, and often present challenging management dilemmas. The purpose of this chapter is to review the current information concern-ing arrhythmia management in the elderly.

AGING AND THE CONDUCTION SYSTEM

With normal aging, the cardiac skeleton becomes fibrotic and calci-fied. These changes begin to appear in pathology specimens around 30 to 40 years of age and can lead to the disruption of the atrioventricular (AV) node and bundle branches. Despite the high prevalence of ischemic disease in the Western world, age-related fibrosis is the most common cause of complete AV block *(4,5)*. Amyloid deposition may also play a role in age-related conduction disorders, as 23% of patients over 60 years of age have evidence of amyloid deposition in the atrial myocardium *(6)*.

Similar changes can be observed in the SAN. With age, there is an increase in fibrosis and loss of myocardial fibers in the SAN *(7)*.

ELECTROCARDIOGRAPHIC CHANGES
IN THE ELDERLY

The evaluation of the conduction system in elderly patients begins with a history, physical examination, and a resting 12-lead electrocardiogram (EKG). Despite the proliferation of other diagnostic modalities, the EKG remains an integral noninvasive diagnostic technique for cardiovascular evaluation of elderly individuals.

EKG abnormalities are common in the elderly. Among 5150 adults older than 65 years old enrolled in the Cardiovascular Health Study, 29% had abnormal findings on their EKG *(8)*. Between 0.9% and 6.8% of elderly individuals have first degree AV block consistent with age-related atrophy and fibrosis of the AV node *(9,10)*. With respect to ven-tricular activation, elderly individuals exhibit a leftward shift in the QRS axis and an increased prevalence of bundle branch disease. There is also an increase in subtle, nonspecific repolarization abnormalities, includ-ing decreased T-wave amplitude, and nonspecific flattening of the ST-segment.

When evaluating the elderly, special attention should be given to elec-trocardiographic evidence of left ventricular hypertrophy (LVH) by either the modified Cornell criteria or the Sokolow-Lyon criteria. Although the EKG is not sensitive for the detection of LVH, it is highly specific. The presence of EKG evidence of LVH is an important finding in the elderly because it is a predictor of heart failure and premature cardiovascular death *(11)*.

BRADYARRHYTHMIAS

Sick Sinus Syndrome

Sick sinus syndrome (SSS) is common in elderly populations, accounts for approximately one-half of pacemaker insertions in the United States, and is associated with an increased prevalence of falls in the elderly *(12, 13)*. The term "sick sinus syndrome" was first used by Bernard Lown in 1967 to describe the slow return of sinus node activity following direct current (DC) cardioversion *(14)*. This bradyarrhythmic syndrome is characterized by chronic inappropriate bradycardia accompanied by symptomatic sinus pauses with an inadequate junctional escape rhythm and sinoatrial block. More than half of patients with SSS have AV conduction disturbances and tachyarrhythmias. These patients are said to have tachycardia–bradycardia syndrome. The diagnosis of tachycardia–bradycardia syndrome in a patient with SSS is concerning because tachycardia-mediated overdrive suppression can lead to long sinus pauses following the termination of an atrial arrhythmia.

The bradyarrhythmia in SSS can be the result of either impaired impulse initiation or impaired impulse propagation. SSS can be caused by several pathological processes, including infiltrative disease such as sarcoidosis and amyloidosis, inflammatory pericardial processes, and metabolic disorders such as hypothyroidism, but it is most commonly caused by fibrous replacement of the SAN.

In patients suspected of having a bradyarrhythmia and/or sinus node dysfunction, the chief goal of the evaluation is to determine whether the patient has a symptomatic bradyarrhythmia. This is most readily accomplished with ambulatory monitoring, including the use of an event monitor. Although electrophysiology (EP) testing can also be used to evaluate sinus node function, its sensitivity is low. For this reason, EP testing is typically only used to evaluate sinus node function among patients with syncope in whom an obvious cause of syncope cannot be identified. Pacemaker placement is recommended for treatment of most patients with a symptomatic bradyarrhythmia, unless the bradyarrhythmia is the result of a transient and reversible cause (e.g., recent initiation of β-blocker therapy where the indication for β-blocker therapy is not compelling). Dual-chamber rate-responsive pacemakers or single-chamber atrial pacemakers are recommended for treatment of patients with SSS who have an indication for pacemaker therapy *(15)*.

Atrioventricular Block

Following atrial activation, the electrical impulse must be propagated through the AV node and the bundle of His before it can activate the bundle branches. It has long been observed that AV conduction is prolonged with age. The AV node is the first part of the conduction system to be affected by age-related fibrosis, as fatty infiltrates and collagen interposition in AV nodal tissues begin to appear at 30 years of age *(16)*. Over time, these changes lead to delayed impulse propagation and predispose to the fractionation of AV conduction and subsequent reentry. These age-related delays in AV conduction are primarily localized to the AV node and the proximal portion of the His bundle *(17)*. Although animal models have implicated decreased β-receptor density in the AV node, PR prolongation in humans appears to be independent of β-adrenergic and parasympathetic input *(18,19)*.

Patients with impaired AV conduction may be asymptomatic or may complain of syncope, lightheadedness, and fatigue. AV conduction block can be classified as first-, second-, and third-degree AV block (also known as complete heart block). The differential diagnosis of AV block includes primary and secondary AV block. Conditions associated with secondary AV block include myocardial ischemia, enhanced vagal tone, drug effect (including digitalis intoxication, β-blockers, nondihydropyridine calcium channel blockers [CCBs], and class I anti-arrhythmics), lyme disease, syphilis, calcific aortic stenosis, aortic valve ring abscesses, and infiltrative disorders, which include hemochromotosis, amyloidosis, and sarcoidosis.

First-degree AV block is defined by a PR interval longer than 200 ms. The incidence of primary first-degree heart block increases with age and is associated with a moderate increase in the PR interval (0.2–0.23). Primary first-degree AV block is a benign condition and is not associated with increased mortality *(20)*.

Second-degree AV block includes Mobitz type I and Mobitz type II block. Mobitz type I or Wenckebach block, is characterized by progressive lengthening of the PR interval and intermittent block. In contrast, Mobitz type II second-degree AV block, is associated with intermittent AV block without PR interval lengthening. The key step in evaluating a patient in second-degree heart block is determining whether or not Mobitz type II block is present, as Mobitz type II indicates distal His pathology and a high risk of progression to complete heart block. Because of these high-risk features, Mobitz type II second-degree AV block, like complete heart block, is a class I indication for permanent pacemaker insertion.

Bundle Branch Disease

Bundle branch block (BBB) is highly age dependent with a prevalence of 1.2% among those age 50 and a prevalence of 17% among those age 80 *(21)*. A common dilemma facing clinicians is how to manage patients with chronic bifasicular block. These patients are sometimes said to be "hanging by a fascicle." Fortunately, chronic bifasicular block rarely progresses to complete heart block. In fact, among patients with BBB, only 1% per year progress to complete heart block (22).

Given the low risk of progression to heart block in these patients, it is generally agreed that asymptomatic patients with bifasicular and trifasicular block should not undergo pacemaker implantation. Class I indications for pacemaker insertion in patients with chronic bifasicular and trifasicular block include symptomatic bradycardia, intermittent complete heart block, and intermittent type II second degree AV block. Patients with unexplained syncope who have evidence of underlying conducton system disease should undergo an EP study. Pacemaker placement is indicated for those patients with an H-V interval longer than 100 ms. EP testing is not indicated for the asymptomatic patient with an underling BBB pattern on EKG.

TACHYARRHYTHMIAS

Supraventricular Arrhythmias

Paroxysmal Supraventricular Tachycardia

The term paroxysmal supraventricular tachycardia (PSVT) generally refers to a clinical syndrome characterized by a sustained regular supraventricular arrhythmia of abrupt onset and termination. Two-thirds of all cases of PSVT result from AV nodal re-entrant tachycardia. The remaining one-third of patients with PSVT has an accessory pathway that provides a substrate for AV-reciprocating tachycardia. In very unusual cases, PSVT may result from a re-entrant atrial tachycardia such as sinus node re-entrant tachycardia or from an ectopic atrial focus. Although the incidence of PSVT peaks in the fifth decade, patients 65 years and older have five times the risk of developing PSVT compared with their younger counterparts (23).

The presentation of PSVT can vary dramatically. Some patients complain of palpitations, light-headedness, neck-pounding, and fatigue, others remain asymptomatic, and a few present with syncope. If an episode of PSVT is prolonged, patients may report polyuria owing to atrial stretch-mediated release of atrial natriuretic peptide. Generally, the physical examination has limited diagnostic value in the diagnosis of PSVT. This reflects the fact that most episodes of PSVT terminate spontaneously. Furthermore, in the rare situation when the tachycardia is ongoing, the physical examination is rarely informative.

Evaluation of a patient with PSVT should include a search for possible precipitants including infection, hypoxemia, anemia, and metabolic disturbances. The first step in management includes an assessment of the patient's vital signs. Hemodynamically unstable PSVT, like any unstable tachyarrhythmia should be treated with immediate DC cardioversion; otherwise, attempts should be made to obtain an EKG and to abort the arrhythmia with vagal maneuvers.

If PSVT does not terminate with vagal maneuvers, therapeutic and diagnostic administration of adenosine is recommended. Adenosine should be administered in a rapid bolus with an initial dose of 6 mg. If the tachycardia persists, 12 mg of adenosine should be administered. The only contraindication to adenosine is a history of severe brochospastic pulmonary disease. Adenosine should never be administered unless the patient is being monitored and a defibrillator is present. Rarely, on termination of PSVT, AF appears. If a patient has a rapidly conducting accessory pathway, this may lead to VF. Rarely, adenosine administration will result in persistence of the tachycardia with AV block. This finding excludes an arrhythmia involving the AV node and strongly suggests that the underlying arrhythmia is either atrial tachycardia or atrial flutter. If the arrhythmia does not terminate with adenosine, a CCB or β-blocker can be administered.

Once PSVT is terminated, either spontaneously or following adenosine, a long-term treatment strategy can be developed. In general, the approach to treatment depends on the severity and frequency of symptoms, and patient preference. Catheter ablation is considered an appropriate first-line therapy for PSVT, particularly among patients with frequent tachycardic episodes, hemodynamic intolerance, or for those who have failed an attempt at empiric therapy with a β-blocker or CCB. As discussed later, catheter ablation is also recommended for all patients with PSVT that occurs in the setting of the Wolff-Parkinson-White Syndrome. For patients who are not interested in catheter ablation, alternate treatment strategies include clinical follow-up without specific therapy, empiric treatment with a CCB or β-blocker, or rarely a class 1c anti-arrhythmic agent such as flecainide or propafenone (24).

AV NODAL RE-ENTRANT TACHYCARDIA

AV nodal re-entrant tachycardia (AVNRT) is the most common cause of PSVT in the elderly, accounting for approximately two-thirds of all cases (25,26). The presence of a narrow complex tachycardia with a regular RR interval at a rate of 140 to 250 beats per minute (bpm) without P waves or with retrograde P waves in the ST-segment suggests the presence of AVNRT.

The AV node is a compact bundle of atrial tissue located at the apex of the triangle of Koch. In AVNRT, the presence of a second conducting

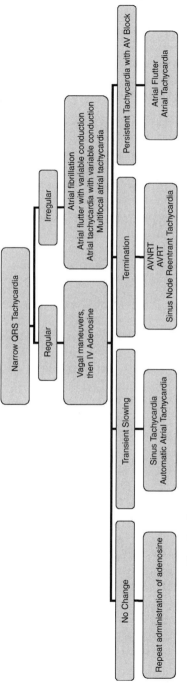

Fig. 1. Diagnostic alogorithm for narrow QRS tachycardias. (Adapted from ref. 24.)

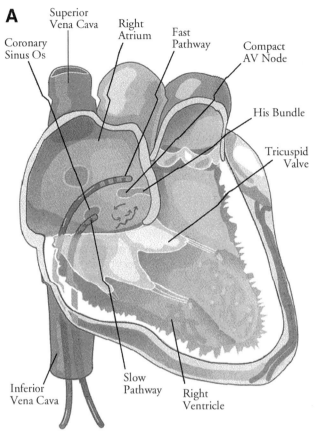

Fig. 2. Catheter ablation of atrioventricular nodal re-entrant tachycardia (AVNRT).
(A) In AVNRT, the presence of a second conducting pathway (with a different
refractory period) adjacent to the AV node, enables unidirectional block and formation of a reentrant circuit between the "fast" and "slow" conducting pathways.
This unique anatomic relationship allows for successful catheter ablation of the
slow pathway in over 95% of cases.

pathway (with a different refractory period) adjacent to the AV node,
enables unidirectional block and formation of a re-entrant circuit involving both the fast and slow pathways. This unique anatomic relationship
enables the adjacent slow pathway to be safely ablated with a success
rate in excess of 95% (27). Because the elderly are at the greatest risk for
adverse events related to long-term oral antiarrhythmic therapy, radiofrequency ablation should be considered first line therapy in all active
elderly individuals who are willing to accept the 1% risk of AV block
associated with catheter ablation of AVNRT.

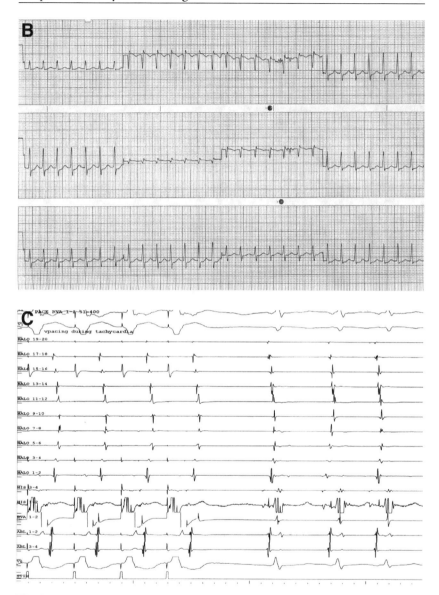

Fig. 2. *(Continued)* Also depicted are **(B)** a 12-lead electrocardiogram of AVNRT and **(C)** an intracardiac electrogram demonstrating AVNRT with termination of the arrhythmia on the fast pathway.

Often, EKG changes are observed during an episode of AVNRT, or shortly thereafter. Significant ST-segment depressions can be seen during the tachycardia in 25%–50% of patients with AVNRT, however, these changes are not predictive of ischemia *(28)*. Additionally, there is no correlation between the rate of tachycardia and the presence or extent of ST segment changes. Other EKG changes may be seen during or after the termination of AVNRT. Newly acquired T-wave inversion after termination of AVNRT, commonly in anterior or inferior leads, can be present in nearly 40% of patients *(29)*. Despite the concern that is often raised with these EKG changes, there is no significant association between AVNRT and underlying structural heart disease.

ACCESSORY PATHWAY TACHYCARDIAS

Accessory pathways are anatomically distinct AV connections that form as a result of incomplete separation of the myocardium during development. These connections bypass the AV node and can lead to premature excitation of the ventricle. Accessory pathways can conduct from the atrium to the ventricle, from the ventricle to the atrium, or both. Accessory pathways that only conduct from the ventricle to the atrium are not apparent on a 12-lead EKG and are referred to as "concealed" pathways. In contrast, anterograde conducting accessory pathways result in premature activation of the ventricle and give the typical pattern of pre-excitation on the EKG. Features of pre-excitation include a short PR interval, a slurred QRS upstroke (δ wave), and a widened QRS complex. The Wolff-Parkinson-White syndrome is an accessory pathway syndrome characterized by the presence of a δ waves on the 12-lead EKG in conjunction with supraventricular arrhythmias. Because patients with Wolff-Parkinson-White syndrome have an increased risk of sudden death, catheter ablation is usually considered the standard of care.

Among patients with an accessory pathway, the most common arrhythmia is orthodromic atrioventricular reciprocating tachycardia (AVRT). This tachycardia involves anterograde conduction through the AV node to the ventricles and retrograde conduction from the ventricles to the atrium via the accessory pathway. Orthodromic AVRT typically presents as a narrow complex tachycardia. Antidromic AVRT, a less common arrhythmia, involves the same reentrant circuit but the wavefront travels anterogradely from the atrium to the ventricle via the accessory pathway. This results in a wide complex tachycardia.

SINUS TACHYCARDIA

Elderly individuals frequently present with sinus tachycardia. Sinus tachycardia is marked by a gradual onset and termination and its diagnosis requires EKG evidence of sinus rhythm. Sinus activation results in a P wave vector between 0 and 90 degrees with positive deflections in leads I, II, and aVF and a negative deflection in lead aVR. The presence of sinus tachycardia almost always represents an appropriate physiological response to a demand stressor. In the elderly, the differential diagnosis is broad, but consideration should be given to hyperthyroidism, occult gastrointestinal bleeding, pulmonary embolism, and infection. Because this rhythm represents an appropriate physiological response, treatment should be directed at the underlying etiology. Inappropriate sinus tachycardia is defined as sinus tachycardia in the absence of a physiological stimulus. This condition is rare and virtually never occurs in the elderly.

MULTIFOCAL ATRIAL TACHYCARDIA

Multifocal atrial tachycardia (MAT) is an uncommon arrhythmia seen in critically ill elderly inpatients, with a mean age at diagnosis of 72 years. MAT is rare, but when is does occur, it is usually in the setting of an intensive care unit admission owing to an exacerbation of underlying pulmonary disease (especially chronic obstructive pulmonary disease [COPD]). MAT portends an ominous prognosis with an in-hospital mortality rate of 45% (30). Clinically, MAT is often mistaken for AF because it is an irregular narrow complex rhythm. The diagnosis of MAT rests on an atrial rate greater than 100 bpm, the presence of three separate P-wave morphologies, and irregular PP intervals. Like sinus tachycardia the treatment is directed at reversing the underlying cause, however, previous studies have shown that metoprolol and verapamil can be useful for rate control.

ATRIAL FLUTTER

Atrial flutter occurs 100 times more often in those aged 80 years and older, as compared to younger persons (31). Risk factors for atrial flutter include advancing age, heart failure, and COPD. Among patients who present with SVT, approximately 10% will have atrial flutter (32). Atrial flutter is a macro-reentrant atrial tachycardia that is distinguished by its atrial rate (typically ranges from 250 to 350 bpm). The re-entrant circuit in atrial flutter is almost always located in the right atrium, commonly involving the cavotricuspid isthmus, an isolated area of slowed conduction anatomically bound by the coronary sinus, the inferior vena cava, the tricuspid annulus, and the eustachian ridge. Also known as typical flutter or type 1 flutter, this common type of atrial flutter is characterized by a counterclockwise wavefront in the right atrium, which gives rise to negative flutter waves in leads II and III and positive atrial deflections in lead V1. Uncommon atrial flutter involves the same re-entrant circuit, but the wavefront travels in a clockwise direction. In contrast to type 1 atrial flutter, atypical or type 2 atrial flutter is a more rapid arrhythmia that results from functional re-entry. Atrial flutter is commonly associated with the presence of structural heart disease, thus patients with no known structural heart disease should undergo an investigative echocardiogram *(33)*.

The management of atrial flutter consists of two main strategies. Because atrial flutter is associated with an increased risk of stroke, systemic anticoagulation is recommended for all patients with atrial flutter who have other risk factors for stroke (including age >75 years). If a patient has symptomatic atrial flutter, treatment to restore sinus rhythm is indicated. This typically involves a cardioversion procedure. If atrial flutter recurs, pharmacological treatment or catheter ablation is recommended to prevent further recurrences. A recent randomized clinical trial demonstrated that catheter ablation is superior to pharmacological therapy in the maintenance of sinus rhythm in patients with atrial flutter *(34)*. For this reason, catheter ablation is considered first-line therapy. Catheter ablation can be performed on an outpatient basis and is associated with a 95% efficacy and less than a 1% risk of major complications. If a patient prefers pharmacological therapy, a class 1A, 1C, or class 3 anti-arrhythmic can be considered. The selection of an anti-arrhythmic agent is generally based on the drug's side-effect profile. Pharmacological therapy is successful in the long-term suppression of atrial flutter in approximately 50% of patients.

ATRIAL FIBRILLATION

AF is a re-entrant supraventricular tachycardia (SVT) that is confined to the atrium. This tachyarrhythmia is characterized by (a) the absence of organized atrial activity, (b) the presence of irregular oscillations or fibrillatory waves, and (c) an irregularly irregular ventricular rate. AF is by far the most common and clinically most important SVT. Among patients undergoing coronary artery bypass grafting, older age is the strongest predictor of postoperative AF *(35)*. Not surprisingly, the prevalence of AF increases with age, such that only 0.1% of adults younger than 55 years of age have AF, but among adults older than 80 years, 9% have AF. It is estimated that 2.3 million Americans have AF, a figure that is expected to increase 2.5 fold over the next 50 years *(36)*. AF is not a benign rhythm and is associated with considerable morbidity and mortality. Most importantly, AF increases the risk of stroke fivefold (approximately 5% per year) and accounts for approximately one-sixth of all strokes in the United States *(37)*. In the Framingham Study, patients with AF had a two- to threefold increase in cardiovascular mortality *(38)*. Although lone AF is not associated with increased cardiovascular morbidity in

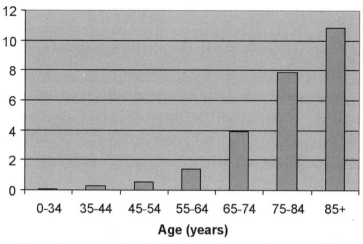

Fig. 3. Prevalence of atrial fibrillation by age. (From ref. *40*.)

younger individuals, patients over the age of 60 with lone AF do have a marked increase in cardiovascular events (*39; see* Fig. 3 *[40]*).

Once initiated, AF is composed of multiple re-entrant circuits with a cycle length between 150 and 300 ms. The decremental conduction properties of the AV node prevent most of these atrial impulses from reaching the ventricle. AF facilitates its own propagation by shortening the atrial refractory period, mostly through reductions in L-type calcium channel current. Previously, it has been taught that the initiation of AF, much like sustained AF, was not a focal process. Associations with hyperthyroidism and ethanol consumption appeared to support this hypothesis. However, it has become clear that the spontaneous initiation of AF is often due to isolated rapidly firing foci, which are found in the right atrium, left atrium, superior vena cava, the coronary sinus, and most commonly, the pulmonary vein ostia *(41)*. In the past several years, it has been demonstrated that ectopic foci in the pulmonary vein ostia are amenable to ablation techniques and that pulmonary vein ablation can be a very effective treatment for AF *(42–44)*.

The management of AF includes the following: (a) evaluation of underlying etiology and risk stratification, (b) selection of a rhythm- vs rate-control strategy, and (c) stroke prophylaxis *(45)*. Patients suspected of having AF should undergo 24-hour ambulatory EKG monitoring. All patients with a new diagnosis of AF should undergo echocardiography to evaluate the presence of any structural heart disease and to identify high-risk features for stroke. Thyroid function should also be assessed, as AF may be the only presenting symptom of thyroid disease in the elderly. The size of the left atrium provides a general assessment of how long a patient has been in AF and what the probability is that sinus rhythm can be restored and maintained. The chance of successful conversion in a patient with a left atrial size greater than 6 cm is extremely small.

When a patient presents with AF, the onset and duration of the arrhythmia should be determined, if possible. Patients who present within 48 hours of onset are candidates for immediate pharmacological or electrical conversion. Patients who present with AF for longer than 48 hours should be anticoagulated for 3 weeks prior to cardioversion. Alternatively, the clinician can pursue transesophageal echocardiography (TEE)-guided cardioversion (46). If a patient has no evidence of left atrial appendage thrombi or spontaneous echo contrast on TEE examination, they can safely undergo cardioversion without increased risk of cardioembolic stroke. Conversely, all patients with AF for longer than 48 hours duration, regardless of their precardioversion care, should be anticoagulated for 4 weeks following resumption of sinus rhythm. This strategy is necessary because there is a paradoxical increase in the rate of stroke in the first 48 hours following cardioversion owing to left atrial stunning (localized tachycardia-mediated atrial cardiomyopathy) following the termination of AF.

Although many debate the relative merits of rate control and rhythm control, it is reasonable to give every patient at least one chance at cardioversion, regardless of their risk for recurrence. Cardioversion has an 86% success rate at 72 hours (47). However, it is important to note that 68% of patients who present with AF of less than 72 hours duration will spontaneously convert to normal sinus rhythm (48). Risk factors for arrhythmia recurrence include age older than 75 years, left atrial diameter greater than 45 mm, AF for more than 4 weeks, presence of heart failure, left ventriuclar systolic dysfunction, and a history of prior cardioversion (49–51). Utilization of a biphasic waveform achieves cardioversion at lower energy levels when compared with monophasic waveform defibrillation (52). Finally, anterior–posterior application of defibrillator leads is associated with increased cardioversion efficacy (53).

A central debate in clinical cardiology is whether patients with AF should be managed with rate control or rhythm-based strategies. As mentioned previously, AF is not a benign rhythm. The presence of AF impairs cardiovascular hemodynamics through several mechanisms. Loss of synchronous atrial contraction results in impaired ventricular filling and elevated left atrial end-diastolic pressures. Inappropriate tachycardia in AF decreases the diastolic filling interval, whereas irregular RR intervals are associated with decreased cardiac output, elevated pulmonary capillary wedge pressures, and elevated right atrial pressures. These alterations can lead to adverse cardiac remodeling and impaired left ventricular function. Older patients with poor vascular compliance and diastolic dysfunction may not tolerate these changes as well as younger individuals, thus leading to impaired ventricular function and heart failure. Maintenance of sinus rhythm has several advantages, including relief of symptoms, and improved hemodynamics. No study to date has demonstrated that restoration and maintenance of sinus rhythm lowers stroke risk. For this reason, the approach to management of AF should be considered independently from the issue of anticoagulation.

Despite the common perception that rate control represents a "simpler" strategy, rate control can often be difficult to achieve, especially in patients with left ventricular dysfunction. Rate control is defined as a mean 24-hour heart rate of 80 bpm or lower as recorded on a Holter monitor. The objective of a rate-control strategy, however, is to control heart-rate variability as well as the average heart rate. Therefore, rate control cannot be assessed with a resting heart rate or at a single point in time. First-line rate-control agents include β-blockers and nondihydropyridine CCBs. Digitalis preparations are rarely adequate as monotherapy, especially in active individuals, because they lower heart rate through a vagotonic mechanism (54).

Pharmacological cardioversion is most successful when attempted within 7 days of AF onset (55). Although several drugs are shown to limit the recurrence of AF, amiodarone appears to be more effective than sotalol and class I agents at maintaining sinus rhythm (56). Selection of an initial anti-arrhythmic agent in AF should focus on the patient's underlying pathophysiology and co-morbidities. For those patients without structural heart disease, flecainide, propafenone, and sotalol are all reasonable choices given their tolerability and lower incidence of complications. The presence of ischemic heart disease is a relative contraindication for a class 1c anti-arrhythmic drug like flecainide or propafenone. In young patients, disopyramide is often recommended as a first-line agent for treatment of vagally mediated AF. It is important to note, however, that norpace may exacerbate bladder outlet obstruction in elderly men and therefore should be avoided in this clinical situation. Similarly, β-blockers should be considered in those patients with adrenergically mediated AF. Amiodarone is generally reserved for patients who have failed other anti-arrhythmic drugs and/or those with significant left ventricular dysfunction. Although amiodarone has been shown to have the greatest efficacy for treatment of AF, it is associated with important side effects including thyroid disease, pulmonary disease, and peripheral neuropathy. Amiodarone may also result in impaired vision. For these reasons, annual screening is required to allow for early detection of amiodarone-induced side effects.

Several randomized, controlled trials have compared a primary strategy of rate control vs rhythm control *(57–60)*. Although these studies are limited by selection bias, exclusion criteria, limited follow-up duration, and varying efficacy in the rhythm-control arm, several common findings have emerged. Most importantly, in the short term (i.e., 1 to 3 years of follow-up), rate control is not inferior to a rhythm-control strategy. It has also been observed that the maintenance of sinus rhythm is difficult to achieve, as only 40% to 60% of the patients in the rhythm-control arms actually were in sinus rhythm at the conclusion of the trials. A rhythm-control strategy is also associated with increased hospitalization rates owing to the need for repeat cardioversion and initiation of pharmacological therapy. Because in several of the trials, most of the cardioembolic events occurred in the rhythm-control groups, patients with risk factors for stroke should continue to receive anticoagulation even after sinus rhythm is achieved. Not unexpectedly, exercise tolerance was better in patients managed with rhythm control.

Consistent with the results of these recent trials, the approach to management of AF is based largely on symptoms. If a patient has asymptomatic AF, rate control and systemic anticoagulation are considered the usual standard of care. One attempt at cardioversion could be considered if this is the patient's first episode of AF. In contrast, medical or catheter-based therapy should be considered for patients with symptomatic AF. Anti-arrhythmic therapy is generally the first step. As discussed previously, the selection of anti-arrhythmic agents is based largely on the drug's side-effect profile and potential for pro-arrhythmia. Amiodarone is an effective pharmacological agent but is associated with many potential side effects. For this reason, it is rarely considered first-line therapy. Catheter ablation of AF has made tremendous strides over the past several years. Catheter ablation is indicated for patients with highly symptomatic AF that has been refractory to attempts at pharmacological therapy. The 1-year efficacy of this procedure for patients with paroxysmal AF is approximately 75%.

VENTRICULAR ARRHYTHMIAS

Monomorphic Ventricular Tachycardia

There are two important types of re-entrant ventricular arrhythmias, ventricular tachycardia (VT) and ventricular fibrillation (VF). VT can be further subdivided based on its morphology into monomorphic VT and polymorphic VT. These descriptive labels are very helpful from a diagnostic standpoint because they shed light on the etiology. To be more specific, monomorphic VT is caused by fixed re-entry and polymorphic VT is caused by dynamic re-entry. Therefore, after examining the patient's rhythm strip, the clinician is immediately clued in to the possible etiologies of the ventricular arrhythmia.

Sustained monomorphic ventricular tachycardia is usually the result of the presence of a fixed re-entrant circuit in the ventricle. Almost all patients with this type of VT have some form of structural heart disease that accounts for the presence of this abnormal re-entrant circuit, most commonly prior myocardial infarction (MI). The border zone of an MI is often characterized by an island of fibrosis surrounded by living tissue. Myocardial scar enables unidirectional block and establishes the milieu necessary for re-entry. Sustained VT in the setting of structural heart disease (and therefore, not idiopathic) is associated with an increased risk of sudden cardiac death. VT requires aggressive evaluation and treatment, often with an implantable cardioverter defibrillator (ICD).

VT must be differentiated from aberrantly conducted supraventricular arrhythmias. EKG features that suggest ventricular origin include AV dissociation (apparent in 30%), QRS complex duration longer than 160 ms, a shift in the QRS axis, and the presence of fusion beats. Although these features are helpful, the patient's history may be more informative. In patients with a history of coronary artery disease (CAD), more than 95% of wide complex tachycardia represents VT.

Polymorphic Ventricular Tachycardia

Polymorphic ventricular tachycardia is a form of VT in which there is variation in the axis and morphology of the QRS complex. Unlike monomorphic VT, which is usually caused by a fixed re-entrant circuit, polymorphic VT is caused by heterogeneity in ventricular repolarization. Polymophic VT is most commonly seen under the following situations: (a) long QT syndrome resulting in torsade de pointes, (b) pro-arrhythmia resulting in a drug-induced prolongation of the QT interval and torsade, (c) severe dilated cardiomyopathy (DCM), and (d) severe ischemic disease with ongoing ischemia (e.g., left main CAD).

Ventricular Fibrillation

VF is a rapid, irregular tachycardia arising in the ventricles that results from multiple re-entrant circuits. The EKG features of VF include a rapid (>250 bpm) and very irregular wide complex tachycardia.

VF may occur as a primary arrhythmia or may result from degeneration of VT. As VF continues, global myocardial ischemia ensues and post-repolarization refractoriness and conduction delay increase *(61)*. Unless terminated, VF results rapidly in sudden cardiac death. The majority of patients who experience VF have cardiac disease, especially CAD. Although VF can occur within 24 hours of an acute MI, the vast majority of VF does not.

Evaluation of Ventricular Arrhythmias in the Elderly

The evaluation of a patient who has experienced a sustained or non-sustained ventricular arrhythmia (NSVT) involves several steps. Perhaps the most important of these is determining whether the arrhythmia is symptomatic or asymptomtic. Whereas treatment is indicated for most symptomatic arrhythmias, treatment is rarely recommended for asymptomatic arrhythmias. The exception to this rule is the patient with asymptomatic ventricular arrhythmias and impaired left ventricular function (ejection fraction [EF] $\leq 35\%$). Recent studies demonstrate that the risk of sudden death is significantly increased in this patient population and that placement of an ICD may prolong the survival. The second step in the evaluation of a patient with a ventricular arrhythmia involves an assessment of their ventricular function and whether they have ischemic heart disease. Elderly patients without structural heart disease or exercise induced NSVT do not appear to have an increased risk of sudden death *(62)*.

Management of Ventricular Arrhythmias

Management of patients with ventricular arrhythmias is focused on assessing the severity of symptoms and risk for sudden death. The role of defibrillator therapy in the primary and secondary prevention of sudden death is discussed later. For patients who are not at high risk of sudden death, the treatment of ventricular arrhythmias is directed at reducing symptoms. Treatment options include pharamacological agents such as β-blockers and anti-arrhythmic agents, as well as catheter ablation. The success of catheter ablation is highly dependent on the arrhythmia being ablated. Among patients with idiopathic VT arising from the right ventricular outflow tract, catheter ablation is associated with an efficacy of greater than 90%. In contrast, catheter ablation is rarely curative for arrhythmias that arise in the setting of significant structural heart disease.

SECONDARY PREVENTION
OF SUDDEN CARDIAC DEATH

In the late 1970s, Michel Mirokski pioneered the development of the ICD at Sinai Hospital in Baltimore, Maryland. His work led to the first implantation of an ICD at the Johns Hopkins Hospital in 1980 *(63)*. Since that time, the numbers of ICDs implanted per year has increased significantly.

Patients with sustained VT and prior MI have a mortality rate of 20% at 2 years *(64)*. These patients are at high risk for future sudden cardiac death. Unfortunately, the survival rate for out-of-hospital cardiac arrest is low; ranging from 2% to 25% *(65)*. The ICD quickly became the focus of several clinical trials aimed at secondary prevention of sudden cardiac death owing to the risk of pro-arrhythmia with drug treatment and the association between time-to-defibrillation and survival. The Anti-arrhythmics Versus Implantable Defibrillators (AVID) trial randomized 1016 survivors of cardiac arrest (455 patients had VT, 561 patients had VF) to conventional anti-arrhythmic treatment vs ICD implantation. When the investigators found a significant reduction in mortality in the ICD group (15.8% vs 24.0%) after 18.2 months of follow-up, the trial was terminated prematurely *(66)*. The mortality benefit in AVID seemed to be restricted to those patients with a left ventricular ejection fraction (LVEF) less than 35%, confirming the predictive power of left ventricular dysfunction for sudden cardiac death. The results of this trial were soon confirmed by two other secondary prevention trials: the Canadian Implantable Defibrillator Study and the Cardiac Arrest Study Hamburg. A meta-analysis of approximately 900 patients enrolled in randomized controlled trials (RCTs) of secondary prevention found a 27% risk reduction for sudden cardiac death after ICD implantation *(67)*.

Consistent with the results of these studies, ICDs are now indicated for the treatment of most sudden death survivors. ICDs are also recommended for treatment of sustained ventricular arrhythmias that occur in the setting of structural heart disease *(15)* (Table 1).

PRIMARY PREVENTION OF SUDDEN CARDIAC DEATH

Although our attempts at secondary prevention have been successful, patients with a history of lethal ventricular arrhythmia account for only 5% to 10% of sudden cardiac death victims in the United States *(68)*. Furthermore, 40% of patients who suffer primary VT have no prior warning arrhythmias *(69)*. Several trials investigated the use of ICD implantation for the primary prevention of sudden cardiac death. From these first trials we learned that ICD implantation in patients (mean age between 62 and 67 years) with ischemic cardiomyopathy, an LVEF less than 40%, evidence of NSVT, and inducible VT at electrophysiology study (EPS) yields a 50% reduction in mortality *(70,71)*. The Multicenter Automatic Defibrillator Implantation Trial (MADIT II) demonstrated the efficacy of

Table 1
Indications for ICD Implantation

Class I
• Cardiac arrest due to VT/VF (not due to a reversible cause)
• Sustained VT
• Syncope of unknown etiology with hemodynamically significant
  ventricular arrhythmia induced at EPS despite anti-arrhythmic therapy
• Nonsustained VT and inducible sustained VT/VF at EPS in the setting
  of ischemic left ventricular dysfunction following MI that is not
  suppressible with class I anti-arrhythmics
Class IIa
• LVEF <30% at least 1 month status post-MI or 3 months status post-
  CABG
Class IIb
• Cardiac arrest presumed secondary to VT/VF when EPS is contraindicated
• Severe symptomatic VT/VF while awaiting cardiac transplantation
• Familial syndromes such as long QT and hypertrophic cardiomyopathy
  with a high-risk of sudden cardiac death
• Nonsustained VT in the setting of coronary artery disease with inducable
  VT/VF at EPS
• Recurrent syncope with left ventricular dysfunction with inducible
  ventricular arrhythmias at EPS when other causes of syncope have been
  excluded
• Syncope with a Brugada pattern on EKG testing
Class III
• Syncope of unknown etiology with a nondiagnostic EPS
• VT/VF storm
• VT/VF amenable to catheter ablation (e.g., WPW)
• VT/VF in the setting of electrolyte disturbances (e.g., hypomagnesemia)
• Patients with class IV NYHA heart failure not responding to pharmaco-
  logical therapy and ineligible for cardiac transplantation

ICD, implantable cardiac defibrillator; VT/VF, ventricular tachycardiac/ventricular
fibrillation; EPS, electrophysiology study; MI, myocardial infarction; LVEF, left ventricular ejection fraction; CABG, coronary artery bypass grafting ; EKG, electrocardiogram; WPW, Wolff-Parkinson-White syndrome; NYHA, New York Heart Association.
(Adapted from ref. 15.)

primary prevention in patients with an LVEF below 30% and prior MI.
The study was more bold in that patients were not required to have either
documented NSVT or an invasive EP study. Notably, the mean age of the
MADIT II population was 65 years.

There is growing evidence to suggest that ICD implantation is also an
effective means of primary prevention in patients with nonischemic DCM.

A retrospective analysis of ICD firing in patients with nonischemic DCM has shown that the incidence of ICD firing (approximatley 30%) is similar in patients, regardless of whether or not they had a prior history of ventricular arrhythmia *(72)*. In addition, recent studies suggest that EP testing may have less predictive value in patients with markedly impaired ventricular function, particularly those with idiopathic DCM. Middlekauff and colleagues have called attention to the strong link between syncope and sudden cardiac death in patients with a history of heart failure *(73–75)*. Their findings reiterate the poor negative predictive value of EP testing in patients with reduced ventricular function. Approximately one-half of patients with nonischemic DCM, syncope, and a negative EPS who undergo ICD implantation will have an appropriate device firing for VT/VF in the ensuing 24 months *(76)*. These findings suggest that more sensitive diagnostic tests are needed to evaluate patients' risk for sudden cardiac death and that those patients with nonischemic DCM will likely benefit from ICD implantation. The recent completion of the Comparison of Medical Therapy, Pacing, and Defibrillation in Heart Failure, Defibrillators in Non-Ischemic Cardiomyopathy Treatment Evaluation, and Sudden Cardiac Death in Heart Failure Trial (SCD-HeFT) trials confirmed the benefit of ICD implantation in patients with reduced EF, regardless of coronary disease *(77–79)*. In the SCD-HeFT trial, defibrillator placement in patients with New York Heart Association class II or III heart failure and impaired left ventricular function (LVEF < 35%), reduced all-cause mortality by 23%. The treatment benefit was independent of heart failure etiology (ischemic heart rate 0.79 vs nonischemic heart rate 0.73) and QRS duration *(78–81)*. Although the present American College of Cardiologists (ACC) guidelines do not reflect the findings of these recently completed trials, they are currently under revision to incorporate these new data.

At the present time, ICDs are recommended for primary prevention in patients with ischemic and nonischemic cardiomyopathy and an EF less than 35%. EP testing is indicated for patients with ischemic cardiomyopathy with less severe cardiac dysfunction (EF = 35%–45%).

SYNCOPE

Syncope is a sudden transient loss of consciousness and postural tone with spontaneous recovery. Loss of consciousness results from a reduction of blood flow to the reticular activating system located in the brain stem and does not require electrical or chemical therapy for reversal. Cessation of cerebral blood flow leads to loss of consciousness within approximately 10 seconds. Syncope is important because it is a common, costly,

Table 2
Etiology and Prevalence of Syncope
in Different Elderly Populations[a]

Vasodepressor syncope	37%[b]
Orthostatic hypotension	31%[c]
Unknown etiology	14%[d]
Arrhtyhmia	13%
Sinus bradycardia	<1%
Atrioventricular block	3%[d]
Ventricular tachycardia	<1%
Neurological	5%
Seizure	2%
TIA/stroke	2%
Carotid sinus hypersensitivity	19%[e]
Drug-induced	11%[f]
Myocardial ischemia	1%
Aortic stenosis	<1%
Pulmonary embolism	<1%

[a]Adapted from ref. 85.
[b]Adapted from ref. 86.
[c]Adapted from ref. 87.
[d]Adapted from ref. 88.
[e]Adapted from ref. 89.
[f]Adapted from ref. 90.

and often disabling problem. Syncope may be the only warning sign before sudden cardiac death (82,83). Elderly persons have a 6% annual incidence of syncope and a 30% recurrence rate at 2 years. The annual cost of evaluating and treating patients with syncope has been estimated to be $800 million (84).

The causes of syncope can be classified into four primary groups: vascular, cardiac, neurological/cerebrovascular, and metabolic/miscellaneous (Table 2). Vascular causes of syncope can be further subdivided into anatomical, orthostatic, and reflex-mediated causes. The probable cause of syncope can be identified in approximatley 75% of patients (91). Syncope in elderly individuals is often multifactorial in origin. Vascular causes of syncope, particularly reflex-mediated syncope and orthostatic hypotension, are by far the most common causes of syncope, accounting for at least one-third of all syncopal episodes. When a person stands, 500 to 800 mL of blood is displaced to the abdomen and lower extremities, resulting in an abrupt drop in venous return to the heart. This leads to a decrease in cardiac output and stimulation of aortic, carotid, and cardiopulmonary baroreceptors that trigger a reflex increase in sympathetic outflow. As a result, heart rate, cardiac contractility, and vascular resistance increase to maintain a stable systemic blood pressure (BP) on standing *(92)*. Orthostatic hypotension, which is defined as a 20 mmHg drop in systolic BP (SBP) or a 10 mmHg drop in diastolic BP within 3 minutes of standing, results from a defect in any portion of this BP-control system *(93)*. Orthostatic hypotension may be asymptomatic or may be associated with symptoms such as lightheadedness, dizziness, blurred vision, weakness, palpitations, tremulousness, and syncope. These symptoms are often worse immediately on arising in the morning and/or after meals or exercise. Syncope that occurs after meals, particularly in the elderly, may result from a redistribution of blood to the gut. A decline in SBP of about 20 mmHg approximately 1 hour after eating has been reported in up to one-third of elderly nursing home residents *(94)*. Although usually asymptomatic, it may result in lightheadedness or syncope.

Drugs that either cause volume depletion or result in vasodilation are the most common cause of orthostatic hypotension. Elderly patients are particularly susceptible to the hypotensive effects of drugs because of reduced baroreceptor sensitivity, decreased cerebral blood flow, renal sodium wasting, and an age-associated impaired thirst mechanism *(95)*. Orthostatic hypotension may also result from neurogenic causes, including primary and secondary autonomic failure.

Postural orthostatic tachycardia syndrome (POTS) is a milder form of chronic autonomic failure and orthostatic intolerance characterized by the presence of symptoms of orthostatic intolerance, a 28 bpm or greater increase in heart rate, and the absence of a significant change in BP within 5 minutes of standing or upright tilt *(96)*. POTS appears to result from a failure of the peripheral vasculature to appropriately vasoconstrict under orthostatic stress.

Reflex-Mediated Syncope

Reflex-mediated syncopal syndromes (*see* Table 2) are characterized by increased vagal tone and the withdrawal of peripheral sympathetic tone, which lead to bradycardia, vasodilation, and, ultimately, hypotension, presyncope, or syncope. What distinguishes these causes of syncope are the specific triggers. For example, micturition syncope results from activation of mechanoreceptors in the bladder; defecation syncope results from neural inputs from gut wall tension receptors; and swallowing syncope results from afferent neural impulses arising from the upper gastrointestinal tract. The two most common types of reflex-mediated syncope are carotid sinus hypersensitivity and neurally mediated hypotension.

Neurally mediated hypotension/syncope also known as neurocardiogenic, vasodepressor, and vasovagal syncope and as "fainting" has been used to describe a common abnormality of BP regulation characterized by the abrupt onset of hypotension with or without bradycardia. Triggers associated with the development of neurally mediated syncope are those that either reduce ventricular filling (prolonged standing, a warm environment, or hot shower) or increase catecholamine secretion (sight of blood, pain, and stressful situations). Under these types of situations, patients with this condition develop severe lightheadedness and/or syncope. It has been proposed that these clinical phenomena result from a paradoxical reflex that is initiated when ventricular preload is reduced by venous pooling. This leads to a reduction in cardiac output and BP, which is sensed by arterial baroreceptors. The resultant increased catecholamine levels, combined with reduced venous filling, leads to a vigorously contracting volume-depleted ventricle (97). Neurally mediated syncope is far more common among young individuals than among the elderly.

Syncope as a result of carotid sinus hypersensitivity results from stimulation of carotid sinus baroreceptors. Carotid sinus hypersensitivity is diagnosed by applying gentle pressure over the carotid pulsation just below the angle of the jaw, where the carotid bifurcation is located. After listening for a carotid bruit, pressure should be applied unilaterally for approximately 5 seconds. It has recently been reported that the sensitivity of diagnosing carotid sinus hypersensitivity can be increased, with no change in specificity, by performing carotid sinus massage during 60- or 70-degree upright tilt (98,99). The normal response to carotid sinus massage is a transient decrease in the sinus rate and/or slowing of AV conduction. Three types of abnormal responses are: (a) the cardioinhibitory response, characterized by marked bradycardia (>3-second pause); (b) the vasodepressor type, characterized by a 50 mmHg fall in the SBP in the absence of bradycardia; and (c) the mixed response. It is important to recognize that carotid sinus hypersensitivity is also commonly observed in asymptomatic elderly patients, with carotid sinus hypersensitivity identified in one study in more than one-third of asymptomatic patients undergoing cardiac catheterization for CAD. Because of this, the diagnosis of carotid sinus hypersensitivity should be approached cautiously after excluding alternative causes of syncope.

Cardiac Syncope

Cardiac causes of syncope, particularly tachyarrhythmias and bradyarrhythmias, are the second most common causes, accounting for 10% to 20% of syncopal episodes. VT is the most common tachyarrhythmia that causes syncope. Supraventricular arrhythmias can also cause syncope, although the great majority of patients with supraventricular arrhythmias present with less severe symptoms such as palpitations, dyspnea, and lightheadedness. Bradyarrhythmias that can result in syncope include SSS as well as AV block. Anatomical causes of syncope result from obstruction to blood flow, such as a massive pulmonary embolus, an atrial myxoma, and aortic stenosis.

Neurological Causes of Syncope

Neurological causes of syncope are surprisingly uncommon, accounting for less than 10% of all cases of syncope. The majority of patients in whom a "neurological" cause of syncope is established are found in fact to have had a seizure rather than true syncope *(100)*. Syncope, as an isolated symptom, rarely results from a neurological cause. As a result, widespread use of tests to screen for neurological conditions rarely are diagnostic. In many institutions, computed tomography, electroencephalography, and carotid duplex scans are overused, being obtained in more than 50% of patients with syncope. A diagnosis is almost never uncovered that was not first suspected based on a careful history and neurological examination *(101)*. One study indicated that 29% of patients with treatment-resistant epilepsy or suspected nonepileptic seizures have an underlying cardiovascular cause of syncope such as neurally mediated hypotension, carotid sinus hypersensitivity, or transient AV block *(102)*.

Metabolic/Miscellaneous Causes of Syncope

Metabolic causes of syncope are rare, accounting for less than 5% of syncopal episodes. The most common metabolic causes of syncope are hypoglycemia, hypoxia, and hyperventilation. The establishment of hypoglycemia as the cause of syncope requires demonstration of hypoglycemia during the syncopal episode. Psychiatric disorders may also cause syncope. It has been reported that up to 25% of patients with syncope of unknown origin may have psychiatric disorders for which syncope is one of the presenting symptoms *(103)*.

Prognosis in Syncope

The prognosis of patients with syncope varies greatly with etiology. Syncope of unknown origin or syncope due to a noncardiac etiology (including reflex-mediated syncope) is generally associated with a benign prognosis. In contrast, syncope owing to a cardiac cause is associated with a 30% mortality at 1 year.

DIAGNOSTIC TESTING

Identification of the precise cause of syncope is often challenging. The history and physical examination are the most important components of the evaluation of a patient with syncope *(104)*. When taking a clinical history, particular attention should focus on (a) determining if the patient experienced true syncope as compared with a transient alteration in consciousness without loss of postural tone; (b) determining if the patient has a history of cardiac disease and, if a family history of cardiac disease, syncope, or sudden death exists; (c) identifying medications that may have played a role in syncope; (d) quantifying the number and chronicity of prior episodes; (e) identifying precipitating factors including body position; and (f) quantifying the type and duration of prodromal and recovery symptoms. After obtaining a careful history, evaluation should continue with a physical examination including the determination of orthostatic vital signs, defining the patient's level of hydration, and a thorough neurological examination *(105)*.

Tilt-table testing is a standard diagnostic test for evaluating patients with syncope *(106)*. Despite its limitations, tilt-table testing is generally considered the "gold standard" for establishing a diagnosis of neurally mediated syncope. Upright tilt-table testing is performed for 30 to 45 minutes at an angle of approximately 70 degrees. In general, a positive response to tilt-table testing is defined as the development of syncope or presyncope in association with hypotension and/or bradycardia. The sensitivity of the test can be increased, with an associated fall in specificity, by the use of longer tilt durations, steeper tilt angles, and provocative agents such as isoproterenol, nitroglycerin, or edrophonium. In the absence of pharmacological provocation, the specificity of the test has been estimated to be 90% *(107)*. There is general agreement that upright tilt-table testing is indicated in patients with (a) recurrent syncope or a single syncopal episode in a high-risk patient who either has no evidence of structural heart disease or in whom other causes of syncope have been excluded, (b) evaluation of patients in whom the causes of syncope have been determined (e.g., asystole) but in whom the presence of neurally mediated syncope on upright tilt would influence treatment, and (c) as part of the evaluation of patients with exercise-related syncope. There is also general agreement that upright tilt-table testing is not necessary for patients who have experienced only a single syncopal episode that was highly typical for neurally mediated syncope and during which no injury occurred. Tilt-table testing is not useful in establishing a diagnosis of situation syncope (i.e., postmicturition syncope) *(108)*. Although echocardiograms are commonly used in the evaluation of patients with syncope, little objective evidence exists to support their use in patients with a normal physical examination and a normal EKG *(109,110)*. The rationale for obtaining an echocardiogram in patients with syncope is to risk stratify the patient by excluding the possibility of occult cardiac disease not apparent after the history, physical examination, and EKG. If detected, the presence of impaired ventricular function or significant valvular dysfunction would suggest a cardiac cause of syncope and therefore a worse long-term prognosis.

Myocardial ischemia is an unlikely cause of syncope and, when present, is usually accompanied by angina. The use of stress tests in the evaluation of a patient with syncope is best reserved for patients in whom the clinical suspicion of ischemia is high, that is, syncope or presyncope that occurred during or immediately after exertion or in association with chest pain. Even among patients with syncope during exertion it is highly unlikely that exercise stress testing will trigger another event. Patients suspected of having severe aortic stenosis or obstructive hypertrophic cardiomyopathy should not undergo exercise stress testing, because it may precipitate a cardiac arrest.

The 12-lead EKG is a standard component in the work-up of a patient with syncope and will lead to a diagnosis in approximately 10% of patients. Specific findings that may identify the probable cause of syncope include QT prolongation (long QT syndrome), the presence of a short PR interval and a δ wave (Wolff-Parkinson-White syndrome), and evidence of an acute MI, and high-grade AV block. Less-specific findings that may suggest potential causes of syncope include evidence of a prior MI, BBB, ventricular hypertrophy, and ventricular premature beats. These findings can be confirmed later with direct testing. T-wave inversion in the right precordial leads with an incomplete right BBB (RBBB) pattern, suggests a diagnosis of right ventricular dysplasia. Persistent ST-segment elevation in leads V_1 to V_3 with an incomplete RBBB pattern suggests a diagnosis of the Brugada syndrome. These hereditary disorders are associated with a high incidence of sudden cardiac death. Although more common in younger patients, they can present in the elderly (111). The finding of a normal EKG suggests that a cardiac cause of syncope is unlikely.

Continuous EKG monitoring using telemetry and/or Holter recording is commonly performed in patients with syncope. The information provided by EKG recording at the time of syncope is extremely valuable because it allows an arrhythmic cause of syncope to be established or excluded. However, because of the infrequent and sporadic nature of syncope, the diagnostic yield of Holter recording is low. The likelihood of experiencing an episode of syncope while wearing a Holter recorder in an unselected population of patients with syncope is approximately 0.1%. Although detection of asymptomatic sinus bradycardia, AV block, or nonsustained supraventricular or ventricular arrhythmias can suggest an arrhythmic cause of syncope, it is important to recognize that unless syncope or presyncope accompanies these arrhythmias they are likely to be incidental findings and should not be assumed to be the cause of syncope. Another inherent limitation of Holter recording is that it requires that the patient experience another episode of syncope to establish a diagnosis. For these reasons, the clinical situation in which Holter recording is most likely to be diagnostic is the occasional patient with very frequent (i.e., daily) episodes of syncope or presyncope. Alternatively, event recorders are especially useful for patients with infrequent episodes of presyncope or syncope, particularly once potentially malignant causes of syncope have been excluded *(112)*.

Electrophysiology Testing

The results of EP testing can be useful in establishing a diagnosis of SSS, heart block, SVT, or VT in patients with syncope. The indications for EP testing in the evaluation of patients with syncope have recently been established based on an ACC/American Heart Association Task Force report *(113)*. There is general agreement that EP testing should be performed in patients with suspected structural heart disease and unexplained syncope (class I indication) and that it should not be performed in patients with a known cause of syncope for whom treatment will not be influenced by the findings of the test (class III indication). The role of EP testing in evaluating patients with recurrent unexplained syncope who do not have structural heart disease and have had a negative tilt-test remains controversial.

MANAGEMENT OF THE PATIENT WITH SYNCOPE

The approach to treatment of a patient with syncope largely depends on the diagnosis that is established. For example, the appropriate treatment of a patient with syncope as a result of AV block or SSS would likely involve placement of a permanent pacemaker; treatment of a patient with syncope owing to the Wolff-Parkinson-White syndrome would likely involve catheter ablation; and treatment of a patient with syncope caused by VT would likely involve placement of an ICD. For other types of syncope, optimal patient management may involve discontinuation of an offending pharmacological agent, an increase in salt intake, or patient education.

Special Issues in Management

ANTICOAGULATION IN THE ELDERLY

Anticoagulation for stroke prophylaxis represents a special challenge in the elderly. Although the aged benefit the most from anticoagulation, they also are at the highest risk for bleeding events, including intracranial bleeding.

AF is an independent risk factor for stroke and is associated with a sixfold increased risk of stroke *(114)*. AF leads to atrial stasis and formation of left atrial thrombi, which have a tendency to embolize to the cerebral vasculature. Among patients with AF, the risk of stroke is approximately 5% per year. Both paroxysmal AF and persistent AF are associated with similar stroke rates *(115,116)*.

Risk stratification and cardioembolic stroke prophylaxis represent a cornerstone in the management of AF patients. Patients at a high risk of stroke benefit the most from systemic anticoagulation. A multivariate analysis in the Stroke Prophylaxis in Atrial Fibrillation I Trial (SPAF I) identified several risk factors for stroke in AF, including hypertension, heart failure, transient ischemic attacks, evidence of systemic embolism, and a history of stroke *(117)*.

The SPAF trials suggested that patients at low risk for stroke should receive aspirin, whereas patients older than 75 years or those with moderate to high risk of stroke should receive anticoagulation. There are now several RCTs that have demonstrated the efficacy of warfarin in the prevention of stroke in patients with nonvalvular AF and one or more risk factors for cerebrovascular emboli *(37,118)*. Adjusted-dose warfarin was associated with a 74% relative risk reduction ($p < 0.001$) in stroke in the SPAF III trial *(119)*. However, this risk reduction comes at a price. Anticoagulation increases bleeding risk and doubles the risk of intracranial hemorrhage *(120)*.

Multiple authorities have questioned the role of anticoagulation in the oldest old (those 85 years and older), especially since many RCTs have not been adequately powered to assess the risk–benefit ratio in this age group *(121)*. Clearly, more RCTs of anticoagulation in octogenarians are needed. In the meantime, stroke prophylaxis should be tailored to the individual patient and guided by the patient's risk profile and functional status. If the patient has both high risk and good functional status (i.e., their quality of life would be impaired by a disabling stroke), then they should be anticoagulated, regardless of their age. Unfortunately, many elderly patients with nonvalvular AF who are at high risk for future stroke and have no contraindications to anticoagulation are not on warfarin (approximately 50%). Among those who are taking warfarin, only half of these patients have international normalized ratios in the therapeutic range *(122)*. Coordinating patient care with anticoagulation clinics improves patient outcomes, with respect to both complications and stroke reduction *(123)*.

ANTI-ARRHYTHMICS IN THE ELDERLY

Elderly patients are more likely to suffer complications and side effects from anti-arrhythmic medications. For example, in the Cardiac Arrhythmia Suppression Trial, older age was an independent predictor of adverse events in patients taking flecainide *(124)*. Furthermore, prior research has shown that the elderly are less likely to be prescribed anti-arrhythmic (especially β-blockers) therapy when compared to younger patients with the same therapeutic indications. Not surprisingly, lower rates of therapy in the elderly are associated with increased adverse outcomes *(125)*.

There are several age-associated changes that make pharmacotherapy in the elderly more challenging. Glomerular filtration rate declines with age, limiting therapeutic options in many elderly patients. Decreased drug clearance and decreases in lean body mass lead to an increased half-life and volume of distribution of amiodarone in elderly patients *(126)*. With regard to amiodarone, it is important to remember that its side effects include corneal deposits and photosensitivity in addition to the better known thyroid, hepatic, and pulmonary complications. Routine monitoring for patients on amiodarone should include thyroid function testing, serum transaminase determination and a chest x-ray at baseline and every 6 months. Pulmonary function testing is the most sensitive test for amiodarone associated pulmonary fibrosis and should be performed annually or whenever patients complain of dyspnea on exertion *(127)* (Table 3).

RADIOFREQUENCY ABLATION

Radiofrequency (RF) ablation destroys arrhythmogenic tissue through the thermal disruption of cardiac membranes. Although RF catheter ablation is an invasive procedure and is associated with procedural risk, RF termination often liberates patients from anti-arrhythmic medications that carry significant side effects, especially in the elderly population. At the present time, a significant number of ablation procedures are carried out in elderly patients. The 1998 North American Society of Pacing and Electrophysiology (NASPE) prospective catheter ablation registry revealed that patients undergoing RF ablation for atrial flutter had a mean age of 61 ± 14 years and that 28% of the cohort were older than 70 years *(27)*.

Although some studies suggest that older age and the presence of systemic illness increase the risk for RF ablation procedure complications *(128)*, a review of three recent large-scale studies regarding the use of catheter ablation in elderly patients with SVT demonstrated that there is no difference in success rate or adverse events between older and younger individuals *(129)*. Accordingly, RF ablation therapy should not be avoided in active, elderly individuals whose quality of life will be benefited by the termination of their arrhythmias *(130,131)*.

According to the NASPE guidelines, class I recommendations for RF ablation in patients who have failed one or more trials of anti-arrhythmic

Table 3
Recommended Monitoring and Testing for Patients Taking Amiodarone

Test	Testing interval	Toxicity
Electrocardiogram	Baseline and every 6 months	Evaluate for QTc prolongation and impaired atrioventricular conduction.
Pulmonary function testing (with DLCO)	Baseline, yearly, and with complaints of new or progressive dyspnea	Very important in patients with underlying pulmonary disease. A reduced DLCO (>15%) is the most sensitive finding of early amiodarone toxicity.
T4 and TSH	Baseline and every 6 months	Thyroid dysfunction occurs in 22% of patients (hyperthyroidism or hypothyroidism.)
Liver function tests	Baseline and every 6 months	Evaluate for transaminitis and discontinue if ALT/AST is 2x normal.
Chest x-ray	Baseline and annually	Evaluate for interstitial pneumonitis (early) and pulmonary fibrosis (late).
Ophthalmological evaluation	Baseline, annually, and with visual complaints	Corneal deposits (common) and optic neuritis (rare).

DLCO, diffusing capacity for carbon monoxide; TSH, thyroid-stimulating hormone. (Adapted from ref. *127*.)

therapy include slow pathway ablation in AVNRT, AV re-entry, AV nodal ablation in patients with SVT in whom the rate cannot be controlled with maximal medical therapy, atrial tachycardia, and isthmus-dependent atrial flutter. Similarly, RF ablation of AVNRT, AV junction, isthmus-dependent atrial flutter, and accessory pathways have success rates in excess of 85% *(132)* (Table 4).

DEVICE THERAPY IN THE ELDERLY

The incidence of sinus node dysfunction, AV block, heart failure, and sudden cardiac death all increase with age. Accordingly, most patients who require pacemaker or ICD implantation are older. Given the finite resources of our health care system and the disproportionate expenditure of health care dollars in the later years of life, many have examined the efficacy of device therapy in the elderly. Several studies have shown that

Table 4
Arrhythmias Amenable to Catheter Ablation: Success Rates and Recurrence

Arrhythmia	Success rate	Recurrence
Focal atrial tachycardia	95%	5%
AVRT (accessory pathway)[1]	95%	3%
AVNRT (slow pathway ablation)	97%	3%
Isthmus-dependent atrial flutter	97%	15%
Nonisthmus dependent Flutter	70%	20%
Atrial fibrillation (pulmonary vein ablation)	70%	20%

AVRT, atrioventricular reciprocating tachycardia; AVNRT, atrioventricular nodal re-entrant tachycardia. (From ref. *132*.)

device therapy in the elderly is both safe and effective and that advanced age alone should not be a contraindication to device therapy *(134–136)*. Among octagenarians and nonagenarians, AV block, SSS, and chronic AF complicated by bradycardia are the most common indications for pacemaker placement. Pacemaker implantation relieves symptoms in 75% of these patients. Much like any therapeutic intervention, treatment should be tailored to the individual patient after consideration of the potential risks and benefits. Although the majority of those 80 years and older do well after ICD and pacemaker implantation, some patients experience functional decline or require nursing home placement. Although device therapy is a safe and effective intervention in the functional elderly patient, more research is needed regarding patient selection among the oldest old.

CONCLUSION

The prevalence of cardiac arrhythmias and conduction disorders increase with age and impart significant morbidity and mortality in the elderly population, especially among those with compromised left ventricular function and heart failure. Fortunately, over the past decade, numerous safe and effective therapies have been developed to treat dysrrhythmia and prevent sudden cardiac death. As with any condition, treatment should be tailored to the individual patient. However, age should not preclude functional elderly patients from catheter ablation, device therapy, and other interventional strategies. These patients have much to gain from symptomatic relief and stand to benefit the most from avoiding side effects of anti-arrhythmic medications.

REFERENCES

1. Clarke JM, Hamer J, Shelton JR, Taylor S, Venning GR. The rhythm of the normal human heart. Lancet 1976;1(7984):508–512.

2. Kantelip JP, Sage E, Duchene-Marullaz P. Findings on ambulatory electrocardiographic monitoring in subjects older than 80 years. Am J Cardiol 1986;57(6): 398–401.

3. Baine WB, Yu W, Weis KA. Trends and outcomes in the hospitalization of older Americans for cardiac conduction disorders or arrhythmias, 1991–1998. J Am Geriatr Soc 2001;49(6):763–770.

4. Lev M. Anatomic basis for atrioventricular block. Am J Med 1964;37:742.

5. Davies MJ. Pathology of chronic AV Block. Acta Cardiol Suppl 1976;21:19–30.

6. Hodkinson HM, Pomerance A. The clinical significance of senile cardiac amyloidosis: a prospective clinico-pathological study. Q J Med 1977;46(183):381–387.

7. Lev M. Aging changes in the human sinoatrial node. J Gerontol 1954;9:1–8.

8. Furberg CD, Manolio TA, Psaty BM, et al. Major electrocardiographic abnormalities in persons aged 65 years and older (the Cardiovascular Health Study). Cardiovascular Health Study Collaborative Research Group. Am J Cardiol 1992;69(16): 1329–1335.

9. Caird FI, Campbell A, Jackson TF. Significance of abnormalities of electrocardiogram in old people. Br Heart J 1974;36(10):1012–1018.

10. Ostor E, Schnohr P, Jensen G, Nyboe J, Hansen AT. Electrocardiographic findings and their association with mortality in the Copenhagen City Heart Study. Eur Heart J 1981;2(4):317–328.

11. Kannel WB, Dannenberg AL, Levy D. Population implications of electrocardiographic left ventricular hypertrophy. Am J Cardiol 1987;60(17):85I–93I.

12. Seifer C, Kenny RA. The prevalence of falls in older persons paced for atrioventricular block and sick sinus syndrome. Am J Geriatr Cardiol 2003;12:298–305.

13. Lamas GA, Pashos CL, Normand SL, McNeil B. Permanent pacemaker selection and subsequent survival in elderly Medicare pacemaker recipients. Circulation 1995; 91:1063–1069.

14. Lown B. Electrical reversion of cardiac arrhythmias. Br Heart J 1967;29:469.

15. Gregoratos G, Abrams J, Epstein AE, et al. ACC/AHA/NASPE 2002 Guideline Update for Implantation of Cardiac Pacemakers and Antiarrhythmia Devices— summary article: a report of the American College of Cardiology/American Heart Association Task Force on Practice Guidelines (ACC/AHA/NASPE Committee to Update the 1998 Pacemaker Guidelines). J Am Coll Cardiol 2002; 40:1703–1719.

16. Song Y, Yao Q, Zhu J, Luo B, Liang S. Age-related variation in the interstitial tissues of the cardiac conduction system; and autopsy study of 230 Han Chinese. Forensic Sci Int 1999;104:133–142.

17. Fleg JL, Das DN, Wright J, Lakatta EG. Age-associated changes in the components of atrioventricular conduction in apparently healthy volunteers. J Gertol 1990;45: M95–M100.

18. Kusumoto FM, Lurie KG, Dutton J, Capili H, Schwartz JB. Effects of aging on AV nodal and ventricular beta-adrenergic receptors in the Fischer 344 rat. Am J Physiol 1994;266:H1408–H1415.

19. Craft N, Schwartz JB. Effects of age on intrinsic heart rate, heart rate variability, AV conduction in healthy humans. Am J Physiol 1995;268:H1441–H1452.

20. Mymin D, Mathewson FA, Tate RB, Manfreda J. The natural history of primary first-degree atrioventricular heart block. N Engl J Med 1986;315:1183–1187.

21. Eriksson P, Hansson PO, Eriksson H, Dellborg M. Bundle-branch block in a general male population: the study of men born 1913. Circulation 1998;98:2494–2500.

22. McAnulty JH, Rahimtoola SH, Murphy E, et al. Natural history of "high-risk" bundle-branch block: final report of a prospective study. N Engl J Med 1982;307: 137–143.

23. Orejarena LA, Vidaillet H Jr, DeStefano F, et al. Paroxysmal supraventricular tachycardia in the general population. J Am Coll Cardiol 1998;31:150–157.
24. Blomstrom-Lundqvist C, Scheinman MM, Aliot EM, et al. European Society of Cardiology Committee, NASPE-Heart Rhythm Society. ACC/AHA/ESC guidelines for the management of patients with supraventricular arrhythmias—executive summary. a report of the American college of cardiology/American heart association task force on practice guidelines and the European society of cardiology committee for practice guidelines (writing committee to develop guidelines for the management of patients with supraventricular arrhythmias) developed in collaboration with NASPE-Heart Rhythm Society. J Am Coll Cardiol 2003;42:1493–1531.
25. Wu D, Denes P, Amat-y-Leon F, et al. Clinical, electrocardiographic and electrophysiologic observations in patients with paroxysmal supraventricular tachycardia. Am J Cardiol 1978;41:1045–1051.
26. Brembilla-Perrot B, Houriez P, Beurrier D, et al. Influence of age on the electrophysiological mechanism of paroxysmal supraventricular tachycardias. Int J Cardiol 2001;78(3):293–298.
27. Scheinman MM, Huang S. The 1998 NASPE prospective catheter ablation registry. Pacing Clin Electrophysiol 2000;23:1020–1028.
28. Nelson SD, Kou WH, Annesley T, DeBuitleir M, Morady F. Significance of ST segment depression during paroxysmal supraventricular tachycardia. J Am Coll Cardiol 1988;12:383–387.
29. Paparella N, Ouyang F, Fuca G. Significance of newly acquired negative T waves after interruption of paroxysmal reentrant supraventricular tachycardia with narrow QRS complex. Am J Cardiol 2000;85:261–263.
30. McCord J, Borzak S. Multifocal atrial tachycardia. Chest 2004;113:203–209.
31. Granada J, Uribe W, Chyou PH, et al. Incidence and predictors of atrial flutter in the general population. J Am Coll Cardiol 2004;36:2242–2246.
32. Bialy D, Lehman MH. Hospitalization for arrhythmias in the United States: importance of atrial fibrillation. J Am Coll Cardiol 1992;19:716.
33. Wellens HJJ. Contemporary management of atrial flutter. Circulation 2002;106: 649–652.
34. Natale A, Newby KH, Pisano E, et al. Prospective randomized comparison of antiarrhythmic therapy versus first-line radiofrequency ablation in patients with atrial flutter. J Am Coll Cardiol 2000;35:1898–1904.
35. Amar D, Zhang H, Leung DH, Roistacher N, Kadish AH. Older age is the strongest predictor of postoperative atrial fibrillation. Anesthesiology 2002;96:352–356.
36. Go AS, Hylek EM, Phillips KA, et al. Prevalence of diagnosed atrial fibrillation in adults—National implications for rhythm management and stroke prevention: the AnTicoagulation and Risk Factors in Atrial Fibrillation (ATRIA) Study. JAMA 2001;285:2370–2375.
37. Risk factors for stroke and efficacy of antithrombotic therapy in atrial fibrillation. Analysis of pooled data from five randomized controlled trials. Arch Intern Med 1994;154:1449–1467.
38. Kannel WB, Abbott RD, Savage DD, McNamara PM. Epidemiologic features of chronic atrial fibrillation: the Framingham study. N Engl J Med 1982;306(17): 1018–1022.
39. Kopecky SL, Gersh BJ, McGoon MD, et al. Lone atrial fibrillation in elderly persons: a marker for cardiovascular risk. Arch Intern Med 1999;159:1118–1122.
40. Majeed A, Moser K, Carroll K. Trends in the prevalence and management of atrial fibrillation in general practice in England and Wales, 1994–1998: analysis of data from the general practice research database. Heart 2001;86(3):284–286.

41. Haissaguerre M, Jais P, Shah DC, et al. Spontaneous initiation of atrial fibrillation by ectopic beats originating in the pulmonary veins. N Engl J Med 1998;339: 659–666.

42. Pappone C, Rosanio S, Augello G, et al. Mortality, morbidity, and quality of life after circumferential pulmonary vein ablation for atrial fibrillation: outcomes from a controlled nonrandomized long-term study. J Am Coll Cardiol 2003;42:185–197.

43. Oral H, Scharf C, Chugh A, et al. Catheter ablation for paroxysmal atrial fibrillation: segmental pulmonary vein ostial ablation versus left atrial ablation. Circulation. 2003;108:2355–2360.

44. Kato R, Lickfett L, Meininger G, et al. Pulmonary vein anatomy in patients undergoing catheter ablation of atrial fibrillation: lessons learned by use of magnetic resonance imaging. Circulation 2003;107:2004–2010.

45. Fuster V, Ryden LE, Asinger RW, et al. ACC/AHA/ESC Guidelines for the Management of Patients With Atrial Fibrillation: Executive Summary A Report of the American College of Cardiology/American Heart Association Task Force on Practice Guidelines and the European Society of Cardiology Committee for Practice Guidelines and Policy Conferences (Committee to Develop Guidelines for the Management of Patients With Atrial Fibrillation) Developed in Collaboration With the North American Society of Pacing and Electrophysiology. Circulation 2001; 104:2118–2150.

46. Klein AL, Grimm RA, Murray RD, et al. Assessment of Cardioversion Using Transesophageal Echocardiography Investigators. Use of transesophageal echocardiography to guide cardioversion in patients with atrial fibrillation. N Engl J Med 2001; 344:1411–1420.

47. Lundstrom T, Ryden L. Chronic atrial fibrillation. Long-term results of direct current conversion. Acta Med Scand 1988;223:53–59.

48. Danias PG, Caulfield TA, Weigner MJ, Silverman DI, Manning WJ. Likelihood of spontaneous conversion of atrial fibrillation to sinus rhythm. J Am Coll Cardiol 1998;31:588–592.

49. Flaker GC, Fletcher KA, Rothbart RM, Halperin JL, Hart RG. Clinical and echocardiographic features of intermittent atrial fibrillation that predict recurrent atrial fibrillation. Stroke Prevention in Atrial Fibrillation (SPAF) Investigators. Am J Cardiol 1995;76:355–358.

50. Dittrich HC, Pearce LA, Asinger RW, et al. Left atrial diameter in nonvalvular atrial fibrillation: An echocardiographic study. Stroke Prevention in Atrial Fibrillation Investigators. Am Heart J 1999;137:494–499.

51. Duytschaever M, Haerynck F, Tavernier R, Jordaens L. Factors influencing long term persistence of sinus rhythm after a first electrical cardioversion for atrial fibrillation. Pacing Clin Electrophysiol 1998;21:284–287.

52. Mittal S, Ayati S, Stein KM, et al. Transthoracic cardioversion of atrial fibrillation: comparison of rectilinear biphasic versus damped sine wave monophasic shocks. Circulation 2000;101(11):1282–1287.

53. Kirchhof P, Eckardt L, Loh P, et al. Anterior–posterior versus anterior–lateral electrode positions for external cardioversion of atrial fibrillation: a randomised trial. Lancet 2002;360:1275–1279.

54. Farshi R, Kistner D, Sarma JS, Longmate JA, Singh BN. Ventricular rate control in chronic atrial fibrillation during daily activity and programmed exercise: a crossover open-label study of five drug regimens. J Am Coll Cardiol 1999;33:304–310.

55. Kochiadakis GE, Igoumenidis NE, Solomou MC, Kaleboubas MD, Chlouverakis GI, Vardas PE. Efficacy of amiodarone for the termination of persistent atrial fibrillation. Am J Cardiol 1999;83:58–61.

56. AFFIRM First Antiarrhythmic Drug Substudy Investigators. Maintenance of sinus rhythm in patients with atrial fibrillation: an AFFIRM substudy of the first antiarrhythmic drug. J Am Coll Cardiol 2003;42:20–29.
57. Hohnloser SH, Kuck KH, Lilienthal J. Rhythm or rate control in atrial fibrillation—Pharmacological Intervention in Atrial Fibrillation (PIAF): a randomised trial. Lancet 2000;356:1789–1794.
58. Carlsson J, Miketic S, Windeler J, et al. STAF Investigators. Randomized trial of rate-control versus rhythm-control in persistent atrial fibrillation: the Strategies of Treatment of Atrial Fibrillation (STAF) study. J Am Coll Cardiol 2003;41:1690–1696.
59. Wyse DG, Waldo AL, DiMarco JP, et al. A comparison of rate control and rhythm control in patients with atrial fibrillation. N Engl J Med 2002;347:1825–1833.
60. Van Gelder IC, Hagens VE, Bosker HA, et al. Rate Control versus Electrical Cardioversion for Persistent Atrial Fibrillation Study Group. A comparison of rate control and rhythm control in patients with recurrent persistent atrial fibrillation. N Engl J Med 2002;347:1834–1840.
61. Kimura S, Bassett AL, Kohya T, et al. Simultaneous recording of action potentials from endocardium and epicardium during ischemia in the isolated cat ventricle: relation of temporal electrophysiologic heterogenaieties to arrhythmias. Circulation 1986;74:401–409.
62. Fleg JL, Lakatta EG. Prevalence and prognosis of exercise-induced nonsustained ventricular tachycardia in apparently healthy volunteers. Am J Cardiol 1984;54:762–764.
63. Mirowski M, Reid PK, Mower MM, et al. Termination of malignant ventricular arrhythmias with an implanted automatic defibrillator in human beings. N Engl J Med 1980;303:322–324.
64. Mitchel LB. Clinical trials of antiarrhythmic drugs in patients with sustained ventricular tachycardia. Curr Opin Cardiol 1997;12:33–40.
65. Eisenberg MS, Horwood BT, Cummins RO, Reynolds-Haertle R, Hearne TR. Cardiac arrest and resuscitation: a tale of 29 cities. Ann Emerg Med 1990;19(2):179–186.
66. AVID Investigators. A comparison of antiarrhythmic-drug therapy with implantable defibrillators in patients resuscitated from near-fatal ventricular arrhythmias. The Antiarrhythmics versus Implantable Defibrillators (AVID) Investigators. N Engl J Med 1997;337:1576–1583.
67. Connolly SJ, Hallstrom AP, Cappato R, et al. Meta-analysis of the implantable cardioverter defibrillator secondary prevention trials. AVID, CASH and CIDS studies. Antiarrhythmics vs Implantable Defibrillator study. Cardiac Arrest Study Hamburg. Canadian Implantable Defibrillator Study. Eur Heart J 2000;21(24):2071–2078.
68. Myerburg RJ, Interian A Jr, Mitrani RM, Kessler KM, Castellanos A. Frequency of sudden cardiac death and profiles of risk. Am J Cardiol 1997;80(5B):10F–19F.
69. Lie KI, Wellens HJJ, Downar E, Durrer D. Observations on patients with primary ventricular fibrillation complicating acute myocardial infarction. Circulation 1975;52(5):755–759.
70. Buxton AE, Lee KL, Fisher JD, Josephson ME, Prystowsky EN, Hafley G. A randomized study of the prevention of sudden death in patients with coronary artery disease. Multicenter Unsustained Tachycardia Trial Investigators. N Engl J Med 1999;341(25):1882–1890.
71. Moss AJ, Hall WJ, Cannom DS, et al. Improved survival with an implanted defibrillator in patients with coronary disease at high risk for ventricular arrhythmia. Multicenter Automatic Defibrillator Implantation Trial Investigators. N Engl J Med 1996;335(26):1933–1940.

72. Grimm W, Hoffmann JJ, Muller HH, Maisch B. Implantable defibrillator event rates in patients with idiopathic dilated cardiomyopathy, nonsustained ventricular tachycardia on Holter and a left ventricular ejection fraction below 30%. J Am Coll Cardiol 2002;39:780–787.
73. Middlekauff HR, Stevenson WG, Saxon LA. Prognosis after syncope: impact of left ventricular function. Am Heart J 1993;125:121–127.
74. Middlekauff HR, Stevenson WG, Stevenson LW, Saxon LA. Syncope in advanced heart failure: high risk of sudden death regardless of origin of syncope. J Am Coll Cardiol 1993;21:110–116.
75. Brilakis ES, Shen WK, Hammill SC, et al. Role of programmed ventricular stimulation and implantable cardioverter defibrillators in patients with idiopathic dilated cardiomyopathy and syncope. Pacing Clin Electrophysiol 2001;24:1623–1630.
76. Knight BP, Goyal R, Pelosi F, et al. Outcome of patients with nonischemic dilated cardiomyopathy and unexplained syncope treated with an implantable defibrillator. J Am Coll Cardiol 1999;33:1964–1970.
77. Bristow MR, Saxon LA, Boehmer J, et al. Cardiac-Resynchronization Therapy with or without an Implantable Defibrillator in Advanced Chronic Heart Failure. N Engl J Med 2004;350:2140–2150.
78. Kadish A, Dyer A, Daubert JP, et al. Prophylactic defibrillator implantation in patients with nonischemic dilated cardiomyopathy. N Engl J Med 2004;350(21): 2151–2158.
79. Bardy G, Lee K, Mark D, et al. The Sudden Cardiac Death in Heart Failure Trial. American College of Cardiology 2004 Scientific Sessions. 2004;3–8- Ref Type: Abstract
80. Poole JE, Anderson J, Johnson G, et al. Baseline EKG Data and Outcome in SCD-HeFT. Heart Rhythm Society 2004 Annual Scientific Session. 2004. Ref Type: Abstract
81. Klein H, Auricchio A, Reek S, Geller C. New primary prevention trials of sudden cardiac death in patients with left ventricular dysfunction: SCD-HEFT and MADIT-II. Am J Cardiol 1999;83:91D–97D.
82. Kapoor W. Evaluation and management of syncope. JAMA 1992;268:2553–2560.
83. Calkins H, Byrne M, El-Atassi R, et al. The economic burden of unrecognized vasodepressor syncope. Am J Med 1993;95:473–479.
84. Nyman JA, Krahn AD, Bland PC, et al. The costs of recurrent syncope of unknown origin in elderly patients. Pacing Clin Electrophysiol 1999;22:1386–1394.
85. Getchell WS, Larsen GC, Morris CD, McAnulty JH. Epidemiology of syncope in hospitalized patients. Gen Intern Med 1999;14(11):677–687.
86. Sarasin FP, Louis-Simonet M, Carballo D, et al. Prospective evaluation of patients with syncope: a population-based study. Am J Med 2001;111(3):177–184.
87. Marangoni E, Zucchi A, Lissoni F, et al. Tilt test results in young and elderly patients with syncope of unknown origin. Aging (Milano). 1996;8(6):409–416.
88. Kapoor W, Snustad D, Peterson J, Wieand HS, Cha R, Karpf M. Syncope in the elderly. Am J Med 1986;80(3):419–428.
89. Kenny RA, Richardson DA, Steen N, Bexton RS, Shaw FE, Bond J. Carotid sinus syndrome: a modifiable risk factor for nonaccidental falls in older adults (SAFE PACE). J Am Coll Cardiol 2001;38(5):1491–1496.
90. Lipsitz LA, Wei JY, Rowe JW. Syncope in an elderly, institutionalised population: prevalence, incidence, and associated risk. Q J Med 1985;55(216):45–54.
91. Sra JS, Anderson AJ, Sheikh SH, et al. Unexplained syncope evaluated by electrophysiologic studies and head-up tilt testing. Ann Intern Med 1991;114:1013–1019.

92. Wieling W, van Lieshout JJ. Maintenance of postural normotension in humans. In: Low P (ed.), Clinical Autonomic Disorders. Boston: Little, Brown, 1993, pp. 69–75.
93. The Consensus Committee of the American Autonomic Society and the American Academy of Neurology. Consensus statement on the definition of orthostatic hypotension, pure autonomic failure, and multiple system atrophy. Neurology 1996;46: 1470–1471.
94. Vaitkevicius PV, Esserwein DM, Maynard AK, et al. Frequency and importance of postprandial blood pressure reduction in elderly nursing-home patients. Ann Intern Med 1991;115:865.
95. Kapoor WN. Syncope in the older person. J Am Geriatr Soc 1994;42:426.
96. Low P, Opfer-Gehrking T, Textor S, et al. Postural tachycardia syndrome (POTS). Neurology 1995;45:519–525.
97. Abboud FM. Neurocardiogenic syncope. N Engl J Med 1993;328:1117–1119.
98. Morillo CA, Camacho ME, Wood MA, et al. Diagnostic utility of mechanical, pharmacological and orthostatic stimulation of the carotid sinus in patients with unexplained syncope. J Am Coll Cardiol 1999;34:1587–1594.
99. Parry SW, Richardson DA, O'Shea D, Kenny RA. Diagnosis of carotid sinus hypersensitivity in older adults: Carotid sinus massage in the upright position is essential. Heart 2000;83:22–23.
100. Kapoor WN. Evaluation and outcome of patients with syncope. Medicine 1990;69: 160–175.
101. Davis TL, Freemon FR. Electroencephalography should not be routine in the evaluation of syncope in adults. Arch Intern Med 1990;150:2027–2029.
102. Zaidi A, Crampton S, Clough P, et al. Misdiagnosis of epilepsy-many seizure-like episodes have a cardiovascular cause. PACE 1999;22(2):815.
103. Kapoor WN, Fortunato M, Hanusa BH, Schulberg HC. Psychiatric illnesses in patients with syncope. Am J Med 1995;99:505–512.
104. Calkins H, Shyr Y, Frumin H, et al. The value of the clinical history in the differentiation of syncope due to ventricular tachycardia, atrioventricular block, and neurocardiogenic syncope. Am J Med 1995;98:365–373.
105. Brignole M, Alboni P, Benditt D, et al. Guidelines on management (diagnosis and treatment) of syncope. Eur Heart J 2001;22:1256–1306.
106. Benditt DG, Ferguson DW, Grubb BP, et al. Tilt table testing for assessing syncope. J Am Coll Cardiol 1996;28:263–275.
107. Natale A, Akhtar M, Jazayeri M, et al. Provocation of hypotension during head-up tilt testing in subjects with no history of syncope or presyncope. Circulation 1995; 92:54–58.
108. Sumiyoshi M, Nakata Y, Yoriaki M, et al. Response to head-up tilt testing in patients with situational syncope. Am J Cardiol 1998;82:1117–1118.
109. Panther R, Mahmood S, Gal R. Echocardiography in the diagnostic evaluation of syncope. J Am Soc Echocardiogr 1998;11:294–298.
110. Recchia D, Barzilai B. Echocardiography in the evaluation of patients with syncope. J Gen Intern Med 1995;10:649–655.
111. More D, O'Brien K, Shaw J. Arrhythmogenic right ventricular dysplasia in the elderly. Pacing Clin Electrophysiol 2002;25:1266–1269.
112. Fogel RI, Evans JJ, Prystowsky EN. Utility and cost of event recorders in the diagnosis of palpitations, presyncope, and syncope. Am J Cardiol 1997;79:207–208.
113. Zipes DP, DiMarco JP, Gillette PC, et al. Guidelines for clinical intracardiac electrophysiological and catheter ablation procedures. J Am Coll Cardiol 1995;26: 555–573.

114. Hart RG, Halperin JL, Pearce LA, et al. Lessons from the Stroke Prevention in Atrial Fibrillation trials. Ann Intern Med 2003;138:831–838.

115. Hart RG, Pearce LA, Rothbart RM, et al. Stroke with intermittent atrial fibrillation: incidence and predictors during aspirin therapy. Stroke Prevention in Atrial Fibrillation Investigators. J Am Coll Cardiol 2000;35(1):183–187.

116. Hart RG, Benavente O, McBride R, Pearce LA. Antithrombotic therapy to prevent stroke in patients with atrial fibrillation: a meta-analysis. Ann Intern Med 1999;131: 492–501.

117. Stroke Prevention in Atrial Fibrillation Study. Final results. Circulation 1991;84: 527–539.

118. EAFT (European Atrial Fibrillation Trial) Study Group. Secondary prevention in non-rheumatic atrial fibrillation after transient ischaemic attack or minor stroke. Lancet 1993;342(8882):1255–1262.

119. Adjusted-dose warfarin versus low-intensity, fixed-dose warfarin plus aspirin for high-risk patients with atrial fibrillation: Stroke Prevention in Atrial Fibrillation III randomised clinical trial. Lancet 1996;348:633–638.

120. Liu M, Counsell C, Sandercock P. Anticoagulants for preventing recurrence following ischemic stroke or transient ischemic attack. (Cochrane Review). (1). 2002. Oxford. The Cochrane Library: Update Software. Ref Type: Serial (Book, Monograph)

121. Desbiens NA. Deciding on anticoagulating the oldest old with atrial fibrillation: insights from cost-effectiveness analysis. J Am Geriatr Soc 2002;50(5):863–869.

122. McCormick D, Gurwitz JH, Goldberg RJ, et al. Prevalence and quality of warfarin use for patients with atrial fibrillation in the long-term care setting. Arch Intern Med 2001;161:2458–2463.

123. Chiquette E, Amato MG, Bussey HI. Comparison of an anticoagulation clinic with usual medical care: anticoagulation control, patient outcomes, and health care costs. Arch Intern Med 1998;158(15):1641–1647.

124. Echt DS, Liebson PR, Mitchell LB, et al. Mortality and morbidity in patients receiving encainide, flecainide, or placebo. The Cardiac Arrhythmia Suppression Trial. N Engl J Med 1991;324:781–788.

125. Soumerai SB, McLaughlin TJ, Spiegelman D, Hertzmark E, Thibault G, Goldman L. Adverse outcomes of underuse of beta-blockers in elderly survivors of acute myocardial infarction. JAMA 1997;277:115–121.

126. Zimmerman JJ, Klamerus KJ, Giel S. Clin Pharmacol Ther 1993;53:201.

127. Goldschlager N, Epstein AE, Naccarelli G, Olshansky B, Singh B. Practical guidelines for clinicians who treat patients with amiodarone. Practice Guidelines Subcommittee, North American Society of Pacing and Electrophysiology. Arch Intern Med 2000;160:1741–1748.

128. Chen SA, Chiang CE, Tai CT, et al. Complications of diagnostic electrophysiologic studies and radiofrequency catheter ablation in patients with tachyarrhythmias: an eight-year survey of 3,966 consecutive procedures in a tertiary referral center. Am J Cardiol 1996;77(1):41–46.

129. Scheinman MM. Nonpharmacologic Management of Supraventricular Tachycardia. Am J Geriatr Cardiol 2000;9(3):159–161.

130. Calkins H, Yong P, Miller JM, et al. Catheter ablation of accessory pathways, atrioventricular nodal reentrant tachycardia, and the atrioventricular junction: final results of a prospective, multicenter clinical trial. The Atakr Multicenter Investigators Group. Circulation 1999;99:262–270.

131. Calkins H, Bigger JT Jr, Ackerman SJ, et al. Cost-effectiveness of catheter ablation in patients with ventricular tachycardia. Circulation 2000;101:280–288.

132. Scheinman M, Calkins H, Gillette P, et al. NASPE policy statement on catheter ablation: personnel, policy, procedures, and therapeutic recommendations. Pacing Clin Electrophysiol 2003;26:789–799.
133. Zhou L, Keane D, Reed G, Ruskin J. Thromboembolic complications of cardiac radiofrequency catheter ablation: a review of the reported incidence, pathogenesis and current research directions. J Cardiovasc Electrophysiol 1999;10:611–620.
134. Strauss HD, Berman ND. Permanent pacing in the elderly. Pacing Clin Electrophysiol 1978;1:458–464.
135. Breivik K, Ohm OJ. Permanent pacemaker treatment in older age groups. Acta Med Scand 1984;216:119–125.
136. Geelen P, Lorga Filho A, Primo J, Wellens F, Brugada P. Experience with implantable cardioverter defibrillator therapy in elderly patients. Eur Heart J 1997;18:1339–1342.

12 Peripheral Arterial Disease in the Elderly

Emile R. Mohler III, MD
and William R. Hiatt, MD

CONTENTS

INTRODUCTION

Peripheral arterial disease (PAD) is most commonly caused by atherosclerotic lesions developing in the intimal region of arteries in the lower and upper extremities. The term also includes patients with aortoiliac disease. Claudication, the Latin word for limp, denotes pain or discomfort in a specific muscle group of an extremity with exercise and occurs in approximately one-third of patients with PAD. It is estimated that 8 million people in the United States have PAD and the majority who have claudication are elderly *(1,2)*. The PAD Awareness, Risk and Treatment: New Resources for Survival (PARTNERS) study involved screening patients older than age 70 and older than age 50 years if there was a history of smoking or diabetes *(3)*. The prevalence of PAD alone was 13% and the combination of PAD and coronary artery disease (CAD)

From: *Contemporary Cardiology: Cardiovascular Disease in the Elderly*
Edited by: G. Gerstenblith © Humana Press Inc., Totowa, NJ

was 29% in PARTNERS. The following details the diagnosis and management of PAD.

CLINICAL HISTORY

The medical history is very important in assessing whether a patient has claudication from PAD. If the patient complains of discomfort with ambulation, the history should focus on whether one or both legs are involved, the location of discomfort, the distance walked at which discomfort begins, and whether the discomfort is relieved with rest. The history should also include whether the patient has a history of back pain and if the discomfort is relieved with slight flexion of the back as occurs when pushing a shopping cart through the grocery store (suggesting a neurological cause). Patients should be questioned as to whether there is discomfort at rest, which may distinguish patients with stable claudication from those with critical limb ischemia.

The majority of patients with claudication have a stable course in the leg, as 25% have worsening claudication and approximately 5% undergo amputation within 5 years *(4)*. Patients with critical limb ischemia (ischemic pain in the distal foot, ischemic ulceration, or gangrene) have a more substantial risk of limb loss. The onset of claudication is typically insidious and patients frequently have a difficult time pinpointing the exact time when the onset of symptoms first occurred. Patients presenting with acute arterial occlusion, such as may occur with arterial embolization, are easily distinguished from those with stable claudication, as the limb in patients with acute arterial occlusion is extremely painful at rest and may be associated with acute paralysis. As with all atherosclerotic diseases, risk factors are important to assess. Major risk factors for PAD include cigarette smoking, diabetes mellitus (DM), hypertension, hyperlipidemia, and hyperhomocysteinemia (Table 1). PAD is considered a cardiovascular risk equivalent given the systemic nature of atherosclerosis and thus patients with PAD should be carefully assessed for modifiable risk factors. In this regard, the natural history is much more severe. Whereas the limb outcomes are relatively benign, after 5 years follow-up, 50% of patients with PAD will suffer a myocardial infarction (MI), ischemic stroke, or vascular death *(5)*.

PHYSICAL EXAMINATION

Physical examination for PAD should include evaluation of the entire arterial system with special attention to the extremities. The examination should include palpation of all major pulses including the radial, brachial,

Table 1
Peripheral Artery Disease Risk Factors

Smoking
Diabetes
Hypertension
Hypercholesterolemia
Homocysteinemia
C-reactive protein

carotid, femoral, popliteal, posterior tibial, and dorsalis pedal pulses. The bell of the stethoscope should be used to assess for bruits in the neck, subclavian region, all quadrants of the abdomen and over the femoral artery in the groin.

The examination of lower extremities typically first begins with palpation of the femoral pulses with subsequent pulses distally. The popliteal pulse requires some skill in localization, but it is best done when the knees are flexed at approximately 10 to 15 degrees. The fingers and the hands should be placed in the popliteal space with the thumb on the knee pointed to the head. The popliteal artery lies at the lateral edge of the patella and directly below it. A key aspect of the examination that assists with locating the popliteal artery is firm pressure applied to the popliteal space. The shoes should next be removed and assessment of the soles of the feet including the spaces between the toes should be carefully examined for any ischemic lesions. The posterior tibial artery is behind the medial ankle and lies posterior and inferior to the medial maleolus. The right posterior tibial pulse is typically palpated with the left hand because the left fingers fit well into the ankle space. The right hand should be used to keep the foot at a right angle. A light touch is needed to palpate the foot pulses as too much pressure can cause one to falsely feel their own pulse. Pulses in the feet should be graded as normal, diminished, or absent. The dorsalis pedis pulse usually lies along the line between the first and second metatarsal space on the dorsum of the foot. Similarly, the foot should be kept a right angle and a light touch used with the pads of the fingers to palpate this artery. Approximately 5% to 10% of people do not have a dorsalis pedal pulse, but the anterior tibial pulse may be palpated higher up above the ankle (Fig. 1).

Several maneuvers have been described that assist with determining whether hemodynamically significant PAD is present. The maneuver of "pallor on elevation" is accomplished with both feet in the air and gently milking the feet to remove color in the soles of the foot. Next, wait 30–

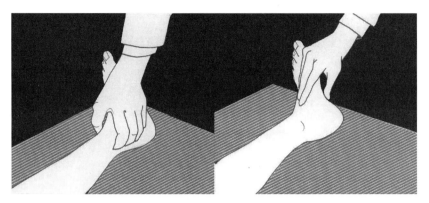

Fig. 1. Palpation of femoral, popliteal, posterier tibial pulses, and dorsalis pedis. The dorsalis pedis (left) and posterior tibial (right) pulses are examined and graded as 0 (absent), 1 (diminished), and 2 (normal). Fingers are kept flat for the dorsalis pedis and fingertips are used for the posterior tibia; as shown, the thumb applies counterpressure.

50 seconds to see whether color reappears. If the patient has significant arterial disease, significant pallor on elevation will be observed. The amount of pallor should be graded from 0 to 4 with, 0 meaning no pallor and 4+ meaning marked pallor. Next, the patient sits up and the time it takes for the first vein of the foot to fill is determined. Veins should fill in approximately 10–15 seconds. If the patient has hemodynamically significant PAD, then a delayed filling of the foot veins will occur with some patients taking up to 30–60 seconds. The time it takes for rubor in the feet to occur on dependency should also be noted. If PAD is present, there will likely be a significant amount of rubor or redness on dependency.

An assessment of the pressure in the extremities is a simple and reliable method to determine whether hemodynamically significant lesions are present. All patients should have blood pressures (BP) obtained in both arms; a 20 mmHg difference indicates disease in the upper extremities. The lower extremity pressure is best assessed using a hand-held Doppler device that utilizes ultrasonography to detect the first systolic sound. BP cuffs should be wrapped at both ankles and after the arm pressures are obtained with hand-held Doppler, the dorsalis pedal and posterior tibial pulses should be assessed. Select the higher of the two arm pressures as a denominator for both the right and left ankle-brachial index (ABI). The higher of the ankle dorsalis pedal/posterior tibial pulses is used as the numerator for calculating the ABI. The normal ABI is considered higher than 0.90 but less than 1.30, mild disease 0.70 to 0.90, moderate disease 0.50 to 0.70, and severe disease less than 0.50 with critical disease less than 0.40. Patients with stable claudication commonly have an ABI ranging from 0.41 to 0.90 and those with critical limb ischemia typically have an ABI of less than 0.40.

VASCULAR LABORATORY TESTING

The ABI, although useful for screening, does not localize the arterial occlusions or assess whether an artery is patent. The goal of vascular laboratory testing is to confirm the clinical diagnosis and to further define the level and extent of arterial obstruction. A variety of algorithms are used to noninvasively diagnose PAD and include segmental limb pressures with pulse volume plethysmography, exercise treadmill testing and arterial ultrasonography.

Segmental limb pressures are commonly measured to evaluate for PAD and are accomplished using pneumatic cuffs, appropriately sized to the diameter of the limb segment under study *(6)*. The patient is initially placed in the supine position for at least 10 minutes and cuffs are automatically inflated to above the systolic pressure. A Doppler instrument (transducer frequency 4–8 MHz) is used to detect the systolic pressure. Many laboratories use a four-cuff method where cuffs are positioned at the high thigh, low thigh above the patella, at the mid-calf, and at the ankle levels. The cuffs proximal to the ankle are inflated individually and pressures of these regions are recorded at the ankle level. The ABI is next calculated and indices are also generated for the calf and thigh regions. Patients with a normal resting ABI, but who nevertheless are believed to clinically manifest claudication, may demonstrate a decrease of the ABI after treadmill testing, which may uncover a subcritical stenosis. Patients with a super normal ABI (>1.30) may have medial artery calcification as typically occurs in patients with diabetes, and may make pressures in the lower extremities not interpretable.

Pulse volume recordings (plethysmography), usually used in conjunction with segmental pressures, are obtained by occluding venous flow and not arterial flow, and provide useful, accurate information even in patients with medial artery calcification *(7)*. Plethysmography, derived from the Greek meaning "increase," describes a change in volume of a limb occurring in response to blood flow in or out of that limb. The amplitude of volume expansion is determined by the rate at which blood simultaneously flows in and out of the segment. After occlusion of venous blood flow, blood entering the venous system results in expansion of the limb, which is responsible for a steep, ascending systolic reflection of the pulse volume recording. After peak expansion of the limb is achieved, blood exits more rapidly than it enters, resulting in a return to end-diastolic or pre-expansion volume. This results in a descending deflection of the normal pulse volume with a curve generated that is analogous to the arterial pulse pressure. Pulse volume amplitude may, however, be affected by such factors as ventricular stroke volume, BP, arrhythmia, and position of the limb. If a hemodynamically significant stenosis is present, dissipation of energy occurs owing to arterial narrowing and is reflected as a decrease in the amplitude of the pulse volume recording below the area of obstruction. The amount of decrease in the pulse volume recording amplitude reflects the severity of disease. Mild PAD is characterized by the absence of a dicrotic notch, whereas in moderate disease the upstroke and downstroke become equal. Severe disease is heralded by a flat waveform.

The advantage of segmental pressures and pulse volume recordings is the noninvasive and relatively rapid technique. The anatomic level and grade of disease can easily be assessed with this technique. A limitation of this study is that multiple vessels located at or above the level of the pneumatic cuff may not be separated and the patency of the vessel cannot be assessed directly.

Duplex Doppler ultrasound is also used in the vascular laboratory to assess anatomic and physiological blood vessel function. A color image, so-called "color Doppler," is used to provide an assessment of normal and abnormal flow states while mapping the arterial system in the extremity. Laminar flow indicates normal physiology, whereas turbulence and aliasing are present at sites of significant disease. When an abnormal color pattern is detected, pulsed (spectral) Doppler is utilized to assess the degree of stenosis. The pulsed Doppler generates a peak systolic velocity and waveform analyses are primary parameters used to quantify localized disease. Peak velocity measurements are typically obtained from arterial segments proximal and distal to the lesion and other Doppler samples are obtained at various locations in the arterial system to establish a baseline flow profile.

The normal Doppler waveform is a narrow, sharply defined tracing that indicates blood cells are moving at an equivalent speed at any time in the cardiac cycle. When flow is no longer uniform or laminar in the vessel, the waveform may broaden with partial or complete filling-in of the area under the spectral waveform. The configuration of the normal waveform is typically tri-phasic with the first phase occurring becuase of initial high-velocity forward flow during ventricular systole, the second phase from early diastolic reversal of flow as the left ventricular pressure falls below the aortic pressure prior to aortic valve closure and the third phase owing to forward flow during diastole that reflects elastic recoil of the vessel walls. With an increase in stenosis of the vessel, there is an increase in the peak systolic velocity and increased spectral broadening. The pulse Doppler at the level of the hemodynamically significant stenosis (e.g., >50%) reveals a monophasic waveform with a peak systolic velocity that is more than double the velocity measured in the proximal segment. Duplex Doppler ultrasound is also useful in assessing the patency of lower extremity bypass grafts and therapeutic interventions such as angioplasty and stent placement.

Some laboratories use segmental pressures and pulse volume recordings exclusively as the initial evaluation, whereas others will measure the ABI and if abnormal use Duplex Doppler ultrasound to assess for disease. Duplex Doppler ultrasound takes longer to accomplish than segmental pressures and pulse volume recordings.

MEDICAL TREATMENT OF DISEASE

All patients with PAD are at risk of fatal and nonfatal cardiovascular events. Thus, the primary goal of medical therapy is to reduce the risk of these events by risk-factor modification and antiplatelet therapy. Once that is accomplished, the next goal for the patient with claudication is to improve ischemic symptoms and thus enhance quality of life. Patients with critical limb ischemia have the added goal of healing an ischemic ulcer, if present, and prevention of limb loss. The comprehensive discussion of medical and treatment therapies for diseases is beyond the scope of this chapter and, thus, only important issues are discussed. Several reviews and consensus publications are available for more detailed review (8).

Risk-Factor Modification

The identification and modification of atherosclerotic risk factors in patients with PAD is essential in order to slow progression of disease in the extremities and also prevent cardiovascular events in this high-risk population (Table 1). It is estimated that more than 90% of patients referred to vascular clinics have a history of cigarette smoking, a statistic that continues to confirm Erb's initial report in 1911 that intermittent claudication occurred three to six times more frequently in patients who smoked cigarettes (9). Studies indicate that patients who stop smoking have a decreased progression to critical limb ischemia and amputation (10). It is uncertain whether smoking cessation will lead to decreased claudication symptoms and improved walking distance. One nonrandomized study showed that patients with claudication improved maximum walking distance by 47 meters (10); however, meta-analysis of nonrandomized studies do not report a significant improvement in maximum treadmill walking distance *(11)*. A prospective cohort study of smokers with coronary heart disease who quit showed a 36% reduction in relative risk of mortality. All smokers should be encouraged to enter a smoking-cessation program, and offered nicotine replacement therapy and/or the use of antidepressant drugs such as bupropion.

Diabetes is a strong risk factor for the development of PAD and also is estimated to accelerate atherosclerosis by 200% to 400% *(12)*. Half of all lower extremity amputations in the United States are attributed to diabetes with a relative risk ranging from 12 to 40 times that of nondiabetic patients *(12)*. There is no published evidence indicating that strict control of diabetes decreases the development of claudication or critical limb ischemia. However, results of studies such as the United Kingdom Prospective Diabetes Study indicate that intensive drug therapy reduces microvascular complications such as retinopathy and nephropathy *(13)*. Thus, all patients with diabetes should have strict glucose control and be monitored closely for microvascular complications.

Hypertension is a recognized independent risk factor for the development of PAD *(14,15)*. It is less clear whether treatment will alter the progression of disease or risk of claudication. Patients with PAD enrolled in the Heart Outcomes Prevention Evaluation had reduced rates of death and MI with angiotensin-converting enzyme inhibition compared to placebo *(16)*. Modification of the renin–angiotensin system in patients with PAD and hypertension is considered beneficial. In the past, the use of β-adrenergic antagonist drugs has been controversial in patients with claudication as some case reports indicated decreased blood flow in patients taking these medications. A meta-analysis of studies with β-adrenergic antagonist drugs indicates that these medications are safe and do not significantly impact claudication; however, caution was advised in those with severe disease *(17)*. Patients with stable claudication undergoing surgical procedures should be offered β-adrenergic antagonists to reduce the risk of periprocedure cardiovascular events *(18)*.

Dyslipidemia has emerged as a risk factor for PAD as several components of the lipid profile including total cholesterol (TC), low-density lipoprotein (LDL) cholesterol, triglycerides and lipoprotein (a) [Lp(a)] elevate the risk of PAD *(19–23)*. Alternatively, patients with increased high-density lipoprotein cholesterol and apolipoprotein A1 have a reduced incidence of PAD *(24,25)*. Patients with type III hyperlipidemia, with similarly elevated TC and triglyceride levels have a particular preponderance toward developing claudication *(26)*.

Clinical trials evaluating the effects of lipid modification on atherosclerosis in peripheral vessels indicate a beneficial effect on femoral atherosclerosis *(27,28)*. One study addressed whether plasma apheresis reduction of Lp(a) concentration would improve peripheral arterial endpoints as assessed with duplex ultrasonographic imaging of the femoral and tibial vessels *(29)*. Patients were randomized to simvastatin plus apheresis or simvastatin alone and followed for 2 years. The patients in the simvastatin-alone group with hemodynamically significant stenoses increased from 6 to 13 as compared with a decrease from 9 to 7 patients in the simvastatin plus apheresis group, suggesting that Lp(a) is an important factor in the development of PAD.

The data are clear that lipid modification reduces cardiovascular events in patients with a history of a cardiovascular event and those at high risk for developing one *(30)*. The Heart Protection Study, a prospective study of simvastatin that prospectively included patients with PAD, found a significant reduction in cardiovascular events among patients with PAD and even in those with an LDL of lower than 120 mg/dL *(31)*.

Studies also indicate that lipid modification improves claudication symptoms. The Program on the Surgical Control of the Hyperlipidemias investigated whether a reduction in cholesterol via ileal bypass surgery improved cardiovascular outcomes *(32)*. After 5 years, the relative risk of claudication or limb-threatening ischemia was reduced by 30% compared with a control group. A *post hoc* analysis of a large clinical study of patients with a previous heart attack demonstrated fewer new or worsening claudication symptoms in patients with PAD taking an hydroxymethylglutaryl-coenzyme A reductase inhibitor (statin) *(33)*. In one relatively small study, patients receiving 40 mg of simvastatin had improved pain-free walking time (time when pain first begins) and maximum walking time (time when patient stops walking) at both 3 and 6 months after initiation of treatment *(34)*. A larger study of 354 patients with claudication and randomized to 80 mg or 10 mg atorvastatin or placebo found that although maximum walking time did not statistically improve, the pain-free walking time improved in the 80 mg atorvastatin treatment group at 12 months *(35)*.

The current guidelines from the National Cholesterol Education Program ATPIII recommend that patients with PAD be considered at equivalent risk to those patients with a history of a heart attack or stroke. The primary LDL goal is less than 100 mg/dL, which will frequently necessitate the use of pharmacological therapy. The initial recommendation of therapy is with a statin drug, although for those patients who do not achieve the LDL cholesterol goal with statin treatment, a second agent such as ezetimibe (inhibitor of cholesterol absorption at the brush border of the small intestine) or bile-acid sequestering resin should be considered to achieve this goal. Also, a secondary target for patients with PAD and a triglyceride of more than 200 mg/dL include a non-HDL cholesterol of less than 130 mg/dL. Pharmacological therapy with fibrates or niacin should be considered along with dietary changes to achieve these secondary goals.

A high serum homocysteine concentration is also an independent risk factor for the development of PAD as well as cardiovascular events *(36, 37)*. Elevated homocysteine levels are implicated in endothelial dysfunction and proliferation of vascular smooth muscle cells owing to promotion of reactive oxygen species leading to acceleration of atherosclerosis *(38)*. There are no clinical trials evaluating whether a reduction in serum homocysteine concentration is beneficial in patients with PAD. However, given the relatively benign risk of treating patients with folic acid and B vitamins, these supplements should be considered in patients with PAD and elevated homocysteine levels.

An important component of the atherosclerosic process is inflammation *(39)*. C-reactive protein (CRP), a marker of inflammation, has emerged as a predictor of MI and thromboembolic stroke in apparently healthy individuals *(40)*. In a case–control design, baseline levels of CRP were reviewed in 144 apparently healthy men participating in the Physicians' Health Study who subsequently developed symptomatic PAD (intermittent claudication or need for revascularization) and in an equal number of control subjects matched on the basis of age and smoking habit who remained free of vascular disease during a follow-up period of 60 months *(41)*. The median CRP levels at baseline were significantly higher among those who subsequently developed PAD (1.34 vs 0.99 mg/L; $p = 0.04$). Thus, baseline levels of CRP predict the risk of developing symptomatic PAD. Higher CRP levels are also associated with poorer 6-minute walk performance and a lower summary performance score of physical parameters among participants with PAD *(42)*.

Antiplatelet Drug Therapy

The development of a thrombus in association with an atherosclerotic plaque in the peripheral arterial system, although not well studied, is generally thought to be important in the pathological process. Similar to the recommendations for antiplatelet therapy in patients with a history of heart attack or stroke, antiplatelet therapy is advocated in patients with PAD (Table 2). The choices of antiplatelet therapy include aspirin, adenosine diphosphate (ADP) receptor antagonists and the combination of dipyridamole with aspirin. Although aspirin is not approved by the Food and Drug Administration (FDA), it is commonly used in patients with PAD to prevent heart attack and stroke. The effectiveness of antiplatelet therapy in patients with PAD was studied in the Anti-Platelet Trialists' collaboration, which included a subgroup of 3295 patients with claudi-

Table 2
Medical Treatment of Peripheral Artery Disease

Antiplatelet drug(s)
Risk-factor modification
- Smoking cessation
- Blood pressure control
- Lipid modification (statin drugs as first line treatment)
- Tight glucose control if diabetic
- Treat elevated homocysteine
Supervised exercise rehabilitation
Cilostazol (Pletal®)
Foot hygiene

cation (43). For those taking aspirin, there was a reduction of 18% in risk of MI, stroke, or death from vascular causes after a mean follow-up of 27 months, but this reduction was not statistically significant. In this meta-analysis, a subgroup of 1928 patients who had received peripheral arterial grafts or had undergone peripheral angioplasty showed a nonsignificant reduction in mortality. However, the Anti-Platelet Trialists' collaboration did note that aspirin significantly decreased graft occlusion by 43% in 3226 patients with PAD who were treated with bypass surgery or peripheral angioplasty and followed for an average of 19 months (44). In this subgroup analysis, aspirin alone was as effective as the combination of aspirin and dipyridamole or ticlopidine in preventing graft occlusion with high-dose aspirin (600–1500 mg per day) as effective as low-dose aspirin (75–325 mg per day).

The thienopyridine drugs (such as ticlopidine and clopidogrel) are ADP receptor antagonists and have also been studied in patients with PAD. One study of ticlopidine vs placebo reported a significant reduction in the risk of fatal or nonfatal MI or stroke (45). Other studies indicate that ticlopidine may reduce the severity of claudication and the need for vascular surgery (46). Another thienopyridine drug, clopidogrel, is generally preferred over ticlopidine because of significantly lower risk of thrombocytopenia, neutropenia, and thrombotic thrombocytopenic purpura (TTP). A large prospective trial, Clopidogrel vs Aspirin in Patients at Risk of Ischemic Events Trial of 19,000 patients compared a daily dose of 75 mg of clopidogrel with 325 mg of aspirin per day in patients with recent MI, recent ischemic stroke, or PAD ($n = 6502$ patients). The patients with PAD had a history of claudication and at least moderately severe disease. An overall reduction of 8.7% was shown in patients with clopidogrel for the primary endpoint of fatal or nonfatal ischemic stroke, fatal or nonfatal MI, or death from other causes ($p = 0.04$). There is no hematological monitoring needed with clopidogrel, although a report did describe TTP occurring in approximately 4 per 1 million patients. The FDA has approved clopidogrel for the secondary prevention of atherosclerotic events in patients with atherosclerosis including those with PAD, heart attack, and stroke.

Other antiplatelet drugs such as picotamide, an inhibitor of thromboxane A_2 synthase and a blocker of thromboxane A_2 receptors and ketanserin, an antagonist of S_2 serotonin receptors, did not significantly reduce ischemic events in patients with PAD. In conclusion, aspirin and clopidogrel should be considered for antiplatelet treatment of patients with PAD and one study indicates that prevention of ischemic events in patients with PAD with clopidogrel may be more effective than aspirin in PAD patients.

TREATMENT OF CLAUDICATION

The perceived disability from claudication symptoms varies from patient to patient, but in general the severity of lifestyle impairment is similar to that of patients with New York Heart Association class III heart failure. The initial treatment of patients with stable intermittent claudication involves exercise therapy aimed at improving mobility and quality of life (Table 2). More than 20 randomized trials indicate that exercise improves treadmill walking distance as well as quality of life *(47)*. One meta-analysis of exercise training found that maximum treadmill walking distance will improve by approximately 180 meters. To obtain the most optimal results from exercise, patients should be referred to a supervised setting and followed on a regular basis as the improvement will be lost if exercise is discontinued for long periods of time. In the past, one limitation to widespread use of exercise programs was a lack of coverage by medical insurance; however, there is now a CPT code, 93668, for this therapy.

Pharmacological Therapy for Claudication

There are two drugs approved by the FDA for claudication symptoms; pentoxifylline (Trental®) and cilostazol (Pletal®). Pentoxifylline is a methylxanthine derivative that improves red cell deformability, lowers plasma fibrinogen, and has minor antiplatelet effects. The results of clinical studies varied significantly regarding the benefit of this medication in patients with claudication. Meta-analyses of pentoxifylline studies show a clinically small effect on improvement in walking distance *(11,48,49)*. Therefore, current data do not support the routine clinical use of this compound.

Cilostazol (pletal) is a phosphodiesterase type III inhibitor that increases intracellular concentrations of cyclic adenosine monophosphate. A myriad of mechanistic actions are reported, including inhibition of platelet aggregation, vasodilatation, inhibition of smooth muscle proliferation, and modification of the lipoprotein profile to explain the benefit in claudication symptoms *(50)*. Because antiplatelet agents and vasodilators have not been shown to improve exercise performance, the mechanism of the salutary effect of cilostazol on symptoms of claudication is unclear. The data from four randomized, placebo-controlled trials of cilostazol enrolling 1534 patients demonstrate improvement in both pain-free and maximum walking distance compared with placebo *(51–54)*. The most optimal dose for improvement in claudication symptoms, as evident from the studies, was 100 mg twice a day, taken at least 30 minutes before or 2 hours after breakfast and dinner. Because of extensive hepatic metabolism by the cytochrome P450 (CYP) system in the liver, a lower 50 mg twice a day dose is recommended when co-administered with inhibitors of CY34A, such as ketoconazole, itraconazole, erythromycin and diltiazem and during the co-administration of such inhibitors of CYP2C19 as omeprazole *(50)*. Cilostazol can be safely given with aspirin or clopidogrel, at the 100 mg twice-a-day dose, but a 50 mg twice-a-day dose is suggested for patients taking warfarin. The predominant side-effect profile of cilostazol includes headache, transient diarrhea, and palpitations *(50)*. A black box in the FDA package insert warns, because of negative experience with other phosphodiesterase inhibitors, that cilostazol should not be given to patients with claudication and a history of congestive heart failure.

INVASIVE THERAPEUTIC APPROACHES

The majority of patients with PAD and claudication do not have significant progression to critical limb ischemia. According to the Trans-Atlantic Inter-Society Consensus (TASC) working group, an intervention by endovascular procedure or surgery is only indicated in selected patients with intermittent claudication in whom exercise and pharmacological therapy have been unsuccessful *(8)*. The management of patients with endovascular therapy is difficult to categorize because of a large number of clinical factors; however, the TASC Working Group defined four lesion groups as follows: type A lesions, for which an endovascular approach is the treatment of choice; type B lesions, for which endovascular treatments are more commonly used; type C lesions, for which surgical treatment is more commonly used; and type D lesions, for which surgery is the treatment of choice. Long-term patency rates are acceptable for angioplasty and/or stent placement of aortoilliac types A and B lesions. When femoropopliteal lesions are considered for revascularization, endovascular treatment is indicated for type A lesions and surgery for type D lesions. The treatment of types B and C femoral lesions is controversial and more evidence is needed before definitive recommendations can be made. Although technology is rapidly changing in regards to infra-inguinal endovascular treatment, femoral stenting as a primary approach for the treatment of claudication or critical limb ischemia is not indicated *(8)*. Of note, placement of a stent may have a limited role in the salvage of acute angioplasty failures or complications. Endovascular therapy for infra-popliteal vessels is reserved for patients with critical acute or chronic limb ischemia. A review of 4662 published angioplasty procedures indicates an overall complication rate of 5.6%, where surgery was required in 2.5%, limb loss observed in 0.2%, and mortality in 0.2% *(55)*. In this same report, minor complications were observed in 4.6%.

Surgery for PAD is usually reserved for patients with critical limb ischemia as it is rarely necessary in patients with intermittent claudication. As with endovascular treatment, surgery should be offered to treat severe symptoms only after other forms of medical therapy have been recommended and have either failed or are not feasible. The preferred operation for aortoilliac disease is an aortofemoral (usually bilateral) bypass or an extended endarterectomy. The operative mortality rate for this procedure is 1%–4% with a 5-year patency of approximately 85% *(56)*. Patients with intermittent claudication and infra-inguinal occlusive disease rarely need bypass to the infrapopliteal arteries. In rare instances, patients with severe lifestyle-limiting disease confined to the superficial femoral artery and with distal vessels relatively free of disease may benefit from surgical bypass. The optimal bypass conduit for below the knee bypass is an autogenous vein, whereas that for above-knee bypass is less clear with some favoring autogenous vein and others favoring a prosthetic bypass graft *(57)*. Patients who have undergone lower extremity bypass graft surgery should have careful surveillance in the noninvasive vascular laboratory for impending graft failure. Surveillance of this nature has been shown to reduce the risk of graft complications *(58–61)*. Also, patients developing worsening symptoms with or without a history of a revascularization procedure should be referred to the vascular laboratory for evaluation.

SUMMARY

The presence of atherosclerotic disease causing ischemia to the limbs is a disease of the aged. The clinician should be astute in identifying atherosclerotic risk factors in this population so that appropriate modifications can be made to prevent not only progression of disease in the extremities, but also heart attack and stroke. The treatment of claudication symptoms involves supervised exercise rehabilitation either with or without pharmacological therapy to improve pain-free walking symptoms. Patients with severe disease limited to the aortoilliac or femoral artery regions may benefit from elective revascularization after failing medical treatment. Most infra-inguinal revascularization is however, reserved for those with limb-threatening ischemia (such as rest pain or a foot ulcer that does not heal) especially in patients with diabetes. All patients should be considered for antiplatelet agents, cholesterol-modifying drugs, and agents that affect the renin–angiotensin system to modify disease progression and associated cardiovascular events.

REFERENCES

1. Criqui MH, Fronek A, Barrett-Connor E, Klauber MR, Gabriel S, Goodman D. The prevalence of peripheral arterial disease in a defined population. Circulation 1985; 71:510–515.
2. Hiatt WR, Hoag S, Hamman RF. Effect of diagnostic criteria on the prevalence of peripheral arterial disease. The San Luis Valley Diabetes Study. Circulation 1995; 91(5):1472–1479.
3. Hirsch AT, Criqui MH, Treat-Jacobson D, et al. Peripheral arterial disease detection, awareness, and treatment in primary care. JAMA 2001;286(11):1317–1324.
4. Imparato AM, Kim GE, Davidson T, Crowley JG. Intermittent claudication: its natural course. Surgery 1975;78:795–799.
5. Weitz JI, Byrne J, Clagett GP, et al. Diagnosis and treatment of chronic arterial insufficiency of the lower extremities: a critical review. Circulation 1996;94:3026–3049.
6. Heintz SE, Bone GE, Slaymaker EE, Hayes AC, Barnes RW. Value of arterial pressure measurements in the proximal and distal part of the thigh in arterial occlusive disease. Surg Gynecol Obstet 1978;146:337–343.
7. Raines JK, Jaffrin MY, Rao S. Quantitative segmental pulse volume recorder: a clinical tool. Surgery 1972;72:873–877.
8. Dormandy JA, Rutherford RB. Management of peripheral arterial disease (PAD). TASC Working Group. TransAtlantic Inter-Society Concensus (TASC). J Vasc Surg 2000;31(1 Pt 2):S1–S296.
9. Erb W. Beiträge zur Pathologie des intermittierenden Hinkens. Münch Med Wschr 1911;2:2487.
10. Quick CR, Cotton LT. The measured effect of stopping smoking on intermittent claudication. Br J Surg 1982;69 Suppl:S24–S26.
11. Girolami B, Bernardi E, Prins MH, et al. Treatment of intermittent claudication with physical training, smoking cessation, pentoxifylline, or nafronyl: a meta-analysis. Arch Intern Med 1999;159:337–345.
12. Beckman JA, Creager MA, Libby P. Diabetes and atherosclerosis: epidemiology, pathophysiology, and management. JAMA 2002;287(19):2570–2581.
13. UK Prospective Diabetes Study Group. UKPDS Blood Pressure Study. Br Med J 1998;317:703–713.
14. Fowkes FG, Housley E, Riemersma RA, et al. Smoking, lipids, glucose intolerance, and blood pressure as risk factors for peripheral atherosclerosis compared with

ischemic heart disease in the Edinburgh Artery Study. Am J Epidemiol 1992;135(4): 331–340.

15. Murabito JM, D'Agostino RB, Silbershatz H, Wilson WF. Intermittent claudication. A risk profile from The Framingham Heart Study. Circulation 1997;96:44–49.

16. Heart Outcomes Prevention Evaluation Study Investigators. Effects of ramipril on cardiovascular and microvascular outcomes in people with diabetes mellitus: results of the HOPE study and MICRO-HOPE substudy. Lancet 2000;355(9200):253–259.

17. Radack K, Deck C. Beta-adrenergic blocker therapy does not worsen intermittent claudication in subjects with peripheral arterial disease. A meta-analysis of randomized controlled trials [see comments]. Arch Intern Med 1991;151:1769–1776.

18. Eagle KA, Berger PB, Calkins H, et al. ACC/AHA Guideline Update for Perioperative Cardiovascular Evaluation for Noncardiac Surgery-Executive Summary: A Report of the American College of Cardiology/American Heart Association Task Force on Practice Guidelines (Committee to Update the 1996 Guidelines on Perioperative Cardiovascular Evaluation for Noncardiac Surgery). Anesth Analg 2002; 94(5):1052–1064.

19. Hughson WG, Mann JI, Garrod A. Intermittent claudication: prevalence and risk factors. Br Med J 1978;1(6124):1379–1381.

20. Gofin R, Kark JD, Friedlander Y, et al. Peripheral vascular disease in a middle-aged population sample. The Jerusalem Lipid Research Clinic Prevalence Study. Isr J Med Sci 1987;23(3):157–167.

21. Bowlin SJ, Medalie JH, Flocke SA, Zyzanski SJ, Goldbourt U. Epidemiology of intermittent claudication in middle-aged men. Am J Epidemiol 1994;140(5): 418–430.

22. Cantin B, Moorjani S, Dagenais GR, Lupien PJ. Lipoprotein(a) distribution in a French Canadian population and its relation to intermittent claudication (the Quebec Cardiovascular Study). Am J Cardiol 1995;75:1224–1228.

23. Johansson J, Egberg N, Johnsson H, Carlson LA. Serum lipoproteins and hemostatic function in intermittent claudication. Arterioscler Thromb 1993;13(10):1441–1448.

24. Mowat BF, Skinner ER, Wilson HM, Leng GC, Fowkes FG, Horrobin D. Alterations in plasma lipids, lipoproteins and high density lipoprotein subfractions in peripheral arterial disease. Athero 1997;131(2):161–166.

25. Bradby GV, Valente AJ, Walton KW. Serum high-density lipoproteins in peripheral vascular disease. Lancet 1978;2:1271–1274.

26. Brewer HB Jr, Zech LA, Gregg RE, Schwartz D, Schaefer EJ. NIH conference. Type III hyperlipoproteinemia: diagnosis, molecular defects, pathology, and treatment. Ann Intern Med 1983;98(5 Pt 1):623–640.

27. Blankenhorn DH, Azen SP, Crawford DW, et al. Effects of colestipol-niacin therapy on human femoral atherosclerosis. Circulation 1991;83:438–447.

28. Lewis B. Randomised controlled trial of the treatment of hyperlipidaemia on progression of atherosclerosis. Acta Med Scand Suppl 1985;701:53–57.

29. Kroon AA, van Asten WN, Stalenhoef AF. Effect of apheresis of low-density lipoprotein on peripheral vascular disease in hypercholesterolemic patients with coronary artery disease. Ann Intern Med 1996;125(12):945–954.

30. LaRosa JC, He J, Vupputuri S. Effect of statins on risk of coronary disease: a meta-analysis of randomized controlled trials. JAMA 1999;282(24):2340–2346.

31. MRC/BHF Heart Protection Study of cholesterol lowering with simvastatin in 20,536 high-risk individuals: a randomised placebo-controlled trial. Lancet 2002; 360(9326):7–22.

32. Buchwald H, Bourdages HR, Campos CT, Nguyen P, Williams SE, Boen JR. Impact of cholesterol reduction on peripheral arterial disease in the Program on the Surgical Control of the Hyperlipidemias (POSCH). Surgery 1996;120:672–679.

33. Pedersen TR, Kjekshus J, Pyorala K, et al. Effect of simvastatin on ischemic signs and symptoms in the Scandinavian simvastatin survival study (4S). Am J Cardiol 1998;81:333–335.

34. Mondillo S, Ballo P, Barbati R, et al. Effects of simvastatin on walking performance and symptoms of intermittent claudication in hypercholesterolemic patients with peripheral vascular disease. Am J Med 2003;114(5):359–364.

35. Mohler ER, III, Hiatt WR, Creager MA. Cholesterol reduction with atorvastatin improves walking distance in patients with peripheral arterial disease. Circulation 2003;108(12):1481–1486.

36. Malinow MR, Kang SS, Taylor LM, et al. Prevalence of hyperhomocyst(e)inemia in patients with peripheral arterial occlusive disease. Circulation 1989;79(6):1180–1188.

37. Kang SS, Wong PW, Malinow MR. Hyperhomocyst(e)inemia as a risk factor for occlusive vascular disease. Annu Rev Nutr 1992;12:279–298.

38. Tawakol A, Omland T, Gerhard M, Wu JT, Creager MA. Hyperhomocyst(e)inemia is associated with impaired endothelium-dependent vasodilation in humans. Circulation 1997;95(5):1119–1121.

39. Ross R. Atherosclerosis—an inflammatory disease. N Engl J Med 1999;340(2):115–126.

40. Ridker PM. Clinical application of C-reactive protein for cardiovascular disease detection and prevention. Circulation 2003;107(3):363–369.

41. Ridker PM, Cushman M, Stampfer MJ, Tracy RP, Hennekens CH. Plasma concentration of C-reactive protein and risk of developing peripheral vascular disease. Circulation 1998;97(5):425–428.

42. McDermott MM, Greenland P, Green D, et al. D-dimer, inflammatory markers, and lower extremity functioning in patients with and without peripheral arterial disease. Circulation 2003;107(25):3191–3198.

43. Antiplatelet Trialists' Collaboration. Collaborative overview of randomised trials of antiplatelet therapy—I: Prevention of death, myocardial infarction, and stroke by prolonged antiplatelet therapy in various categories of patients. BMJ 1994;308:81–106.

44. Antiplatelet Trialists' Collaboration. Collaborative overview of randomised trials of antiplatelet therapy—II: Maintenance of vascular graft or arterial patency by antiplatelet therapy. BMJ 1994;308:159–168.

45. Janzon L, Bergqvist D, Boberg J, et al. Prevention of myocardial infarction and stroke in patients with intermittent claudication; effects of ticlopidine. Results from STIMS, the Swedish Ticlopidine Multicentre Study. J Intern Med 1990;227:301–308.

46. Balsano F, Coccheri S, Libretti A, et al. Ticlopidine in the treatment of intermittent claudication: a 21-month double-blind trial. J Lab Clin Med 1989;114:84–91.

47. Stewart KJ, Hiatt WR, Regensteiner JG, Hirsch AT. Exercise training for claudication. N Engl J Med 2002;347(24):1941–1951.

48. Hood SC, Moher D, Barber GG. Management of intermittent claudication with pentoxifylline: meta-analysis of randomized controlled trials. CMAJ 1996;155(8):1053–1059.

49. Radack K, Wyderski RJ. Conservative management of intermittent claudication. Ann Intern Med 1990;113:135–146.

50. Reilly MP, Mohler ER, III. Cilostazol: treatment of intermittent claudication. Ann Pharmacother 2001;35(1):48–56.

51. Beebe HG, Dawson DL, Cutler BS, et al. A new pharmacological treatment for intermittent claudication: results of a randomized, multicenter trial. Arch Intern Med 1999;159(17):2041–2050.

52. Dawson DL, Cutler BS, Meissner MH, Strandness DEJ. Cilostazol has beneficial effects in treatment of intermittent claudication: results from a multicenter, randomized, prospective, double-blind trial. Circulation 1998;98:678–686.

53. Money SR, Herd JA, Isaacsohn JL, et al. Effect of cilostazol on walking distances in patients with intermittent claudication caused by peripheral vascular disease. J Vasc Surg 1998;27:267–274.

54. Dawson DL, Cutler BS, Hiatt WR, et al. A comparison of cilostazol and pentoxifylline for treating intermittent claudication. AM J Med 2000;109(7):523–530.

55. Becker GJ, Katzen BT, Dake MD. Noncoronary angioplasty. Radiology 1989;170(3 Pt 2):921–940.

56. Brewster DC. Current controversies in the management of aortoiliac occlusive disease. J Vasc Surg 1997;25(2):365–379.

57. Veith FJ, Gupta SK, Ascer E, et al. Six-year prospective multicenter randomized comparison of autologous saphenous vein and expanded polytetrafluoroethylene grafts in infrainguinal arterial reconstructions. J Vasc Surg 1986;3(1):104–114.

58. Mills JL, Fujitani RM, Taylor SM. The characteristics and anatomic distribution of lesions that cause reversed vein graft failure: a five-year prospective study. J Vasc Surg 1993;17(1):195–204.

59. Chang BB, Leather RP, Kaufman JL, Kupinski AM, Leopold PW, Shah DM. Hemodynamic characteristics of failing infrainguinal in situ vein bypass. J Vasc Surg 1990; 12(5):596–600.

60. Calligaro KD, Musser DJ, Chen AY, et al. Duplex ultrasonography to diagnose failing arterial prosthetic grafts. Surgery 1996;120(3):455–459.

61. Woodburn KR, Murtagh A, Breslin P, et al. Insonation and impedance analysis in graft surveillance. Br J Surg 1995;82(9):1222–1225.

13 Cardiac Rehabilitation in Older Cardiac Patients

Philip A. Ades, MD

CONTENTS

INTRODUCTION

"Cardiac rehabilitation services are comprehensive, long-term programs involving medical evaluation, prescribed exercise, cardiac risk factor modification, education and counseling. These programs are designed to limit the physiologic and psychologic effects of cardiac illness, reduce the risk for sudden death or reinfarction, control cardiac symptoms, stabilize or reverse the atherosclerotic process, and enhance the psychosocial and vocational status of patients with coronary heart disease" *(1)*. Although meta-analyses of randomized trials of cardiac rehabilitation, including over 4000 patients, document a 25% decreased mortality over an average follow-up of 3 years after cardiac rehabilitation *(2–4)*, these studies are limited by the inclusion of few patients over the age of 65 years and none over the age of 75 years.

DISABILITY IN OLDER CORONARY PATIENTS

The goals of cardiac rehabilitation and exercise training in older coronary populations are to decrease cardiac disability, to improve health-

From: *Contemporary Cardiology: Cardiovascular Disease in the Elderly*
Edited by: G. Gerstenblith © Humana Press Inc., Totowa, NJ

related quality of life, and to extend disability-free survival. Compared with younger patients with coronary heart disease (CHD), older patients have higher rates of disability and mobility limitations and a diminished exercise capacity *(5–7)*. Coronary artery disease (CAD) in the elderly is also characterized by a greater severity of angiographic disease *(8)*, more severe and more diffuse left ventricular systolic dysfunction *(9)*, and increased levels of peripheral vascular and left ventricular stiffness, also termed "diastolic dysfunction," compared with younger cardiac patients *(10)*. The higher rates of diastolic dysfunction results in the fact that dyspnea is a more common symptom than chest pain in older patients suffering myocardial infarction (MI) *(11,12)*. In women, compared with men, CHD is often a disease of elderly women, with a higher prevalence of chronic heart failure, a greater prevalence of coronary risk factors, and a more complex clinical course *(13)*. Despite the fact that primary prevention has resulted in a lower prevalence of CAD in the elderly, the rapidly increasing size of the older population is such that the absolute number of older patients with CHD is increasing *(14,15)*. Cardiac rehabilitation exercise training, designed to decrease disability in older CHD patients, will assume an increasingly important role as the size of the older CHD population continues to grow.

The Social Security Administration has no guidelines or definitions for cardiac disability for patients over the age of 65 years because at this age, disability pensions are simply converted to "old-age" pensions *(16)*. In practice, disability in older CHD patients is defined by limitations in physical activity, mobility and ability to perform activities of daily living (ADLs), with an underlying psychological component. Data from the Framingham Disability Study provide insight on the effects of various CHD manifestations on disability and mobility in older populations *(5)*. The Framingham Disability Study included 2576 participants and yielded a quantitative assessment of levels of physical and social disability, in older adults, based on self-reported information. The measures of disability were primarily based on three questions: "Are you able to walk up and down stairs to the second floor without help?" "Are you able to walk a half mile without help?" and "Are you able to do heavy work around the house, like shoveling snow or washing windows, walls, or floors without help?" The presence of any positive responses determined a component of physical disability.

At a given age, women were more likely to report disability than men and the presence of CHD was a major predictor of activity limitations in both men and women (Table 1). In the 55- to 69-year age group, 49% of men and 67% of women with CHD were disabled as compared with 9% of men and 25% of women without CHD. In coronary patients over the

Table 1
Framingham Disability Study
by Age and Coronary Disease Status: Age 55–69 Years

	Percent with disability	N
No CAD or CHF		
Women	25%	829
Men	9%	574
CHD		
Women	67%	88
Men	49%	127
Angina pectoris		
Women	67%	67
Men	57%	81
CHF		
Women	80%	15
Men	43%	7

CAD, coronary artery disease; CHF, chronic heart failure; CHD, coronary heart disease. (Adapted from ref. 5.)

Table 2
Framingham Disability Study
by Age and Coronary Disease Status: Age 70–88 Years

	Percent with disability	N
No CAD or CHF		
Women	49%	471
Men	27%	273
CHD		
Women	79%	121
Men	49%	103
Angina pectoris		
Women	84%	83
Men	56%	59
CHF		
Women	88%	25
Men	57%	14

CAD, coronary artery disease; CHF, chronic heart failure; CHD, coronary heart disease. (Adapted from ref. 5.)

age of 70 years with symptoms of angina pectoris or chronic heart failure, disability was reported by more than 80% of women and 55% of men. The presence of CHD in the "oldest old" was particularly ominous, with estimated disability rates of up to 76% in men 75 years of age and older (Table 2).

Other studies on this topic are complementary to the Framingham Study. In the Medical Outcomes Study, angina was related to the total physical activity activity score in older patients although past MI was not *(17)*. Chirikos and Nickel studied 976 men and women hospitalized for acute coronary syndromes (MI or unstable angina) and found by multivariate analysis that the presence of cardiac disease, in particular angina pectoris, was predictive of disability at 6, 18, and 24 months of follow-up *(18)*. In a subsequent analysis, they found that angina was more disabling in older women than older men, supporting the findings of the Framingham Study *(6)*.

Data from our laboratory provide further insight into the determinants of physical functional capacity in older coronary patients *(19)*. A group of 51 men and women over the age of 65 years with established chronic CHD underwent comprehensive evaluations with exercise echocardiography, measurement of peak aerobic capacity, strength and body composition along with detailed clinical histories, and self-reported measures of physical function and mental depression. Univariate predictors of physical function score included peak aerobic capacity, depression score *(20)*, hand-grip strength, gender, and co-morbidity score. By multivariate analysis, the only independent predictors of physical function score were peak aerobic capacity and mental depression score. Left ventricular systolic function, which varies inversely with infarct size, was not related to physical function score *(19)*.

In summary, the presence of clinical CHD is a powerful predictor of disability and mobility limitations in the elderly. Disability rates are highest in women, the oldest old and in the presence of angina pectoris, chronic heart failure, and mental depression.

EXERCISE TRAINING

Again, the goals of exercise training in older coronary populations are to decrease cardiac disability and to extend disability-free survival. This is accomplished by a program that will increase aerobic capacity, muscle strength, and flexibility and by a program that will provide associated psychosocial and perceptual benefits. Exercise-training programs in the elderly, however, need to take into account commonly associated co-morbidities, which can alter the modalities and intensities of the exercise stimulus that is required. These include, but are not limited to, chronic heart failure, arthritis, chronic lung disease, diabetes, osteoporosis, and peripheral and cerebrovascular disease. In middle-aged coronary patients, and in patients with chronic heart failure, reduced cardiovascular fitness as indexed by VO_2 max is a primary clinical predictor of impaired physical function and of diminished survival rates *(21,22)*. Training-induced increases in peak aerobic capacity are associated with a lower mortality rate *(23)*. In older coronary patients, there are no definitive randomized clinical trial data assessing whether exercise conditioning prolongs life. Therefore, the goals of rehabilitation in the elderly should focus on improving physical functioning, health-related quality of life, and extending disability-free survival. The British Regional Heart Study, a large observational study of almost 6000 men with established CHD, found that regular light to moderate physical activity was associated with a lower 5-year all-cause mortality *(24)*. Secondly, exercise rehabilitation plays an important role in coordination of coronary risk-factor therapy including management of hypertension, lipid abnormalities, insulin resistance, and obesity *(1)*.

The cardiac rehabilitation literature and clinical experience of rehabilitation centers clearly support the safety and efficacy of exercise-training regimens in older coronary patients *(7,25–28)*. Compared with younger coronary patients, older patients are significantly less fit at entry into a rehabilitation program 1 to 3 months after suffering a major coronary event such as an MI or coronary bypass surgery *(7)*. However, after 3 months of aerobic conditioning, older coronary patients derive a similar relative training benefit as do younger patients with peak VO_2 increasing 16%–20%, and effectively distancing themselves from mobility limitations and disability. Training programs have been extended to a year and longer with long-term maintenance of exercise-related benefits *(27,29)*.

A recently published randomized controlled trial of cardiac rehabilitation (CR) from Italy extends findings from middle-aged coronary patients (46–65 years), to older (66–75 years), and very old (>75 years) patients after MI *(30)*. Patients were randomized to 2 months of hospital-based CR, home-based CR, or control status and results were analyzed immediately after CR and at 6 and 12 months of follow-up. When results were analyzed immediately after CR, patients in all three age categories increased work capacity compared with control patients. Interestingly, at 12 months of follow-up, patients in the very old group retained a significant increase in work capacity if they had been randomized to the home-exercise group but not to the hospital-based group or to the control group. This suggests that patients in the home-exercise group may have learned skills to help them maintain a long-term home-based exercise program compared with patients whose first 2 months of rehabilitation were hospital-based. Finally, health-related quality of life increased in the very old patients assigned to either exercise group at 2, 6, and 12 months.

The effects of aerobic exercise-training programs on *submaximal* exercise response in older coronary patients is more relevant to the performance of ADLs than the maximal exercise response. In a study of 45 older coronary patients, mean age 69 ± 6 years, who underwent a 3-month aerobic conditioning program, submaximal indices of exercise performance were closely studied *(31)*. Training effects were assessed during an exhaustive submaximal exercise protocol, with patients exercising at a steady intensity of 80% of a previously measured peak aerobic capacity. Outcome measures included endurance time, serum lactate, perceived exertion, heart rate, blood pressure (BP), and expired ventilatory measures. Exhaustive endurance time increased by more than 40% after conditioning, with associated decreases in serum lactate, perceived exertion, minute ventilation, heart rate, and systolic BP during relatively steady-state exercise. The respiratory exchange ratio during steady-state exercise, an indicator of substrate utilization, decreased, indicating a shift toward greater use of free fatty acids as a more efficient metabolic fuel. Activities that were exhaustive before training became sustainable for extended periods of time at a lower perceived exertion.

The mechanisms of physiological adaptations to aerobic exercise conditioning in the elderly may differ somewhat from those seen in younger (i.e., middle-aged) coronary patients. In younger patients, physiological responses to training include both peripheral adaptations (skeletal muscle and vascular) that result in a widened arteriovenous (AV) oxygen difference at maximal exercise *(32,33)*, and cardiac adaptations, which include increases in cardiac dimensions, stroke work, cardiac output, and afterload-corrected indices of left ventricular function *(34–37)*. In older coronary patients, coronary and peripheral vascular disease are superimposed on "age-related" increases in left ventricular and arterial wall thickness and stiffness *(10,38,39)*, which may reduce their adaptability to remodeling. We found that after 3 months of intensive aerobic conditioning in 60 older coronary patients (mean age 68 ± 5 years, range 62–82 years), conditioning-induced adaptations were localized almost exclusively to the periphery *(40)*. Peak exercise cardiac output, hyperemic calf blood flow, and vascular conductance were unaffected by the conditioning program. In contrast, at 3 and 12 months, AV oxygen difference at peak exercise was increased in intervention subjects but not in age-matched controls, explaining the 16% increase in peak aerobic capacity. Histological analysis of skeletal muscle documented a 34% increase in capillary density and a 23% increase in oxidative enzyme capacity after 3 months. After 12 months, an increase in individual fiber area was seen compared with baseline measures. Thus, even after 12 months of aerobic exercise, in contrast with middle-aged coronary patients, we found no discernible improvements in cardiac output or calf blood flow. It is acknowledged, however, that the absolute amount of exercise performed by older coronary patients is less than that performed by younger patients and this may potentially confound comparisons of physiological responses to training by age group.

Practical issues related to the implementation of exercise-training programs in older coronary patients include that training regimens often need to be adjusted to accommodate the presence of co-morbidities such as arthritis, diabetes, and peripheral vascular disease. The least-fit individuals are often unable to sustain exercise for extended periods and do well with repeated intermittent brief bouts of exercise (often termed "interval-training"), which are gradually extended. Some authors recommend longer term exercise programs for the elderly, partly related to their low baseline functional capacity *(29)*. It should be noted, however, that even patients who use canes and walkers can perform an exercise test, and can train on a treadmill with surround bars or on a cycle ergometer.

Despite the documented value of exercise regimens in older patients and the low baseline measures of functional capacity, older coronary patients are far less likely than younger patients to participate in cardiac rehabilitation *(41)*. Our data documented a 21% participation rate in cardiac rehabilitation for patients over the age of 62 years who recently suffered a coronary event and who lived within 1 hour of the rehabilitation center, compared with a 46% participation rate in younger patients *(41)*. By far the most powerful predictor of cardiac rehabilitation participation in the clinical setting was the strength of the primary physician's recommendation for participation as described by the patient. The physician's recommendation was scored on a scale, ranging from 1 (*no encouragement to participate*) to 5 (*strong encouragement to participate*). When the recommendation was weak (scores of 1–3), a 2% participation rate was noted, compared to a strong recommendation for participation (score of 4 or 5) where a 66% participation rate was noted (Fig. 1). Older women had a lower participation rate than men (15% vs 25%, $p = 0.06$). This was primarily related to lower physician-recommendation scores for women than men, although it is also possible that older women would participate less even with an equivalent recommendation score *(42)*. Other factors weighing against participation for women include more co-morbid conditions, more difficulty with transportation, less likely to be married, and more likely to have a dependent spouse at home.

Resistance training has been advocated as a particularly useful intervention in older coronary patients for several reasons *(43–45)*. First and foremost, even "normal" aging is associated with a significant loss of muscle mass and strength, related both to diminished activity profiles

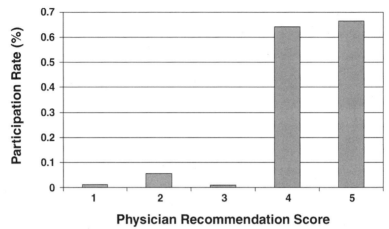

Fig.1. Cardiac rehabilitation participation rates in older coronary patients. 1 = no encouragement, 5 = strong encouragement. (Adapted from ref. *41*.)

and to decreased rates of muscle protein synthesis that actually begins in middle age *(43,46–48)*. Furthermore, in healthy community-living elders and in institutionalized octogenarians, resistance training is demonstrated to improve walking endurance, muscle mass, and strength *(49, 50)*. In coronary patients, aging-related musculoskeletal abnormalities are superimposed on activity restrictions related to chronic disease *(51)*, and diminished muscle mass and strength termed "sarcopenia," is even more severe.

In a study that focused on resistance training in older CAD patients who had recently suffered an MI, relative increases in strength were found to be similar to increases seen in younger CAD patients *(44)*. In older women with chronic CHD in whom the negative effects of age, gender, and chronic disease all result is a severe loss of strength and function *(19)*, the effects of strength training have recently been studied *(52)*. Brochu et al. assessed the effects of 6 months of resistance training on strength, endurance, and on a physical performance test designed to assess physical function during practical household activities in 30 older women, mean age 71 ± 5 years *(52,53)*. Compared with patients randomized to a control group, strength training resulted in increased strength, endurance, and capacity to perform a wide range of household activities such as carrying groceries and climbing stairs. The increase in strength after resistance training correlated with improvements in the overall physical function score (Fig. 2) Maximal power for activities that involved weight-bearing over a distance increased by $40\% < (p < 0.05$ vs controls) *(54)*.

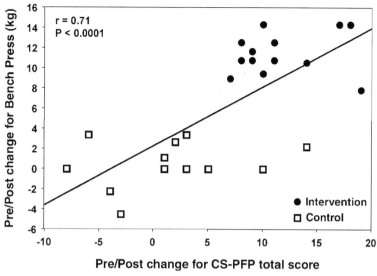

Fig. 2. Association between percent changes in total Continuous Scale Physical Functional Performance test score (CS-PFP) and percent changes in maximal strength on the bench press before and after strength training in older women with coronary heart disease *(52)*.

Finally, in older patients with chronic heart failure, the common presence of sarcopenia and diminished physical function warrants serious consideration of the inclusion of resistance-training to aerobic-training regimens. In a study by Pu et al. of older women (mean age 77 years) with chronic heart failure, a 10-week program of resistance training was associated with a 43% increase in muscle strength and a significant increase in 6-minute walk distance *(55)*. There were no associated changes in cardiac function, nor in peak aerobic capacity suggesting that the beneficial effects were entirely the result of direct effects on skeletal muscle.

From a practical point of view, the onset of upper body resistance training should be delayed until 3 months after coronary bypass surgery to allow for full sternal healing, whereas it can commence as soon as 1 month after MI, after performance of a satisfactory baseline exercise tolerance test. The resistance-training program should include training of the leg extensor muscles to assist with walking and stair-climbing, and upper body training to aid in the lifting and pushing required for the performance of daily household activities. Training is based on the performance of a single repetition maximal lift (1-RM) supplemented by a Borg scale for perceived exertion *(56)*. Patients begin their resistance training with 8 to

10 repetitions of each exercise at 40% to 50% of their 1-RM for a given exercise and gradually increase exercise intensity, as tolerated, to 50% to 80% of updated 1-RMs.

Optimally, older coronary patients begin exercise training only after a careful screening process that should include an EKG monitored exercise tolerance test, strength measures, and a clinical review including an analysis of disease severity, co-morbidities, and questionnaire- or interview-derived data regarding physical functioning and psychosocial function. Diagnostic categories appropriate for consideration of cardiac rehabilitation exercise training in older cardiac patients include the following:

1. Myocardial infarction
2. Coronary bypass surgery
3. Intracoronary revascularization (angioplasty, stenting, rotoblador etc.)
4. Stable angina pectoris
5. Valve replacement
6. Chronic heart failure

Exercise modalities should include options for aerobic exercise, resistance exercise, and flexibility. Aerobic choices include treadmills, a walking course, cycles, airdynes, and rowers. Aerobic exercise is often guided by an exercise heart-rate range and/or scales of perceived exertion such as the Borg scale. A gradual increment of exercise heart rate from 60% to 65% of maximal attained heart rate to higher levels of up to 85% is balanced against the greater risk of injury at higher levels and past demonstration of measurable benefits even with low levels of exercise *(57)*. It has been observed that older coronary patients are less likely to exercise to a physiological maximum at their baseline exercise test than are younger patients, therefore, a strict adherence to an exercise heart-rate range is often inappropriate *(7)*. As mentioned previously, utilization of a perceived exertion scale is a useful guide to exercise intensity in these patients. Duration of the exercise stimulus can begin with very brief, intermittent bouts of exercise, gradually increasing to 20 to 25 minutes or longer. Special considerations in the elderly include that training regimens often need to be adjusted to accommodate the presence of co-morbidities. For example, patients with hip arthritis may do better with cycling or a rowing exercise to avoid the weight bearing of treadmill walking. However, in general, walking is a preferred modality owing to its direct relevance to daily activities. Finally, it should be noted that for many elders, flexibility, or lack thereof, can be an exercise-limiting factor. Flexibility exercises can be as simple as 5 to 10 minutes of stretching per day to more complex protocols of yoga and ti-chi.

GENDER-RELATED ISSUES

Healthy older women have lower levels of habitual physical activity and lower levels of physical functioning than older men, explained in part by lower strength and muscle mass *(58–60)*. Older women with CAD further curtail their activities because of apprehension regarding the safety of specific physical activities, compounding their frailty deconditioning. Following a coronary event, women have lower fitness levels than men, yet are less likely to be referred to an exercise-based rehabilitation program by their physicians *(42)*. This may relate in part to the older age of women after MI, compared with men, or to higher rates of angina pectoris but is most likely related to physician misunderstanding regarding the benefits of rehabilitation in the most severely debilitated patients and/or patient preferences. Women achieve improvements in aerobic fitness and in muscular strength that are similar to men in rehabilitation programs *(42,44)*. The current model of cardiac rehabilitation was developed primarily in middle-aged male coronary patients in the 1960s and 1970s. The differing clinical profile of women in cardiac rehabilitation may require a different model relevant to their older age, their increased prevalence of co-morbid conditions, their more prominent cardiac risk-factor profiles, their higher rates of recurrent coronary events, their higher rates of mental depression, and their differing personal preferences *(61–64)*.

HOME REHABILITATION

Only 15% of eligible patients in the United States receive cardiac rehabilitation services, with the lowest participation rates noted in older patients *(1,41)*. In many cases, cardiac rehabilitation programs are not geographically available, whereas in other cases, patients are unable to travel, or formal rehabilitation is not recommended by the primary physician. Although cardiac rehabilitation services have classically been delivered on-site at a well-defined exercise-training facility, a need to expand preventive cardiology services to include the majority of eligible patients, in a cost-effective manner, necessitates a redefinition of this classical model. In fact, in the study of Marchionni et al. of rehabilitation after MI in the elderly, patients over the age of 75 years who participated in home-based rehabilitation actually had better 1-year fitness levels than patients randomized to perform the first 2 months of their rehabilitation program at the hospital *(30)*.

The development of alternate approaches to delivery of cardiac rehabilitation services is an ongoing process, with a goal of expanding the base of patients who receive services, at the lowest possible health care cost.

Case management, that is, evaluation and management of the exercise program and risk factors for the individual patient by a nurse "case-manager" allows for the individualization of preventive care in health care delivery systems that focus on efficiency and outcomes. Exercise programs can be individualized, with moderate and higher risk patients, and patients at highest risk of disability, referred to a rehabilitation program for closer supervision and monitoring.

PREVENTIVE CARDIOLOGY IN THE ELDERLY

Exercise plays an adjunctive role in the management of blood lipid levels, weight control, and BP control. In older coronary populations exercise rehabilitation has metabolic benefits that include improved blood lipid values, decreased body fat, improved glucose tolerance, and lower BP along with decreased measures of depression and anxiety (28, 65–69). These constitute important outcome measures for older CHD patients engaging in therapeutic exercise. Pharmalogical therapy for these conditions is often indicated and can also be coordinated in the cardiac rehabilitation setting. The benefits of lipid lowering, smoking cessation, angiotensin-converting enzyme (ACE) inhibition, antiplatelet agents and β-adrenergic blockade have all been demonstrated in appropriately selected older patients (70,71).

As the older cardiac population continues to grow in size and complexity much research remains to be done. The effects of aerobic and resistance-training protocols on measures of physical functioning need to be better studied in older coronary populations with inclusion of patients disabled by angina or chronic heart failure. Whether training regimens can improve physical functioning in the most severely disabled patients is of particular importance, although *preventing* disability in the less severely affected "younger old" is also a priority. Effects of exercise regimens on other important outcomes including lipid levels, BP measures, insulin levels, body composition, and body fat distribution need to be better studied to more clearly define the expected benefits of rehabilitation. Finally, whether training regimens can affect the economics of health care is crucial, especially if costly hospitalizations and/or home care services can be minimized.

In summary, although the older coronary population is, in general, a disabled group it is also quite heterogeneous as to physical functioning and disease severity. Exercise rehabilitation training programs are demonstrated to be safe and to improve aerobic fitness capacity and muscular strength. Exercise training may, in fact, reverse and prevent cardiac disability. Thus, cardiac rehabilitation exercise-training programs may pay great medical, social, and economic dividends in the older coronary population.

REFERENCES

1. Wenger NK, Froehlicher ES, Smith LK, et al. (Agency for Health Care Policy and Research and the National Heart, Lung and Blood Institute). Cardiac Rehabilitation. Clinical Practice Guidelines. October, 1995. Report No. AHCPR Publication No. 96-0672.
2. O'Connor GT, Buring JE, Yusuf S, et al. An overview of randomized trials of rehabilitation with exercise after myocardial infarction. Circulation 1989;80:234–244.
3. Oldridge NB, Guyatt GH, Fischer ME, Rimm AA. Cardiac rehabilitation after myocardial infarction: combined experience of randomized clinical trials. JAMA 1988; 260:945–950.
4. Jolliffe J, Rees K, Taylor R, Thompson D, Oldridge N, Ebrahim S. Exercise-based rehabilitation for coronary heart disease. Cochrane Database Syst Rev 2001;1: CD001800.
5. Pinsky JL, Jette AM, Branch LG, Kannel WB, Feinleib M. The Framingham Disability Study: Relationship of various coronary heart disease manifestations to disability in older persons living in the community. Am J Pub Health 1990;80:1363–1368.
6. Nickel JT, Chirikos TN. Functional disability of elderly patients with long-term coronary heart disease: A sex-stratified analysis. J Geront 1990;45:560–568.
7. Ades PA, Grunvald MH. Cardiopulmonary exercise testing before and after conditioning in older coronary patients. Am Heart J 1990;120:585–589.
8. Sugiura M, Hiraoka K, Ohkawa S. Severity of coronary sclerosis in the aged: A pathological study of 968 consecutive autopsy cases. Japan Heart J 1976;17:471–478.
9. Hochman J, Boland J, Sleeper L. Current spectrum of cardiogenic shock and effect of early revascularization on mortality: results of an international registry. Circulation 1995;91:873–881.
10. Rockman HA, Lew W. Left ventricular remodeling and diastolic dysfunction in chronic ischemic heart disease. In: Gaasch WH, LeWinter MM (eds.), Left Ventricular Diastolic Dysfunction and Heart Failure. Lea and Febiger, Philadelphia, 1994, pp. 306–324.
11. Bayer A, Chadha J, Farad R, et al. Changing presentation of myocardial infarction with increasing old age. J Am Geriatr Soc 1986;34:263–266.
12. Solomon C, Lee T, Cook E, et al. Comparison of clinical presentation of acute myocardial infarction in patients older than 65 years of age to younger patients: the multicenter chest pain study experience. Am J Cardiol 1989;63:772–776.
13. Malacrida R, Genoni M, Maggioni A, et al. A comparison of the early outcome of acute myocardial infarction in women and men. New Engl J Med 1998;338:8–14.
14. Weinstein W, Coxson P, Williams L, Pass T, Stason W, Goldman L. Forcasting coronary heart disease incidence, mortality and cost: The Coronary Heart Disease Policy model. Am J Publ Health 1987;77:1417–1426.
15. Salomaa V, Rosamond W, Mahonen M. Decreasing mortality from acute myocardial infarction: effect of incidence and prognosis. J Cardiovasc Risk 1999;6:69–75.
16. Social Security Administration. (U.S. Department of Health and Human Services). Disability Evaluation Under Social Security. 1992 October 1992. Report No. ICN 468 600.
17. Stewart AL, Hays RD, Ware JE. The MOS short-form general health survey. Reliability and validity in a patient population. Med Care 1988;26:724–735.

18. Chirikos T, Nickel J. Socioeconomic determinants of disablement from chronic disease episodes. Soc Sci Med 1986;22:1329–1335.
19. Ades P, Savage P, Tischler M, Poehlman E, Dee J, Niggel J. Determinants of disability in older coronary patients. Am Heart J 2002;143:151–156.
20. Yesavage JA, Brink TL, Rose TL. Development and validation of a geriatric depression screening scale- a preliminary report. J Psychiatr Res 1983;17:37–49.
21. McNeer J, Margolis J, Lee K, et al. The role of the exercise test in the evaluation of patients for ischemic heart disease. Circulation 1978;57:64–70.
22. Mancini D, Eisen H, Kussmaul W, Mull R, Edmunds L, Wilson J. Value of peak oxygen consumption for optimal timing of cardiac transplantation in ambulatory patients with heart failure. Circulation 1991;83:778–786.
23. Vanhees L, Fagard R, Thijs L, Amery A. Prognostic value of training-induced change in peak exercise capacity in patients with myocardial infarcts and patients with coronary bypass surgery. Am J Cardiol 1995;76:1014–1019.
24. Wannamethee SG, Shaper AG, Walker M. Physical activity and mortality in older men with diagnosed coronary heart disease. Circulation 2000;102(12):1358–1363.
25. Williams MA, Maresh CM, Esterbrooks DJ, Harbrecht J, Sketch MH. Early exercise training in patients older than age 65 years compared with that in younger patients after acute myocardial infarction of coronary bypass grafting. Am J Cardiol 1985;55:263–266.
26. Ades PA, Hanson JS, Gunther PG, Tonino RP. Exercise conditioning in the elderly coronary patient. J Am Geriatr Soc 1987;35:121–124.
27. Ades PA, Waldmann ML, Gillespie C. A controlled trial of exercise training in older coronary patients. J Gerontol 1995;50:M7–M11.
28. Lavie CJ, Milani RV, Littman AB. Benefits of cardiac rehabilitation and exercise training in secondary coronary prevention in the elderly. J Am Coll Cardiol 1993;22:678–683.
29. Williams M, Maresh C, Esterbrooks D, et al. Characteristics of exercise responses following short and long term aerobic training in elderly cardiac patients. J Am Geriatr Soc 1987;35:904–909.
30. Marchionni N, Fattirolli F, Fumagalli S, et al. Improved exercise tolerance and quality of life with cardiac rehabilitation of older patients after myocardial infarction. Circulation 2003;107:2201–2206.
31. Ades PA, Waldmann ML, Poehlman ET, et al. Exercise conditioning in older coronary patients: submaximal lactate response and endurance capacity. Circulation 1993;88:572–577.
32. Detry JMR, Rousseau M, Vandenbroecke O, et al. Increased arteriovenous oxygen difference after physical training in coronary heart disease. Circulation 1971;44:109–118.
33. Clausen JP. Circulatory adjustments to dynamic exercise and effect of physical training in normal subjects and in patients with coronary artery disease. Prog Cardiovasc Dis 1976;18:459–495.
34. Ehsani A, Martin WH, Heath GW, Coyle EF. Cardiac effects of prolonged intense exercise training in patients with coronary artery disease. Am J Cardiol 1982;50:246–254.
35. Hagberg JM, Ehsani AA, Holloszy JO. Effects of 12 months of intense exercise training on stroke volume in patients with coronary artery disease. Circulation 1983;67:1194–1199.
36. Ehsani AA, Biello DR, Schultz J, Sobel BR, Holloszy JO. Improvement of left ventricular contractile function by exercise training in patients with coronary artery disease. Circulation 1986;74:350–358.

37. Hagberg JM. Physiologic adaptations to prolonged high-intensity exercise training in patients with coronary artery disease. Med Sci in Sports 1991;23:661–667.
38. Lakatta E, Mitchell J, Pomerance A, Rowe C. Human aging: changes in cardiac structure and function. J Am Coll Cardiol 1987;10:42A–47A.
39. Vaitkevicius P, Fleg J, Engel J, et al. Effects of age and aerobic capacity on arterial stiffness in healthy adults. Circulation 1993;88:1456–1462.
40. Ades PA, Waldmann ML, Meyer WL, et al. Skeletal muscle and cardiovascular adaptations to exercise conditioning in older coronary patients. Circulation 1996;94: 323–330.
41. Ades PA, Waldmann ML, McCann W, Weaver SO. Predictors of cardiac rehabilitation participation in older coronary patients. Arch Int Med 1992;152:1033–1035.
42. Ades PA, Waldmann ML, Polk D, Coflesky JT. Referral patterns and exercise response in the rehabilitation of female coronary patients aged ≥62 years. Am J Cardiol 1992;69:1422–1425.
43. Brechue W, Pollack M. Exercise training for coronary artery disease in the elderly. Clin Geriatr Med 1996;1:207–229.
44. Fragnoli-Munn K, Savage P, Ades P. Combined resistive-aerobic training in older coronary patients early after myocardial infarction. J Cardiopulm Rehabil 1998;18: 416–420.
45. Squires RW, Muri AJ, Amderson LJ, Allison TG, Miller TD, Gav GT. Weight training during phase II (early outpatient) cardiac rehabilitation: Heart rate and blood pressure responses. J Cardiopulm Rehabil 1991;11:360–364.
46. Frontera W, Meredith CN, O'Reilly KP, Knuttgen HG, Evans WJ. Strength conditioning in older men: skeletal muscle hypertrophy and improved function. J Appl Physiol 1988;64:1038–1044.
47. Frontera WR, Meridith CN, O'Reilly KP, Evans WJ. Strength training and determinants of VO2 max. J Appl Physiol 1990;68:329–333.
48. Balagopal P, Rooyackers O, Adey D, Ades P, Nair K. Effects of aging on In-Vivo synthesis of skeletal muscle myosin heavy chain and sarcoplasmic protein in humans. Am J Physiol 1997;273:E790–E800.
49. Ades PA, Ballor DL, Ashikaga T, Utton JL, Nair KS. Weight training improves walking endurance in the healthy elderly. Ann Int Med 1996;124:568–572.
50. Fiatorone MA, Marks EC, Ryan ND, Meridith CN, Lipsitz LA, Evans WJ. High intensity strength training in nonagenarians: Effects of skeletal muscle. JAMA 1990; 263:3029–3034.
51. Neill WA, Branch LG, DeJong G. Cardiac disability—the impact of coronary disease on patients' daily activities. Arch Int Med 1981;145:1642–1647.
52. Brochu M, Savage P, Lee N, et al. Effects of resistance training on physical function in older disabled women with coronary heart disease. J Appl Physiol. 2002;92:672–678.
53. Cress ME, Buchner DM, Questad KA, Esselman PC, deLateur BJ, Schwartz RS. Continuous-scale physical functional performance in a broad range of older adults: A validation study. Arch Phys Med Rehabil 1996;7:1243–1250.
54. Ades PA, Savage PD, Cress ME, et al. Resistance training on physical performance in disabled older female cardiac patients. Med Sci Sports Exerc. 2003;35:1265–1270
55. Pu CT, Johnson MT, Forman DE, et al. Randomized trial of progressive resistance training to counteract the myopathy of chronic heart failure. J Appl Physiol 2001;90: 2341–2350.
56. Borg GA. Perceived exertion: a note on history and methods. Med Sci in Sports 1973; 5:90–93.

57. Lee JY, Jensen BE, Oberman A, Fletcher GF, Fletcher BJ, Raczynski JM. Adherence in the training levels comparison trial. Med Sci Sports Exerc 1996;28(1):47–52.

58. Reaven PD, McPhillips JB, Barrett-Connor EL, Criqui MH. Leisure time exercise and lipid and lipoprotein levels in an older population. J Am Geriatr Soc 1990;38: 847–854.

59. Cress M. Quantifying Physical Functional Performance in Older Adults. Muscle and Nerve 1997;5:S17–S20.

60. Wells CL, Plowman SA. Sexual differences in athletic performance: Biological or behavioral? Phys Sportsmed 1983;11:52–63.

61. Bueno H. Influence of sex on the short-term outcome of elderly patients with a first acute myocardial infarction. Circulation 1995;92:1133–1140.

62. Cannistra LB, Balady GJ, O'Malley CJ, Weiner DA, Ryan TJ. Comparison of the clinical profile and outcome of women and men in cardiac rehabilitation. Am J Cardiol 1992;69:1274–1279.

63. Rich MW, Bosner MS, Chung MK, Shen J, McKenzie JP. Is age an independent predictor of early and late mortality in patients with acute myocardial infarction? Am J Med 1992;92:7–13.

64. Moore SM, Kramer FM. Women's and men's preferences for cardiac rehabilitation program features. J Cardiopulm Rehabili 1996;16:163–168.

65. Brochu M, Poehlman ET, Savage P, Fragnoli-Munn, Ross S, Ades PA. Modest effects of exercise training alone on coronary risk factors and body composition in coronary patients. J Cardiopulm Rehabil 2000;20:180–188.

66. Dylewicz P, Bienkowska S, Szczesniak S, et al. Beneficial effect of short-term endurance training on glucose metabolism during rehabilitation after coronary bypass surgery. Chest 2000;117:47–51.

67. Kokkinos PF, Papademetriou V. Exercise and hypertension. Coron Artery Dis 2000; 11:99–102.

68. Ades PA, Maloney AE, Savage P, Carhart RL Jr. Determinants of physical function in coronary patients: Response to cardiac rehabilitation. Arch Intern Med 1999;159: 2357–2360.

69. Milani RV, Lavie CJ. Prevalence and effects of cardiac rehabilitation on depression in the elderly with coronary heart disease. Am J Cardiol 1998;81:1233–1236.

70. Schriefer J, Ades PA. Secondary prevention in older coronary patients. Cardiovasc Revs and Reps 1994;14:55–66.

14   Clinical Pharmacology

Janice B. Schwartz, MD

CONTENTS

INTRODUCTION

Advancing age and disease can alter pharmacokinetic processes that determine drug concentration and pharmacodynamic processes that determine drug concentration vs response relationships. The frequency of cardiovascular disorders of hypertension, coronary artery disease (CAD), cerebrovascular disease, atrial fibrillation, heart failure, and peripheral vascular diseases increases with age, as does the frequency of diabetes, arthritis, osteoporosis, depression, and vision, hearing, and memory impairments *(1)*. Thus, older patients with cardiovascular disease (CVD) are more likely to receive care from multiple health care providers, and consume multiple medications. Older patients may also be more likely to consume over-the-counter and nutraceutical compounds. These factors combine to increase the complexities of optimal medication prescribing as well as the risk of adverse drug-related events in older patients. The goal of therapy in patients with CVD evolves from a focus on prevention of disease and prolongation of life to a focus on improvement of the

From: *Contemporary Cardiology: Cardiovascular Disease in the Elderly*
Edited by: G. Gerstenblith © Humana Press Inc., Totowa, NJ

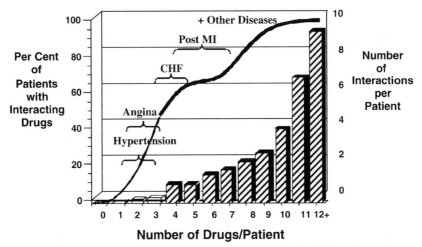

Fig. 1. Relationship between number of drugs consumed and drug interactions. Current recommendations for the pharmacological management of patients with heart failure and for the patient after myocardial infarction place them at high risk for drug interactions. (Reprinted with permission from American College of Cardiology Foundation, 2002, Adult Clinical Cardiology Self-Assessment Module V, Chapter 12).

quality of life at very old ages. With this goal in mind, it is especially important to minimize potential adverse effects of medications in older patients.

ADVERSE DRUG INTERACTIONS

A consistent finding in both the outpatient and inpatient settings is that the strongest risk factor for adverse drug interactions or adverse drug-related events is the number of medications administered (2–7). Most studies suggest that the chronic administration of two drugs is associated with a risk of adverse effects of about 15% and rises to 50% to 60% with the administration of four drugs per day. When the number of drugs co-administered reaches 8 to 10, the likelihood of drug interactions approaches 100% (see Fig. 1). Recognition of the increased chance of adverse outcomes with concomitant administration of 8 to 10 drugs has resulted in regulatory agencies requiring long-term care facilities to report and audit the use of nine or more drugs per patient as an indicator of (poor) quality of medical care.

A recent survey of ambulatory community-dwelling adults in the United States (8) found that medication usage increases with age with 94% of men and 91% of women over age 65 years consuming medications daily.

Fifty-seven percent of women over age 65 consumed 5 or more medications daily, and 12% consumed 10 or more drugs. Forty-four percent of men over age 65 consumed 5 or more medications daily, and 12% consumed 10 or more drugs daily. Although prescription drugs accounted for more than 80% of medications consumed for adults taking fewer than five medications, prescription drugs represented only about 50% of the drugs taken by patients consuming more than five medications per day. The number of medications prescribed to hospitalized or institutionalized elderly are often higher than the number prescribed in the outpatient setting.

Several strategies for reducing the risk of adverse drug interactions exist. Use of the fewest number of drugs is routinely recommended. A goal of prescribing less than four drugs per patient may, however, be an unrealistic goal in many older patients. American College of Cardiologists/American Heart Association guidelines for the pharmacological treatment of patients after uncomplicated myocardial infarction and for management of congestive heart failure recommend use of four to five drugs. Similarly, multidrug regimens are becoming increasingly common for the treatment of hypertension. Because it is likely that multidrug regimens will continue to be used, it is necessary that health care providers anticipate and understand potential medication interactions, that complete medication intake information be available, and that patients be educated to address nonprescription medication risks and benefits.

Adjustment of dosages for age and disease effects and common routes of metabolism of co-administered drugs can help to minimize pharmacokinetic interactions; and consideration of age and disease modifications in sensitivity to drugs as well as combined or antagonistic drug effects can minimize the risk of pharmacodynamic interactions. The following sections review principles of age- and disease-related changes in pharmacokinetic and pharmacodynamic parameters, and suggestions for optimizing drug dosing to avoid adverse effects.

UNDERSTANDING AGING: DEFINITIONS OF ELDERLY

Physiological age-related changes are continuous over time and proceed at differing rates in different individuals, yet, the classification "elderly" is usually based on age in years. World Health Organization uses 60 years of age to define "elderly" and most US classification schema use the age of 65 years. Cardiologists and other clinicians often separate the older population into two groups—patients aged 65–80 years and patients over 80 years of age in recognition that frailty and reduced capacity are more common at more advanced ages.

PHARMACOKINETICS

Pharmacokinetic processes determine the appearance, distribution throughout tissues, and elimination of drug from the body.

Volume of Distribution

Volume of distribution terms relate the amount of drug in the body to the concentration measured. A common way of determining the initial volume of distribution of a drug in humans is to administer an intravenous bolus of a known amount of drug and then measure the concentration immediately following drug administration.

This pharmacokinetic calculation of initial volume of distribution does not represent a "real" volume but the volume if drug were immediately and equally distributed throughout the circulation and highly perfused organs such as the heart, liver, and kidney. In vivo, this is the initial volume of distribution. Additional distribution phases occur related to drug entry into muscle, viscera, skin, fat, and other slowly perfused tissues. The volume of distribution at steady-state is the estimate of drug distribution throughout the body when these processes have reached equilibrium. Drugs that are highly protein-bound in the circulation, in general, have smaller volumes of distribution more closely related to vascular volumes. Drugs that are highly bound to tissue proteins will have large distribution volumes. Examples of drugs with small volumes of distribution include phenytoin and warfarin, whereas examples of drugs with large distribution volumes are digoxin, that distributes into and binds to muscle, and the benzodiazepines that distribute into fat.

The volume of distribution defines the loading dose of a drug as can be seen by its definition:

$$\text{Volume of distribution} = \frac{\text{Drug Dose}}{\text{Concentration}}$$

Modified loading regimens with infusions or multiple doses are often used for drugs with large volume of distributions to avoid higher than desired initial concentrations in the circulation and more rapidly perfused tissues.

AGE-RELATED CHANGES IN VOLUME OF DRUG DISTRIBUTION

Total body weight tends to increase during the adult years from 20 to 60 years of age, but weight decreases after age 60 years, with more marked changes seen after 75 to 80 years of age. In addition to a decrease in total body weight with aging, body composition is altered with decreases in total body water, intravascular volumes, and lean body mass; the relative proportions of upper body and central body fat increases. A smaller distribution volume for a drug in an older person results in a higher drug concentration after a given dose compared to concentrations in a younger or larger person given the same dose. The impact will be most evident when a loading or intravenous bolus dose of a medication is given and for those drugs that have narrow toxic to therapeutic ratios. Lower loading doses of drugs such as aminoglycoside antibiotics or phenytoin (polar drugs that usually distribute only in body water) should be given to older patients. There are more women than men at older ages and body size and volumes are smaller, on average, in women compared with men, further underscoring the need to adjust dosages for body weight in older patients. Weight adjustment for loading doses of the cardiovascular drugs digoxin, lidocaine, and other type I anti-arrhythmic drugs, type III anti-arrhythmic drugs, aminoglycoside antibiotics, chemotherapy regimens, and for unfractionated heparin are standard. When fibrinolytic drugs were administered without weight-based dosage adjustments, increased risk of intracranial hemorrhage was seen in patients of older age, smaller body weight, and female sex (in addition to hypertension and prior cerebrovascular disease) (9,10). Increased risk of bleeding in older patients is also seen after administration of "standard doses" of low-molecular-weight heparins in combination with other lytic agents. In contrast, increased risk of intracranial bleeding in older patients is not seen when weight-based dosing is used (11).

Total protein binding of drugs is not usually altered by aging in healthy individuals and clinically important age-related changes in total drug protein binding are not usually found in patient populations (12–15). Changes in protein binding can, however, result from competition for binding by co-administered drugs. A clinically important example occurs with warfarin that is about 99% protein bound. Displacement from albumin by addition of other highly bound drugs such as amiodarone, acetylsalicylic acid, phenytoin, sulfonamides, fluroquinolones, furosemide, or azole antifungal agents can cause marked increases in anticoagulation. Conversely, discontinuation of such drugs can lead to decreases in anticoagulation.

Bioavailability

Bioavailability is defined as the fraction (F) of drug that reaches the circulation after administration. Intravascular administration of a drug results in a bioavailability of 1 or 100%. Bioavailability for other routes of drug administration is estimated by comparing the area under the curve (AUC) of drug concentration vs time after extravascular administration divided by the AUC of drug concentration vs time data after intravascular dosage (AUC extravascular/AUC intravascular) expressed as a fraction of 1 or percentage. Bioavailability determines dose adjustments between differing routes of drug administration; low bioavailability drugs require greater extravascular vs intravascular. doses, whereas high bioavailability drugs need less dose adjustment between intravascular and extravascular routes of drug adminstration. Studies of traditional oral formulations suggest little clinically significant age-related change in the rate or extent of drug absorption from the gastrointestinal tract.

Low bioavailability may result from low drug permeability through the gut wall (e.g., ezetimibe), oxidative metabolism by cytochrome P450 (CYP)3A enzymes in the gut lumen prior to absorption (e.g., midazolam, propranolol), active transport into the gut lumen by the P-glycoprotein transporter (e.g., digoxin, cyclosporine), or rapid hepatic extraction from blood as it passes through the liver (first-pass effect). Interactions with nutrients and dietary factors are most common for lower bioavailable drugs undergoing CYP3A metabolism. Grapefruit juice has a direct inhibitory effect on gut CYP3A, and has been reported to increase bioavailability of a number of CYP3A substrates including, dihydropyridines (felodipine, nifedipine), verapamil, terfenadine, ethinylestradiol, midazolam, saquinavir, midazolam, cyclosporine a, and most hydroxymethylglutaryl-coenzyme A (HMG-CoA) reductase inhibitor medications (excluding fluvastatin).

Data regarding potential age-related changes in bioavailability after non-oral routes of drug administration are limited.

Clearance

Drugs are eliminated from the body either by metabolism (enzymatic biotransformation in the liver, intestine, or bloodstream) or by excretion (renal or biliary). Total body drug clearance is the net rate of removal of drug from the body described as a unit of volume cleared of drug per unit time (i.e., mL/minute). Clinically, clearance defines the drug-dosing rate per unit time to maintain a stable drug concentration; so, age-related decreases in drug clearance should result in decreases in drug dosages per unit time. The major organs of clearance for currently available drugs are the liver and kidney.

RENAL DRUG CLEARANCE

Elimination by the kidney is influenced by three processes: glomerular filtration, tubular secretion, and tubular reabsorption. Glomerular filtration is often approximated by estimates of creatinine clearance. Renal tubular secretion is detected in vivo when renal clearance of a substance exceeds clearance rates by filtration. Secretion is an active process with separate processes for acids and bases that efficiently eliminates protein-bound drugs. Tubular reabsorption is detected when urinary excretion of a compound is less than filtration rates. For most drugs, reabsorption is passive and can be affected by urine flow and by changes in pH.

Age-Related Changes in Renal Clearance. Renal clearance by all routes (glomerular filtration, renal tubular reabsorption, and secretion) decreases with age and is lower in women compared to men at all ages. Although there is considerable intersubject variability, a general estimate is for a 10% decline in glomerular filtration per decade. It is also key that at all ages, rates are 15%–25% lower in women compared to men.

Reduced lean body muscle mass with aging results in less creatinine production. Thus, serum creatinine concentrations do not accurately reflect creatinine clearance in the elderly. The serum creatinine may be normal when significant reduction of creatinine clearance or glomerular filtration is present. Two commonly used formulae to estimate creatinine clearance or glomerular filtration are:

$$Creatine\ Clearance = \frac{140 - Age\ (Yr) \times Lean\ Body\ Weight\ (kg)^*}{72 \times Serum\ Creatinine}\ (16)\quad (1)$$

*For women multiply by 0.85

Glomerular Filtration = $186.3 \times (Creat)^{-1.154} \times (Age)^{-0.203} \times 1.212$
   (if African American) $\times 0.742$ (if female) per $1.73M^2$ (17) (2)

Note: these estimates are not accurate when the conditions of the patient do not reflect stable physiology

Table 1 presents estimates of creatinine clearance using Eqs. 1 *(16)* and 2 *(17)* for serum creatinine concentrations of 1.0 and 1.2 mg/dL. Although the estimates using the two equations differ somewhat due to the inclusion/exclusion of weight or race, both predict that the average white woman over the age of 65 years will have moderate renal failure or stage 3 renal function (American Kidney Association guidelines) even if the creatinine is normal. Online calculators and kidney function classifications are available at http://www.kidney.org. Algorithms to estimate creatinine clearance or glomerular filtration based on subject age, gender, and serum creatinine should be used before prescribing renally cleared medications, for determining risks for procedures, and before administration of contrast agents or other potentially nephrotoxic agents in older patients, especially older and smaller women.

HEPATIC DRUG CLEARANCE

The rate and extent of hepatic drug metabolism is influenced by hepatic and extrahepatic factors. Hepatic blood flow determines the delivery

Table 1
Estimated Renal Clearance by Age, Gender, and Race

Age (yr)	Rate	Cr = 1					Cr = 1.2				
		45	55	65	75	85	45	55	65	75	85
White men[a]	CrCL	109	100	87	71	55	83	76	65	53	41
	GFR	86	82	80	77	75	70	67	65	63	61
White women	CrCL	75	72	61	50	39	55	51	44	36	28
	GFR	64	61	59	57	56	52	50	48	47	45
Black men	CrCL	107	98	81	69	55	78	71	60	49	39
	GFR	104	100	97	94	91	84	81	78	76	74
Black women	CrCL	88	79	68	56	40	62	56	49	40	29
	GFR	77	74	72	70	68	63	60	58	56	55

Data present average estimated (1) creatinine clearance (CrCL) in mL/minute using the Cockcroft and Gault method (16) based on average weight per age for men and women (source: NHANES) and (2) glomerular filtration rate (GFR) (17,48) in italics for serum creatinine of 1 mg/dL (Cr = 1) and for serum creatinine of 1.2 mg/dL (Cr = 1.2). Bold numbers indicate GFR estimates less than 60 mL/min/1.73m^2 classified as moderate decreases in GFR or stage 3 chronic renal disease. [a]All groups exclude Hispanic.

rate of drug to the liver and enzyme type, numbers, affinity, and activity rate determine hepatic biotransformation rates. In general, hepatic blood flow decreases with aging. Hepatic size has also been shown to decrease with age. Although in vitro experiments with tissues from rodent models of aging show marked and consistent decreases in hepatic enzyme affinity and metabolic rates, similar declines have not been demonstrated in humans. These differences likely result from recognized species differences in hepatic enzyme content, the more heterogeneous genetic composition of human populations, and more complex environmental and pharmacological exposures in humans compared to inbred laboratory animals. Most clinical information is currently presented within the context of the metabolic enzyme pathway involved because this provides a framework for anticipating metabolic drug interactions and the potential impact of genetics on drug metabolism (18–20).

Metabolic biotransformation usually converts drugs to more polar or water-soluble metabolites to facilitate excretion. Administered drugs may also be "pro-drugs" that are biotransformed into biologically active compounds; drugs may also be metabolized to toxic metabolites. Drug metabolism pathways are classified as phase I reactions (i.e., oxidation, reduction, and hydrolysis that usually remove groups from the drug) or phase II, conjugation reactions (i.e., acetylation, glucuronidation, sulfation, and methylation that add groups to the drug) that may occur in any sequence. The cytochrome P450 (CYP) superfamily of heme-containing microsomal enzymes is responsible for the majority of phase I metabolism of drugs, environmental chemicals, a number of hormones, foods, and toxins. A multitude of CYP isoforms have been identified. They are categorized by their amino acid sequences. Sequences with over 40% homology are classed in the same family identified by an Arabic number. Within the family, sequences with more than 55% homology are considered in the same subfamily identified with a letter. Within subfamilies, different forms are further designated with an Arabic numeral. Human CYP protein content is largely 8 to 10 isoforms from three major groups—CYP1, CYP2, and CYP3.

It is estimated that 50% to 55% of therapeutic drugs undergoing phase I metabolism are biotransformed by CYP3A enzymes. CYP3A proteins comprise about 25% of the protein in the liver and are the dominant form in the intestine. No distinct slow or rapid metabolizer phenotypes for this enzyme have been identified. CYP3A metabolizes many β-blockers, calcium channel blockers (CCBs), lidocaine, quinidine, amiodarone, many HMG-CoA reductase inhibitors, most benzodiazepines, estrogens, astemizole, carbamazepine, cisapride, clarithromycin, cortisol, erythromycin, itraconazole, ketoconazole, nefazodone, rifampin, tamoxifen, terfenadine, troglitazone, verapamil, and warfarin among others (*see* Table 2) Putative in vivo probes for the CYP3A pathway include erythromycin clearance, dextromethorphan urinary excretion ratios, urinary excretion ratio of 6-β-hydroxycortisol to free cortisol, urinary dapsone hydroxylation index, plasma ratio of 1-hydroxymidazolam to midazolam, and the lidocaine to monoethylglycinexylidide test. Midazolam is currently considered the purest CYP3A substrate and most studies with midazolam detect age-related decreases in clearance *(21–26)*. Age-related decreases in clearance of cardiovascular medications metabolized by this enzyme have been reported for α-blockers (doxazosin, prazosin, terazosin), some β-blockers (metoprolol, propranolol, timolol), CCBs (dihydropyridines, diltiazem, and verapamil), several HMG-CoA reductase inhibitors (atorvastatin, fluvastatin) and the benzodiazepines (midazolam).

CYP2 has multiple forms found in humans. CYP2D6 is estimated to be responsible for metabolism of 25% of phase I-metabolized drugs. The CYP2D6 enzyme has a number of genetic polymorphisms that can produce distinct phenotypes of ultrarapid, rapid, slow, and ultra-slow drug clearance. Drugs metabolized by this pathway include encainide, metoprolol, warfarin, debrisoquine, dextromethorphan, dehydroepiandosterone, mexiletine, propafenone, the selective serotonin reuptake inhibitor (SSRI) paroxetine, testosterone, most tricyclic antidepressants, and the neuroleptics, haloperidol and risperidone. CYP2C accounts for another 20% of phase I drug metabolism. CYP2C9 metabolizes fluvastatin, losartan, phenytoin, *s*-warfarin (the active enantiomer), and many nonsteroidal anti-inflammatory drugs. CYP2C19 metabolizes the proton pump inhibitors lansoprazole, omeprazole, and pantoprazole. CYP1A2 accounts for the metabolism of about 5% of drugs undergoing oxidative phase I metabolism. Acetaminophen, caffeine, nicotine, tacrine, and theophylline are metabolized via CYP1. It is currently difficult to estimate the clinical impact of genetic polymorphisms of drug-metabolizing enzymes (or receptors) and the relative impact of these variants to age-related, disease-related, or environmental factors in the clinical setting. Routine pharmacogenomic screening is not currently recommended *(27)*.

Age-Related Changes in CYP-Mediated Drug Clearance. CYP-mediated clearance rates vary markedly in human populations. Contributing factors include genetics, varying environmental exposures, enzyme induction or inhibition, multiple pathways for a number of compounds, and certainly additional factors not fully elucidated. Decreases owing to aging have been shown for many CYP substrates, and the CYP3A pathways in particular. Studies of the clearance of antipyrine that is metabolized by multiple CYP enzymes suggest overall decreases with aging.

Table 2
Major Routes of Cytochrome P450 Metabolism of Cardiovascular
and Commonly Administered Pharmacologically Active Agents in the Elderly[a]

Enzyme isoform	Cardiovascular	Other substrates	Inducers[b]	Inhibitors[b]
CYP1A2	Carvedilol	Acetaminophen	Rifampin	Cimetidine
	Fluvastatin	Caffeine (model substrate)	Omeprazole	Grapefruit juice
	Guanabenz	Clozapine	Cigarette smoke	Irbesartan, Losartan
	Mexilitine	Cyclobenzaprine	Charbroiled,	Fluoroquinolones
	Pimobendan	Imipramine	pan-fried Meat	Fluvoxamine
	Propranolol	Mirtazepine	Cruciferous vegetables	Mexiletine
		Nicotine (model substrate)		Ticlodipine
		Tacrine		Cholecalciferol
		Testosterone		
		Theophylline		
CYP2C 8/9 (Polymorphic)	ARBs (irbesartan, losartan)	Acenocoumarol	Dexamethasone	Azole antifungals
	Fluvastatin	Bosentan	Phenobarbital	Amiodarone
	Torsemide	Celecoxib	Phenytoin	Cimetidine
	Warfarin	Fluoxetine	Rifampin	Fluconazole
		Fluvastatin	Secobarbital	Isoniazid
		Glipizide		Sulfaphenazole
		NSAIDs (diclofenac, flurbiprofen Ibuprofen, meloxicam, naproxen, piroxicam)		Ticlodipine
		Phenytoin		
		Tamoxifen		
		Testosterone		
		Tolbutamide		

(continued)

Table 2 (Continued)

Enzyme isoform	Cardiovascular	Other substrates	Inducers[b]	Inhibitors[b]
19 (Polymorphic)		Citalopram Cyclophosphamide Diazepam Lansoprazole Omeprazole, Pantoprazole Phenytoin Progesterone Selegiline Sulfamethoxazole Testosterone Tricyclic antidepressants (amitriptyline, clomipramine) Venlafaxine	Phenobarbital Rifampin	Fluoxetine Fluvoxamine Fluconazole Ketoconazole Lansoprazole Omeprazole Ticlodipine
CYP2D6 (Polymorphic)	β-blockers (carvedilol, metoprolol, propranolol, timolol) Encainide Flecainide Metoprolol Mexiletine Pindolol Procainamide Propafenone	Amitriptylline Codeine Dextromethorphan DHEA Haloperidol Omeprazole Ondansetron Paroxetine Risperidone Some SSRI antidepressants (paroxetine, fluoxetine) Tamoxifen	Dexamethasone Rifampin	Amiodarone Diphenhydramine Clemastine Terfenadine Chloroquine Ticlodipine Quinidine Chlorpheniramine Cimetidine Clomipramine Desipramine Flecainide

CYP3A 4, 5		
Tolterodine	Rifampin	Fluoxetine
Tramadol	Phenytoin	Haloperidol
Tricyclic antidepressants (desipramine, Imipramine)	Bosentan	Lansoprazole
Venlafaxine	Nitric oxide	Methadone
Alprazolam	St. John's Wort	Paroxetine
Astemizole	Carbamazepine	Ketoconazole
Carbamazepine		Itraconazole
Cisapride		Protease Inhibitors
Citalopram		Amiodarone
Colchicine		Nefazodone
Clozapine		Mibefradil
Cyclosporine		Fluvoxamine
Diazepam		Cimetidine
Diclofenac		Grapefruit Juice
Erythromycin		Cyclosporin
Estradiol, ethinylestradiol		Erythromycin
Fentanyl		Verapamil
Itraconazole		Diltiazem
Ketoconazole		Doxorubicin
Medroxyprogesterone		Losartan
Midazolam		Quinidine
Mirtazepine		Antibiotics (fluroquinolones: e.g., ciprofloxacin, macrolides: e.g., clarithromycin, troleandomycin)
Nefazodone		
Omeprazole (partial)		
Paclitaxel		
Protease inhibitors		
β-blockers (bisoprolol, metoprolol)		
Bosentan		
Cilostazol		
Clopidogrel		
Dihydropyridines (nifedipine, amlodipine, felodipine, isradipine, nicardipine, nisoldipine)		
Diltiazem		
Eplerenone		
Fenofibrate		
Flosequinan		
HMG-CoA reductase inhibitors (atorvastatin, lovastatin, pravastatin, simvastatin)		

(continued)

Table 2 (Continued)

Enzyme isoform	Cardiovascular	Other substrates	Inducers[b]	Inhibitors[b]
CYP3A 4, 5 (continued)	Gemfibrozil	Rifampin		
	Lidocaine	Salmeterol		
	Losartan	Sildenafil		
	Propafenone	Sulfinpyrazone		
	Quinidine	Tamoxifen		
	Verapamil	Terfenadine		
	Vesnarinone	Theophylline		
		Triazolam		
		Troglitazone		
		Zolpidem		

[a]Drugs may be substrates of multiple CYP pathways (1). Data are routinely updated and detailed references can be found at www.gentest.com.
[b]In approximate order of potency.
CYP, Cytochrome P450; ARBs, angiotensin receptor blockers; NSAIDs, nonsteroidal anti-inflammatory drugs; DHEA, dehydroepiandrosterone; SSRI, selective serotonin reuptake inhibitors; HMG-CoA, hydroxymethylglutaryl-coenzyme A.

Effects of age that can be demonstrated in carefully controlled investigations of healthy subjects or patients with single disease states may not, however, be detected in clinical populations. In patient groups, variability in clearance due to the effects of disease, gender, smoking or alcohol consumption, and other environmental factors appear to be greater than those of age alone *(13,28)*.

In contrast to the consistent age-related decrease in oxidative biotransformation rates demonstrated in animal models of aging and healthy aging, metabolism by the conjugative reactions of glucuronidation (morphine, diazepam), sulfation (methyldopa), and acetylation (procainamide) do not appear to be affected by aging. Disease states that affect the liver may decrease clearance by these enzymes.

NON-RENAL, NON-HEPATIC DRUG METABOLISM

Some CYP isoforms are found outside the liver. CYP3A is the most common isoform found in the intestine and is recognized as a significant factor in low bioavailability of CYP3A substrates. Hepatic and intestinal CYP3A content and activity appear to be regulated separately. Dietary factors can produce pronounced effects on intestinal CYP3A. Grapefruit juice affects drug availability and resultant clinical effects for high first-pass dihydropyridine calcium channel blockers including nifedipine *(29–32)*. The mechanism of the effect for grapefruit juice is inhibition of gut-mediated CYP3A drug metabolism *(29,30,33)*. Cranberry juice may also decrease intestinal CYP3A activity. Age-related changes in non-renal, non-hepatic drug metabolism have not been elucidated.

Elimination Half-Life

The terminal elimination half-life (t1/2) describes the time it takes for the amount of drug in the body to decrease by half after drug distribution has occurred throughout the body. It is dependent on volume of drug distribution and clearance and is defined as follows:

$$t1/2 = 0.693 \times \frac{\text{Volume of Distribution}}{\text{Clearance}}$$

The half-life defines the time needed for drug concentrations to reach steady-state during both drug initiation and after drug discontinuation with approximately 90% of steady-state reached after 3.3 half-lives. Prior to use of sustained-release drug formulations, the half-life determined the amount of variability seen in drug concentrations among doses and drugs were often dosed at intervals equal to drug half-lives. Sustained-release preparations of drugs alter release characteristics to allow more

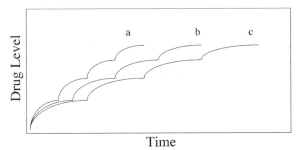

Fig. 2. Example of the changes in time to reach steady-state when the drug elimination half-life increases. The drug elimination half-life increased by 50% from curve a to curve b. Curve c represents an 100% increase in elimination half-life from condition a. For a drug with a half-life of 12 hours at condition a, steady-state for condition a would be approximated at 3.3 half-lives or about 40 hours (dotted line), for condition b this would be reached at about 60 hours, and for condition c this would be reached at about 80 hours. (Reprinted with permission from American College of Cardiology Foundation, 2002, Adult Clinical Cardiology Self-Assessment Module V, Chapter 12).

constant input and less variability in drug concentrations and allow less frequent dosing but do not alter elimination half-lives.

AGE-RELATED CHANGES IN HALF-LIFE

The elimination t1/2 increases with age for a number of drugs. This increase can be the consequence of changes in volumes, clearance rates, or combinations of the two. The clinical consequence is that the time to evaluate effects after drug initiation, after dosage adjustments, or after drug discontinuation should be increased in the older patient compared to younger patients to allow full evaluation of effects. For drugs with longer elimination half-lives, such as digoxin or amiodarone, steady-state concentrations may not be reached during short hospitalizations (*see* Fig. 2).

Summary

In summary, the balance of data suggest that renal clearance and the activity of most enzymes responsible for the majority of oxidative drug biotransformation decrease with aging, with conjugative biotransformation processes generally unaffected by age (*see* Table 3). The general guidelines (*see* Table 4) should be reductions in doses for older patients with routine use of algorithms to estimate renal clearance and understanding of hepatic biotransformation pathways of drugs with longer intervals between dosage change in older patients compared with younger ones.

Table 3
Summary of Age-Related Changes in Pharmacokinetic Parameters

	Decreased	Increased	No change	Unknown
Bioavailability				
Oral			X	
Transdermal				X
Distribution volume[a]				
Water soluble, non-lipophilic	X			
Lipophilic		X[b]		
Protein binding				
Albumin			X	
α-1-acidglycoprotein			X	
Renal clearance				
Glomerular filtration	X			
Tubular secretion	X			
Tubular reabsorption	X			
Enzymatic Clearance				
Phase I: cytochrome P450	X			
Phase II: conjugative			X	
Transporters				X

[a]In general, total volumes are greater in men due to greater body size.
[b]Ages 60–75.

Table 4
Clinical Recommendations for Medication Dosages for Older Patients

Loading doses
- Size matters: dose on a mg/kg basis
- Consult references to identify drugs needing further age-related reductions of 10%–20%
- Use infusions or multiple doses for drugs with large volumes of distribution

Maintenance doses
- Estimate renal clearance for renally eliminated drugs and adjust doses for age, size, gender, and race
- Reduce initial doses of cytochrome P450 cleared drugs by about 30%
- Increase doses at longer intervals and in smaller increments than in younger patients
- Consider potential drug interactions and consult references before prescribing multidrug regimens or when evaluating potential adverse effects
- Obtain complete medication intake information that includes over-the-counter and nutraceutical agents
- Assess compliance adherence routinely

PHARMACOKINETIC DRUG INTERACTIONS

A predictable, and thus considered avoidable, source of drug interactions is competition for the same elimination pathway or administration of an enzyme inhibitor or inducer. Data on CYP-specific routes of metabolism for cardiovascular drugs and common inducers and inhibitors are presented in Table 2. Data on CYP-mediated pathways of drug biotransformation have been extensively reviewed *(20)* but new information appears continually (*see* www.gentest.com; http://medicine.iupui.edu).

Inducibility of hepatic enzyme activity appears to be preserved with aging. Several drugs can produce clinically relevant enzyme induction. Rifampin produces profound increases in CYP-mediated drug clearance in humans. Dosages of drugs cleared by CYP1A and CYP3A, and possibly CYP2D6 that are co-administered with rifampin may need to be increased, and, dosages decreased upon discontinuation of rifampin (*see* Table 2). Other inducers include dexamethasone (CYP2C and possibly CYP2D6), phenytoin (CYP2C), caffeine, cigarette smoke, lansoprazole, and omeprazole (CYP1A), CYP3A, carbamazepine, and St. John's Wort (CYP3A).

Drug enzyme inhibition is also recognized as a source of adverse drug reactions. One of the first inhibitors recognized, cimetidine, inhibits CYP1A2, CYP2C, and CYP3A (in addition to decreasing hepatic blood flow) and can profoundly decrease hepatic drug clearance. Marked ele-vations of serum lidocaine and propranolol concentrations occurred in elderly patients receiving these drugs in combination with cimetidine. Currently, the most potent CYP inhibitors include amiodarone (all CYP isoforms), the azole antifungal drugs itraconazole and ketoconazole (CYP3A), protease inhibitors (CYP3A), erythromycin (CYP3A), and ter-fenadine (CYP3A). Many drugs can produce moderate and lesser enzyme inhibition that may have clinically significant effects depending on the condition of the patient. It is recognized that the risk of myopathy is increased if HMG-CoA reductase inhibitors are administered in combination with gemfibrozil or if CYP3A metabolized HMG-CoA reductase inhibitors (atorvastatin, lovastatin, simvastatin) are co-administered with drugs such as macrolide antibiotics(erythromycin, clarithromycin), nefazodone, cyclosporine, amiodarone, nicotinic acid, or the antifungal azoles that are also metabolized via CYP3A (*see* Table 2). Additional identified risk factors for statin-associated myopathy include age over 80 years (in women more than men), small body frame, frailty, and multisystem disease.

Data on potential drug interactions are currently addressed during the drug-evaluation process prior to marketing but many interactions are not identified until larger numbers of patients are exposed after marketing approval. The volume of data is large, the number of drugs taken by the elderly is higher than younger patients with many of the drugs being unfamiliar to cardiologists. It has become essential to access regularly updated information and guidelines to avoid drug interactions. Many tools are available that range from sophisticated pharmacy medication databases, programs for hand-held devices for individual caregivers to reference texts, and pocket guides. Inclusion of pharmacy-trained individuals in reviewing planned medication regimens can also decrease the incidence of adverse effects *(34)*. Routine use of such tools is recommended. It is pertinent that the only tool shown to be ineffective in reducing medication errors is the retrospective drug utilization review approach *(35)*.

PHARMACODYNAMICS

Pharmacodynamic models relate drug dose or concentration to the intensity of response or "effect." Such pharmacodynamic models assume effects are related to the drug concentration alone. Pharmacodynamic models provide parameters such as maximal effects, concentrations at which half maximal effects are seen, and "sensitivity" or slopes of response vs concentration relationships. These concepts and models are useful experimentally and demonstrate age, disease, and gender-related differences in cardiovascular receptors and physiological responses to pharmacological agents. In vitro experiments, however, may not fully elucidate effects seen in vivo or patients because the net effects are the result of a combination of both "direct" effects of drugs and homeostatic or reflex mechanisms that may counter "direct" drug effects. The contribution or lack of contribution of reflex responses to net drug effect is of especial importance in understanding responses to drugs such as potent vasodilators in the older patient. Age-related changes in the underlying cardiovascular physiology (increased peripheral resistance, altered diastolic filling, slowed AV conduction) or cardiovascular diseases (hypertension, heart failure, CAD) also contribute to altered pharmacodynamic responses. Age-related changes in the autonomic nervous system and reflex responses and changes owing to non-cardiovascular diseases common in the elderly will be briefly summarized here. Changes related to cardiovascular diseases common in the elderly are presented in chapters related to these diseases.

Age-Related Changes in the Adrenergic System

A decline in β-adrenergic responsiveness is perhaps the most consistent age-related findings in all species and tissues. Decreased responses of heart rate, white blood cells, platelets, AV conduction, cardiac contractility, and vasodilation are seen following isoproterenol or other β_1-adrenergic stimuli with aging. Decreased β_1-adrenergic responsiveness shifts the concentration vs response relationship such that higher concentrations are necessary for any given effect. Age-related decreases in β-adrenergic responsiveness result from decreased receptor numbers, altered G protein coupling to the β-adrenergic receptor, and G protein-mediated signal transduction. Important to the older patient with CVD, there are decreased heart rate responses to β-adrenergic stimulation such as exercise or stress and a decrease in the maximal heart rate, and these changes result in blunted baroreflex responses. These changes contribute to postural hypotension with potent vasodilators or intravascular volume depletion and to limited cardiovascular reserve.

In brain tissue from animals, dopaminergic mRNA as well as receptor and transporter content decrease with aging. Positron emission tomography in humans has also demonstrated a consistent decrease in dopaminergic content in the human brain with increasing age. When the loss reaches about 80% of that present in younger individuals in the substantia nigra, Parkinson's disease occurs. Age-related effects on cardiovascular responses to dopaminergic stimulation are more variable. Contractile responses may be blunted with aging, whereas chronotropic and dromotropic responses are preserved or enhanced in models of aging.

Age-related changes of other adrenergic receptor systems are less uniform. For the α-adrenergic system, data from humans support the presence of age-related decreases in α-adrenergic platelet receptors and decreased α-adrenergic mediated arterial vasoreactivity of forearm blood vessels in healthy men that are similar to the decreased β-adrenergic-mediated of responses with aging. In contrast, α-adrenergic responses in veins may not show age-related changes.

Age-Related Changes in the Parasympathetic System

Decreased sensitivity and responses to parasympathetic stimulation are commonly seen in cardiac and vascular tissues with aging. Age-related decreases in vasodilation in response to acetylcholine have been shown in both normal and diseased coronary and peripheral arteries. In contrast, greater central nervous system (CNS) effects following parasympathetic stimulation is frequently seen in older people compared to younger individuals. Physiological consequences are blunted heart-rate responses to atropine but increased anticholinergic CNS effects, including delirium, in older compared to younger subjects. Greater sensitivity may also explain the increased frequency of adverse effects such as urinary retention, constipation, and fecal impaction in the elderly who receive drugs with anticholinergic properties (e.g., disopyramide, verapamil).

Age-Related Changes in Reflex Responses

Blunted responses to vasodilators, vasoconstrictors, postural maneuvers, and the Valsalva maneuver occur with aging. Diseases and deconditioning further decrease reflex responses. Pharmacodynamic alterations at many levels (sensing, signal transmission, central processing, autonomic α-, and β-adrenergic and parasympathetic pathways, and vessel receptor content and responsiveness) contribute to the blunted baroreceptor responses seen with aging. Physiological consequences are greater postural hypotension and even syncope after potent nitrate or vasodilator administration to older patients, with intravascular depletion with diuretics, or with the combination of vasodilation and diuresis. Decreased cardiovascular responses of most adrenergic, parasympathetic, and tissue receptors contribute to decreased responses to pharmacological stimulation or blockade, exercise, physiological stress, and regulatory responses in older patients.

Age-Related Changes in Nonautonomic Vascular Responses

Coronary vascular responses to endothelin are blunted with aging. Vasodilation in response to nonendothelium-dependent agents such as nitrates or nitroprusside are not consistently altered by aging but may vary by vascular bed or be altered by diseases such as hypertension or diabetes that are common in the elderly. Physiological consequences are signs of endothelial dysfunction with aging but preserved responses to nonendothelial vasodilatory responses that are not autonomically mediated.

Age-Related Changes in Central Nervous System Responses

CNS effects or side effects may be more frequent in older patients and may significantly affect quality of life, mentation, and functional status (i.e., long-acting hypnotics, histaminergic and α-blocking drugs, and drugs with anticholinergic effects such as disopyramide and antihistamines). Risks of falls and hip fractures in older patients are associated with the use of psychotropic medications including hypnotic-anxiolytics, tricyclic antidepressants, neuroleptics, and more recently with SSRIs. Altered mental status may be the manifestation of CNS adverse effects in the older patient and a high index of suspicion must always be present (e.g., digitalis excess presenting as altered mental status).

Age-Related Changes in Coagulation

Greater prolongation of prothrombin times and longer duration of anticoagulation are reported in older patients given the same dose of warfarin as younger patients requiring anticoagulation without age-related changes in the pharmacokinetics of warfarin. Age-specific recommendations for anticoagulation have been developed by the American Geriatrics Society that differ somewhat from those published by other organizations (*see* www.americangeriatics.org). Key points are the recommendation for initiation at estimated maintenance doses (usually less than 5 mg) for most older patients and close monitoring of anticoagulation. Use of specialized anticoagulation services can decrease risks of bleeding and potential drug interactions with warfarin. Concentration vs response relationships for aspirin, thrombolytics, and low-molecular-weight heparins in older patients are not elucidated. Ginkgo biloba, a nutraceutical with purported memory and circulatory benefits, has some anticoagulant effect. Effects of garlic are variable.

A less well-recognized risk of chronic warfarin administration is osteoporosis. Vitamin K plays a role in bone metabolism, and anticoagulation with warfarin antagonizes vitamin K. In women receiving chronic oral anticoagulation, increased risk of osteoporosis and higher rates of vertebral and rib fractures were associated with longer than 12 months of oral anticoagulation *(36)*. Administration of unfractionated heparin for more than 3 to 6 months is also associated with increased rates of bone mineral loss *(37)*.

Age-Related Changes in Gastrointestinal Motility

Constipation is a frequent complaint of hospitalized elderly, less-active elderly, and institutionalized elderly patients. Drug-induced constipation is reported more frequently in the elderly compared to younger patients and bowel obstruction has been reported in older patients receiving bile-acid sequestrants, anticholinergic medications, opiates, and verapamil. Bowel hygiene regimens are recommended for elderly patients receiving these drugs and for those who are inactive.

PHARMACODYNAMIC DRUG INTERACTIONS

Pharmacodynamic drug interactions are less well studied than pharmacokinetic drug interactions and can lead to either potentiation of drug action or decreased drug effects. Just as pharmacokinetic interactions are more likely to occur between drugs that are metabolized by the same pathway, it is likely that drugs with pharmacodynamic actions on the same system are more likely to interact. In the elderly, pharmacodynamic interactions of direct vasodilators or nitrates combined with α-blockers, β-blockers, CCBs, angiotensin-converting enzyme (ACE) inhibitors, diuretics, or sildenafil can result in postural hypotension. Additive bradycardia with combinations of amiodarone, β-adrenergic blocking drugs, digoxin, diltiazem, verapamil, or sotalol is another potential pharmacodynamic drug interaction. Interactions related to direct drug effects can be predicted and may also be clinically utilized in designing drug regimens. Several clinically important pharmacodynamic effects that may be more common in the elderly are detailed next.

Potentiating interactions that result in decreased renal function and/or hyperkalemia may have greater consequences in the older patient because of basal age-related decreases in renal function. Several cardiovascular drug classes can reduce renal function in the elderly with ACE inhibitors and angiotensin receptor blocking drugs being among the most widely recognized. Both renal blood flow and production of angiotensin II responsible for dilation of the efferent arteriole can be affected with clinically significant decreases in glomerular filtration and increases in serum potassium in the elderly patient. Nonsteroidal anti-inflammatory agents (NSAIDs) can produce similar effects. In one prospective study of NSAID initiation in elderly long-term care residents, 13% developed azotemia during a short course of therapy (38). Importantly, adverse renal effects are equally common with both cyclooxygenase (COX)-2 selective and nonselective agents in older patients. When NSAIDs and ACE inhibitors are combined, adverse renal effects may be increased. NSAIDs may also decrease potassium excretion and can cause hyperkalemia in the older patient; especially, when given in combination with ACE inhibitors or spironolactone, which also decrease potassium excretion. Diuretic-induced decreases in intravascular volume or congestive heart failure also increase the risk of nonselective and COX-2-selective NSAID renal toxicity. The incidence of hyponatremia appears to be more common in the elderly. This appears to be true for thiazide and nonthiazide diuretics (39) and may also occur with SSRIs.

Examples of pharmacodynamic interactions with an antagonistic effect include loss of anginal control when β-agonists or theophylline are given to angina patients on β-blockers or calcium channel antagonists. Administration of medications with anticholinergic effects may also antagonize effects of anticholinesterase inhibitors.

INAPPROPRIATE PRESCRIBING IN THE ELDERLY

In 1997, Beers introduced the concept of drugs that were potentially "inappropriate" for use in the elderly based on an unfavorable risk to benefit ratio. These criteria were adopted by Center of Medicare Services for use in nursing home regulations *(40)*. Udated versions of "inappropriate" drug use in the elderly have appeared by Beers and others *(41, 42)*. Medications in these lists vary and the nature of the lists criticized, but long-acting benzodiazepines, sedative and hypnotic agents, long-acting oral hypoglycemic agents, selected analgesics, antiemetics, and gastrointestinal antispasmodics are usually included. Other drugs have been included when they are no longer considered appropriate for usage in most populations (e.g., short-acting nifedipine; estrogens in women, testosterone in men). Although doxazosin, clonidine, guanethidine, ethacrynic acid, amiodarone, and reserpine doses over 0.25 mg per day appear on the most recent list by Beers *(42)*, most cardiovascular medications are not considered "inappropriate" for use in the older patient. Recent definitions of "inappropriate drug use," however, extend beyond individual drug choices. By current criteria, it is "inappropriate" to fail to consider drug–disease interactions, fail to adjust drug dosages for age-related changes, fail to avoid drug duplication, fail to consider drug–drug interactions and fail to limit duration of use for medications recommended for short-term administration only. Explicit criteria for "appropriate" prescribing of digoxin, CCBs, and ACE inhibitors in older patients have been developed by expert consensus panels *(43)*. Using these criteria, most drug-utilization review studies conclude that inappropriate drug prescribing occurs in a significant fraction of older patients. It is pertinent to note, however, that data on effective therapies, age-related changes in pharmacokinetics and pharmacodynamics and the risk of drug interactions in patients over 80 years of age are extremely limited. Guidelines and criteria usually refer to patients in the younger old age groups of 65–75. Consideration of the principles outlined in this chapter that highlight the continuous nature of age-related changes and greater effects that disease states may have on some parameters should serve as guides for medication management of the very old patient.

COMPLIANCE

Accutate estimates of compliance on a population basis are not known but cost of medications, poor patient education regarding medications, and cognitive impairment are reported to be major reasons for poor compliance in older patients living alone *(44)*. In one study, medication noncompliance preceded hospitalization for decompensated heart failure in 42% of elderly patients *(45)*. Additional factors that contribute to noncompliance with medication regimens in the older patient include inadequate directions (small print of written directions, hearing impairment, or impaired memory), complex dosing regimens, difficulty with packaging materials, memory impairment, and physician overestimation of compliance. It is estimated that more than 40% of people aged 80 years and older have dementia. Assessment of memory and compliance should be part of a pharmacotherapy plan. Issues related to potential medication noncompliance should be addressed by prescribing health care professionals. Although there are few trials of interventions to improve medication adherence with resources usually available in clinical settings *(46)*, visual or memory aids, medication-dispensing tools, use of geriatric-friendly packaging, assessment of cognitive status and patient understanding, and inclusion of caregivers or family members in discussions regarding medications can be beneficial. It may be difficult to improve compliance for the majority of older patients without recognizing and addressing cost. In the United States in 2000, about 50% of people over age 65 years had after-tax incomes at the poverty level (41% of 65–74 year olds and 56% of those over 75 years of age) *(47)*.

SUMMARY

Age-related changes are reliably found and estimated for renal drug clearance but changes in hepatic drug clearance, half-life, bioavailability, and volume of distribution are less predictable. The current state of knowledge is limited by the paucity of investigations in women, minority groups, the oldest old, and patient populations with multiple diseases. Clinical dosing guidelines suggest reduction of initial drug dosages in elderly patients and titration of drug dosages in smaller increments with greater time between dosage adjustments than in younger patients. Because the co-administration of multiple medications is the single most important factor in the risk for adverse drug effects, the fewest number of drugs possible should be used. When multiple drug regimens are necessary, drug interactions should be anticipated based on metabolic route or mechanism of effect; and, adjustments in drug administration made to avoid adverse drug interactions. Routine utilization of reference sources for drug information can markedly assist in the management of older patients requiring multiple medications. Routine assessment of factors that contribute to poor compliance should also be a part of routine pharmacotherapy in the older patient.

ACKNOWLEDGMENT

This work was supported in part by PHRA National Institute on Aging: RO1 AG 15982.

REFERENCES

1. National Center for Health Statistics. Prevalence of selected conditions by age and sex: United States, 1984–1995 (NHIS). In www.cdc.gov.
2. Denham M. Adverse drug reactions. British Medical Bulletins 1990;46(1):53–62.
3. Nolan L, O'Malley K. Prescribing for the elderly: Part I: Sensitivity of the elderly to adverse drug reactions. J Am Geriatr Soc 1988;36:142–149.
4. Gurwitz J, Sanchez-Cross M, Eckler M, Matulis J. The epidemiology of adverse and unexpected events in the long-term care setting. J Am Geriatr Soc 1994;42:33–38.
5. Gandhi TK, Weingart SN, Borus J, Seger AC, et al. Adverse drug events in ambulatory care. N Eng J Med 2003;348(16):1556–1564.
6. Onder G, Pedone C, Landi F, Cesari M, Della Vedova C, Bernabei R, Gambassi G. Adverse drug reactions as cause of hosptial admission: results from the Italian Group of Pharmacoepidemiology in the Elderly (GIFA). JAGS 2002;50:1962–1968.
7. Field TS, Avorn J, McCormick D, et al. Risk factors for adverse drug events among nursing home residents. Arch Intern Med 2001;161:1629–1634.
8. Kaufman D, Kelly JP, Rosenberg L, Anderson TE, Mitchell AA. Recent patterns of medication use in the ambulatory adult population of the United States. The Slone Survey. JAMA 2002;287:337–344.
9. Gurwitz J, Gore J, Goldberg R, et al. Risk for intracranial hemorrhage after tissue plasminogen activator treatment for acute myocardial infarction. Participants in the National Registry of Myocardial Infarction 2. Ann Intern Med 1998;129(8):597–604.
10. Van de Werf F, Barron H, Armstrong P, et al. Incidence and predictors of bleeding events after fibrinolytic therapy with fibin-specific agents. Eur Heart J 2001;22: 2253–2261.
11. Van de Werf F. ASSENT-3: implications for future trial design and clinical practice. Eur Heart J 2002;23:911–912.
12. Keefe D, Yee Y, Kates R. Verapamil protein binding in patients and in normal subjects. Clin Pharmacol Ther 1981;29:21–26.
13. Krecic-Shepard M, Park K, Barnas C, Slimko J, Kerwin D, Schwartz J. Race and sex influence clearance of nifedipine: results of a population study. Clin Pharmacol Ther 2000;68:130–142.
14. Schwartz J, Troconiz I, Verotta D, Liu S, Capili H. Aging effects on stereoselective pharmacokinetics and pharmacodynamics of verapamil. J Pharmacol Exp Ther 1993; 265:690–698.
15. Benet L, Hoener B. Changes in plasma protein binding have little clinical relevance. Clin Pharmacol Ther 2002;71(3):115–121.
16. Cockcroft DW, Gault MH. Prediction of creatinine clearance from serum creatinine. Nephron 1976;16:31–41.
17. Manjunath G, Sarnak M, Levey A. Prediction equations to estimate glomerular filtration rate: an update. Curr Opin Nephrol Hypertens 2001;10:785–792.
18. Evans W, Relling M. Pharmacogenomics: translating functional genomics into rational therapeutics. Science 1999;286:487–491.
19. Weinshilboum R. Inheritance and drug response. N Engl J Med 2003;348(6):529–537.
20. Rendic S. Summary of information on human CYP enzymes: human P450 metabolism data. Drug Metab Reviews 2002;34(1–2):83–448.
21. Gorski J, Wang Z, Haehner-Daniesl B, Wrighton S, Hall S. The effect of hormone replacement therapy on CYP3A activity. Clin Pharmacol Ther 2000;68:412–417.
22. Greenblatt D, Abernethy D, Locniskar A, Harmatz J, Limjuco R, Shader R. Effect of age, gender, and obesity on midazolam kinetics. Anesthesiology 1984;61(1):27–35.

23. Holazo A, Winkler M, Patel I. Effects of age, gender and oral contraceptives on intramuscular midazolam pharmacokinetics. J Clin Pharmacol 1988;28(11):1040–1045.
24. Smith M, Heazlewood V, Eadie M, Brophy T, Tyrer J. Pharmacokinetics of midazolam in the aged. Eur J Clin Pharmacol 1984;26(3):381–388.
25. Platten H, Schweizer E, Dilger K, Mikus G, Klotz U. Pharmacokinetics and the pharmacodynamic action of midazolam in young and elderly patients undergoing tooth extraction. Clin Pharmacol Ther 1998;63:552–560.
26. Nishiyama T, Matsukawa T, Hanaoka K. The effects of age and gender on the optimal premedication dose of intramuscular midazolam. Anesth Analges 1998;86:1103–1108.
27. Roden D, Brown WJ. Preprescription genotyping: not yet ready for prime time, but getting there. Circulation 2001;103(12):1608–1610.
28. Kang D, Verotta D, Krecic-Shepard ME, Nishit BM, Gupta SK, Schwartz JB. Population analyses of sustained release verapamil in patients: age, race, and sex effects. Clin Pharmacol Ther 2003;71:31–40.
29. Bailey DG, Spence JD, Munoz C, Arnold J. Interaction of citrus juices with felodipine and nifedipine. Lancet 1991;337:268–269.
30. Bailey DG, Arnold JMO, Munoz C, Spence JD. Grapefruit juice–felodipine interaction: mechanism, predictability, and effect of naringin. Clin Pharmacol Ther 1993;53:637–642.
31. Lundahl J, Regardh CG, Johnsson G. Effects of grapefruit juice ingestion—pharmacokinetics and haemodynamics of intravenously and orally administered felodipine in healthy men. Eur J Clin Pharmacol 1997;52(2):139–145.
32. Rashid T, Martin U, Clarke H, Waller D, Renwick A, George C. Factors affecting the absolute bioavailability of nifedipine. Br J Clin Pharmacol 1995;40(1):51–58.
33. Lown KS, Bailey DG, Fontana RJ, et al. Grapefruit juice increases felodipine oral availability in humans by decreasing intestinal CYP3A protein expression. J Clin Invest 1997;99:2545–2553.
34. Freedman J, Becker R, Adams J, et al. Medication errors in acute cardiac care. An American Heart Assoication Scientific Statement from the Council on Clinical Cardiology Subcommittee on Acute Cardiac Care, Council on Cardiopulmonary and Critical Care, Council on Cardiovascular Nursing, and Council on Stroke. Circulation 2002;106:2623–2629.
35. Hennessy S, Bilker W, Zhou L, et al. Retrospective drug utilization review, prescribing errors, and clinical outcomes. JAMA 2003;290:1494–1499.
36. Caraballo P, Heit J, Atkinson E, et al. Long-term use of oral anticoagulants and the risk of fracture. Arch Intern Med 1999;159(15):1750–1756.
37. Hirsh J. Heparin. N Engl J Med 1991;324:1565–1574.
38. Gurwitz JH, Avorn J, Ross-Degnan D, Lipsitz LA. Nonsteroidal anti-inflammatory drug associated azotemia in the very old. JAMA 1990;264:471–475.
39. Chapman M, Hanrahan R, McEwen J, Marley J. Hyponatraemia and hypokalemia due to indapamide. MJA 2002;176:219–221.
40. Beers M. Explicit criteria for determining potentially inappropriate medication by the elderly. Arch Intern Med 1997;157:1531–1536.
41. Hanlon JT, Schmader KE, Boult C, et al. Use of inappropriate prescription drugs by older people. JAGS 2002;50:26–34.
42. Fick D, Cooper J, Wade W, Waller J, Maclean R, Beers M. Updating the Beers criteria for potentially inappropriate medication use in older adults. Results of a US Consensus Panel of Experts. Arch Intern Med 2003;163:2716–2724.

43. Zhan C, Sangl J, Bierman AS, et al. Potentially inappropriate medication use in the community-dwelling elderly: findings from the 1996 Medical Expenditure Panel Survey. JAMA 2001;286(22):2866–2868.
44. Salas M, Veld BA, van der Linden PD, Hofman A, Breteler M, Stricker BH. Impaired cognitive function and compliance with antihypertensive drugs in elderly: the Rotterdam Study. Clin Pharmacol Ther 2001;70:561–566.
45. Michalsen A, Konig G, Thimme W. Preventable causative factors leading to hospital admission with decompensated heart failure. Heart 1998;80(5):437–441.
46. McDonald HP, Garg AX, Haynes RB. Interventions to enhance patient adherence to medication prescriptions. Scientific Review. JAMA 2002;288:2868–2879.
47. U.S. Census Bureau. Income 2001. In. http://www.census.gov/hhes/income ed.
48. Levey A, Bosch J, Lewis J, Greene T, Rogers N, Roth D. A more accurate method to estimate glomerular filtration rate from serum creatinine: a new prediction equation. Ann Intern Med 1999;130(6):461–470.

15 Medical Treatment of the Cardiac Patient Approaching the End of Life

Lofty L. Basta, MD, FRCP, FACC,
W. Daniel Doty, MD, FACC, FAHA,
and Michael D. D. Geldart, ESQ

Contents

From: *Contemporary Cardiology: Cardiovascular Disease in the Elderly*
Edited by: G. Gerstenblith © Humana Press Inc., Totowa, NJ

Last scene of all . . .
    that ends this strange eventful history;
is seemed childishness and mere oblivion,
        sans teeth . . .
        sans eyes . . .
        sans everything
—Shakespeare, As You Like It, 2:7:139

INTRODUCTION

All life ends. This is life's only certainty. Fifty years ago, a family of five saw a loved one die and people accepted the biblical unalterable truth that there is a time for everything under heaven . . . a time to be born and a time to die.

Over the past half-century, we in America, as in the rest of the Western world and Japan, have managed to increase average human longevity from 50 to almost 80 years and decrease infant mortality from 4 in 10 to less than 7 in 1000. By the year 2030, more than 70 million Americans will be over 65 years old, of whom more than 12% will be 85 years or older *(1)*. Of the approximately 2.5 million people who now die each year in America, only 55,000 are children and 80% are Medicare beneficiaries *(2)*.

All Western civilized countries agree on the following general ethical principles in health care when dealing with their elderly, vulnerable, or disabled:

- All human beings have equal worth
- Society has a duty to protect the weakest and most vulnerable among its citizens
- Cost-efficiency and maximum return to society for the amount of money spent on health care should prevail *(3)*.

This means that when there is reasonable hope to stop or reverse a disease process, barring clear, specific instructions to the contrary from a well-informed patient, the treating physician has an obligation to fight for the patient's life. Age *per se* should not be a criterion to forego end-of-life medical treatment because people senesce at different rates *(4)*. Historically, it has been the demented, frail, and elderly who tend to die fast; no matter the cause *(5)*. The past century has brought with it medical technology that can significantly prolong the process of dying. However, it is no great triumph to maintain a mindless existence in a dysfunctional body at an exorbitant cost to the victim and to society.

A TYPICAL AMERICAN DEATH

A common medical situation is that of a catastrophic illness with hospitalization. The family is informed, "everything will be done," confirming their hope that modern medical technology will cure their loved one. The patient is placed in critical care, multiple specialists care for sick organs, high-tech procedures are performed, and drugs and machines support failing bodily functions. Because the patient's illness is too severe, recovery is impossible. Physicians communicate through chart notes, but never discuss the patient collectively. Some physicians eventually reduce the aggressiveness of care for their particular organ system, informing the family that the prognosis is not good. Others treat every complication, informing the family of each small "hopeful" physiological improvement. At times, the patient does not receive sufficient medications to prevent pain and anxiety, owing to concerns that over-sedation may prevent weaning the patient from the ventilator or that the patient may become "addicted." Although the patient suspects death is near, she bravely endures the ongoing discomfort and treatment. When she asks about her prognosis, she is told to "just hang in there." She mourns unresolved personal and family issues and uncompleted life goals, but does not discuss them for fear of upsetting her family. The family does not discuss the possibility of death for fear that it will upset her. As complications worsen, all physicians suspect there is no hope of recovery. Additional "curative" care is withdrawn, but not totally stopped. After weeks of intensive, bedridden care, she finally suffers a cardiac arrest and dies . . . wasted, naked, cold, and alone in an intensive care unit bed. Her last experience is a resuscitation attempt by the code team, including multiple counter shocks and 30 minutes of chest compression, which results in transient return of consciousness and fracture of her osteoporotic ribs and sternum. Physicians and family feel guilty that they may have failed by not attempting "one more thing" to prolong her life.

Virtually all of us have witnessed the "bad death" of a loved one and fear that it could happen to us. What we fear is not so much death itself, but loss of control and dignity. We not only fear severe pain, but also loss of physical, cognitive, and emotional self; and the possibility of becoming a burden to family or friends. Ninety percent of Americans wish to die at home, yet more than 50% die in hospitals, 19% in nursing homes, and only 21% at home *(6)*. Although extraordinary *palliative care* (including complete relief of pain and anxiety) is usually possible, it is rarely provided. Palliative care is often low priority and is adversely impacted by inadequate resources, poor reimbursement, and nursing shortages. In hospitalized patients, "no resuscitation" too often means "no care." Patients are reluctant to report pain for fear of distracting physicians from treating their disease, of not being a "good, brave patient," and of becoming tolerant or addicted to medications. Physicians typically have limited knowledge of pain management, are afraid of scrutiny for use of any (much less adequate) narcotics, confuse terminal comfort through sedation with euthanasia, and avoid early initiation of palliative care because they feel this is perceived as "giving up" on the patient.

FORCES IN THE EVOLUTION
OF FUTILE MEDICAL TREATMENT

With all that can now be accomplished in medicine, why do patients die an undesirable, "bad," technology-driven death within systems that otherwise deliver the best health care in the world? The forces that have led to the futile use of ineffective medical diagnostic tests, treatments, and interventions include (a) the imbalance of scientific knowledge, with extensive knowledge of benefits but typically little knowledge of the limitations of rapidly evolving medical technology; (b) inadequate training of health care workers for providing palliative care in a setting of increasing demands and training to rapidly apply highly technical skill to ever increasing numbers of patients; (c) cultural obstacles to accepting death as a natural part of life; (d) economic forces that promote high-tech futile treatment and inadequately support alternative palliative care; (e) a legal climate that promotes unfounded concerns about liability for not "doing everything" and inadequately supports policies that guard against medically futile treatments; (f) continued debate by medical, legal, and ethical leadership over accurate recognition and management of medical futility and the related disagreement over appropriate allocation of health care resources.

LEGAL RIGHTS OF THE DYING

Yes, the dying have legal rights. It is incumbent on the treating physician to avail him or herself of these before embarking on any medical treatment. The courts at common law have recognized this right to self-determination and control of our own person for a very long time. The US Supreme Court clearly articulated this concept more than 100 years ago: "No right is held more sacred, or is more carefully guarded, by the common law, than the right of every individual to the possession and control of his own person . . ." *(7)*. From this right of freedom of choice over bodily invasion evolved the doctrine of informed consent *(8,9)*.

Informed Consent

The law requires that for consent to be valid, the patient must be properly informed. The patient must have a general understanding of the following key concepts and procedures:

- the procedure or treatment
- the medically acceptable alternative procedures or treatments
- the substantial risks and hazards inherent in the proposed treatment or procedure

LIABILITY IN THE ABSENCE OF INFORMED CONSENT

Failure to obtain informed consent from a patient is a species of medical negligence and also constitutes a technical battery *(10)*. While serving on the Court of Appeals of New York, Justice Cardozo wrote, "Every human being of adult years and sound mind has a right to determine what shall be done with his own body; and a surgeon who performs an operation without his patient's consent commits an assault, for which he is liable in damages" *(11)*. The specific nature of a cause of action for failure to obtain informed consent is somewhat confusing. For example, in Florida, it has been described both as action in trespass or battery and as an action for negligence involving a violation of the physician's duty to use care in treating the patient *(12)*.

The key difference between an action for medical malpractice and an action for failure to obtain informed consent is that in failure to obtain informed consent, the plaintiff does not need to prove that the physician was medically negligent. For example, if during surgery an untoward event occurs that results in damage to the patient, the patient may bring an action for medical malpractice against the physician only by proving that the physician was negligent. However, if a known complication occurs that is not the result of negligence, but the patient was not informed of the potential for the complication, the patient may bring an action for failure to obtain informed consent regardless of whether the event was caused by negligence. Furthermore, in many states an action for failure to obtain informed consent is not limited by the short statute of limitations that applies to medical malpractice actions. Increasingly, plaintiffs have chosen to bring a cause of action for failure to obtain informed consent instead of bringing an action for malpractice.

STATUTES THAT REQUIRE SPECIFIC INFORMED CONSENT

In addition to the general medical consent statute, most states also have special informed consent statutes for specific situations. These specific statutes generally require that some additional information must be provided to the patient. For example, in Florida, some of the statutes that require informed consent are as follows:

1. testing for the HIV *(13)*
2. termination of pregnancies *(14)*
3. treatments to a nursing home resident (there is a specific requirement to advise the resident of the risks of refusing treatment) *(15)*
4. admission to a hospice program *(16)*

EXCEPTIONS TO THE REQUIREMENT OF INFORMED CONSENT

Emergency Situation. Most states recognize that, in a true emergency, there may be no time to try to obtain consent from the patient or surrogate. The health care provider is generally authorized to provide emergency care without informed consent when such an emergency exists. Statutes *(17)* typically protect any persons from civil liability (including medical providers) who gratuitously and in good faith render emergency care or treatment at the scene of an emergency, where the persons act as ordinary reasonably prudent persons would have acted under the same or similar circumstances, as long as there is no objection from the injured victim.

If the patient is inside of a hospital, the statute protects from civil liability any employee of a hospital or person licensed to practice medicine who in good faith renders medical care or treatment necessitated by a sudden, unexpected situation or occurrence resulting in a serious medical condition demanding immediate medical attention, for which the patient enters the hospital through its emergency room or trauma center.

Cardiopulmonary Resuscitation. Many states have legal doctrines that provide that a person is presumed to consent to cardiopulmonary resuscitation (CPR). The rationale for protection from liability for attempting CPR is that emergency medical personnel generally do not have time to determine if the patient or surrogate can consent to CPR. However, a number of states recognize that a patient may legally override this presumption with a Do Not Resuscitate Order (DNRO) or Do Not Attempt Resuscitation Directive *(18)*.

Special Exceptions to Informed Consent. The exceptions include emergency examination and treatment of incapacitated persons *(19)*. Examples include the patient who is intoxicated, under the influence of drugs, or otherwise incapable of providing informed consent; is experiencing an emergency medical condition; and would reasonably, under all the surrounding circumstances, undergo such examination, treatment, or procedure if he or she was advised by a health care provider *(20)*.

Court-Ordered Involuntary Treatment and Examination. Examples of court-ordered involuntary treatment and examination include the

Baker Act (Treatment and Examination for the Mentally Ill) *(21)*, Substance Abuse Services Act *(22)*, examination and treatment for tuberculosis *(23)*, and screening for sexually transmitted disease other than AIDS *(24)*.

THE RIGHT OF A COMPETENT PERSON TO REFUSE MEDICAL CARE

Constitutional Basis. An individual's right to refuse care has a constitutional basis *(25)*.

Overriding the Refusal Through Court Order. The courts are typically reluctant to override a competent adult person's right to refuse care. Generally the court must find that a compelling state interest exists, such as in the preservation of life, protection of innocent third parties, prevention of suicide, or maintenance of the ethical integrity of the medical profession.

The Health Care Provider's Role. In the first half of the 20th century, medical providers and physicians were viewed as the overseers of their patients. People "did what the doctor said." Later, court rulings indicate that, despite concededly good intentions, a health care provider's function is to provide medical treatment in accordance with the patient's wishes and best interests, not as a "substitute parent" supervening the wishes of a competent adult. Accordingly, a health care provider must comply with the wishes of a patient to refuse medical treatment unless ordered to do otherwise by a court of competent jurisdiction *(26)*.

Liability of the Health Care Provider. Many states have laws that provide that when a health care provider, acting in good faith, follows the wishes of a competent and informed patient to refuse medical treatment, the health care provider is acting appropriately and cannot be subjected to civil or criminal liability.

THE RIGHT OF AN INCOMPETENT PERSON TO REFUSE MEDICAL CARE

An incompetent person has the same right to refuse medical treatment as a competent person *(27)*. A surrogate decision maker acting on behalf of the incompetent person in accordance with the incompetent person's wishes must exercise his or her right.

Surrogate Decision Makers.

Written Appointment of Health Care Surrogate. A competent person may designate another person to make decisions when he or she is incapable of making his or her own medical decisions. This designation must be in writing, signed by the individual and two witnesses *(28)*. In the event that the patient has not appointed a surrogate in a written designation, many states provide for a statutory order of priority. For example, in Florida, the following individuals in the following order of priority are authorized to make medical decisions on behalf of the patient *(29)*:

- Judicially appointed guardian. However, this section does not require the appointment of a guardian to make health care decisions.
- The patient's spouse.
- An adult child of the patient, or if the patient has more than one adult child, a majority of the adult children who are reasonably available for consultation.
- A parent of the patient.
- The adult sibling of the patient, or if the patient has more than one sibling, a majority of the adult siblings who are reasonably available for consultation.
- An adult relative of the patient who has exhibited special care and concern for the patient and who is familiar with the patient and who is familiar with the patient's activities, health and religious or moral beliefs.
- A close friend of the patient.

The dissolution or annulment of the marriage of the patient revokes the designation of the patient's former spouse as a surrogate. Generally, most state laws provide that a surrogate's decision to withhold or withdraw life-prolonging procedures must be supported by clear and convincing evidence that the decision would have been the one the patient would have chosen, had he or she been competent *(30)*, and not one that the surrogate might make for him or herself, or that the surrogate might think is in the patient's best interests *(31)*. However, there is a developing body of statutes and cases that allow a surrogate to look at the best interests of the patient in the absence of evidence of the patient's wishes.

The procedure that is generally followed is that, if the attending physician concludes that the patient lacks capacity to make health care decisions, another physician must evaluate the patient's capacity. If the second physician agrees that the patient lacks the capacity to make health care decisions or provide informed consent, the health care facility must enter both physicians' evaluations in the patient's clinical record. The surrogate's authority commences upon the determination and continues until a determination is made that the patient has regained such capacity.

The difficult question arises as to what to do in a case where the patient, while competent, simply never expressed a clear and specific preference as to his or her wishes. The surrogate must consider the patient's prior statements about and reactions to medical issues, all the facets of the patient's personality with which the surrogate is familiar—with of course, particular reference to his or her relevant philosophical, theological, and ethical values—in order to extrapolate what course of medical treatment the patient would choose *(32)*.

Generally the patient's family, the health care facility, the attending physician, or any other interested person who may reasonably be expected to be directly affected by the surrogate's decision, may seek judicial intervention *(33)*, if that person believes:

- the surrogate's decision is not in accord with the patient's known desires
- the advance directive is ambiguous
- the patient has changed his or her mind after execution of the advance directive
- the surrogate was improperly designated or appointed
- the designation of the surrogate is no longer effective
- the designation of the surrogate has been revoked
- the surrogate has failed to discharge duties
- incapacity or illness has rendered the surrogate incapable of discharging his or her duties
- the surrogate has abused powers
- the patient has sufficient capacity to make his or her own health care decisions

The patient may revoke an advance directive or previous designation of a surrogate *(34)* in the following ways:

- by means of a signed, dated writing;
- by means of the physical cancellation or destruction of the advance directive by the patient or by another in the patient's presence and at the patient's direction;
- by means of an oral expression of his or her intent to revoke; or
- by means of a subsequently executed advance directive that is materially different from a previously executed advance directive.

A revocation will be effective when it is communicated to the surrogate, health care provider, or health care facility.

Additional Considerations. Along with the basic elements that must be contained, there are additional matters that should be addressed in an effective designation of a health care surrogate:

1. Nomination of a successor surrogate: provide for a successor if the nominated surrogate is unable or unwilling to serve.
2. A summary of any discussion of the patient with the surrogate: it is essential that the patient discuss his or her preferences and values with the surrogate. An effective designation of health care surrogate can reflect this discussion.
3. Authorization to make anatomical gifts.
4. Authority to seek compliance: a patient may consider granting the surrogate power to seek court intervention for the purposes of securing compliance with the directions of the surrogate and the living will.
5. Statement of the patient's views about life-prolonging measures: for example, the patient may state that "no life-prolonging treatment is to be provided"; or, at the other end of the spectrum, that such treatment "should be afforded to the greatest extent possible, without regard to chances of recovery or quality of life considerations"; or some middle

ground, such as "provide life prolonging treatment only if the expected benefits of the treatment will outweigh the burdens."

Withholding or Withdrawing Life-Prolonging Procedures

LIVING WILLS (ADVANCE DIRECTIVES)

Most states have laws that provide that any competent adult may make a living will or declaration providing for the withholding or withdrawal of life-prolonging procedures in the event such person suffers from a terminal condition *(35)*. The purpose of a living will is to provide written evidence of the patient's intentions and beliefs regarding life-prolonging procedures. It does not eliminate the need to name a health care surrogate. Generally, a living will must be signed by the patient in the presence of two subscribing witnesses, one of whom is neither a spouse nor blood relative of the patient. If the patient is physically unable to sign, one of the witnesses must subscribe the patient's signature in the patient's presence and at the patient's direction *(36)*. A properly executed living will can establish a rebuttal presumption of clear and convincing evidence of the patient's wishes *(37)*. It is the responsibility of the patient or someone acting on behalf of the patient to notify the attending or treating physician that a living will has been made. A treating physician or health care facility that is notified of a living will is required to make the living will or a copy part of the patient's medical records. Before proceeding in accordance with the patient's living will, it must be determined that the patient does not have reasonable probability of recovering competency *(38)*, the patient's physical condition is terminal *(39)*, and that any limitation or conditions expressed orally or in a written declaration have been carefully considered and satisfied *(40)*.

The Patient Self Determination Act of 1990 *(41)* requires health care facilities that participate in the Medicare or Medicaid programs to provide information to adult patients upon admission about their right to make medical decisions and document in the patient's medical record whether or not the patient has executed an advance directive. Facilities may not condition the provision of care or otherwise discriminate against an individual based on whether or not he or she has executed an advance directive, and must provide for the education of staff and the community on issues concerning advance directives.

LIFE-PROLONGING PROCEDURES

Life prolonging procedures include any medical procedure, treatment or intervention that utilizes mechanical or other artificial means to sustain, restore or supplant a spontaneous vital function. When applied to a patient in a terminal condition, such treatment serves only to prolong the process of dying *(42)*. Several courts have held that there is no legal distinction between "supplying oxygen by a mechanical respirator or supplying food and water through a feeding tube" *(43)*. "Artificial hydration and nutrition are viewed as treatment by the medical community and by courts of other jurisdictions" *(44)*.

"Terminal condition" is defined as a condition caused by injury, disease, or illness from which there is no reasonable probability of recovery and which, without treatment, can be expected to cause death; or a persistent vegetative state characterized by a permanent and irreversible condition or unconsciousness *(45)*. In determining whether the patient has a terminal condition or may recover capacity, or whether a medical condition or limitation referred to in an advance directive exists, the patient's attending or treating physician and at least one other consulting physician must separately examine the patient *(46)*. The findings of each physician must be documented in the patient's medical record and signed by each physician before life-prolonging procedures may be withheld or withdrawn. Evidence of the examining physician's signed documentation in the patient's medical record establishing the existence of any such medical condition establishes a rebuttable presumption that the condition exists *(47)*.

PROCEDURE IN THE ABSENCE OF A WRITTEN LIVING WILL

A surrogate may rely on oral statements made by the patient while competent to exercise the patient's right to refuse life-sustaining treatment. Oral evidence, considered alone, may constitute clear and convincing evidence.

The decision to withhold or withdraw life-prolonging procedures from a patient may be made by the designated health care surrogate unless the designation limits the surrogate's authority to exclude consent to the withholding or withdrawing of life-prolonging procedures *(48)*. Before exercising the patient's right to forego treatment, the surrogate must be satisfied that the patient does not have a reasonable probability of recovering competency so that the patient could exercise the right, and the patient's physical condition is terminal *(49)*.

Pre-Hospital Do Not Resuscitate Orders

REASON AND RATIONALE

In Florida, emergency medical technicians (EMTs) and paramedics may not deny pre-hospital treatment or transport for an emergency medical condition, unless the person has an approved DNRO *(50)*. The DNRO must be on a specific state promulgated form. The DNRO in the state of Florida is DCFS Form 1896, which must be printed on yellow paper.

Ethical Considerations, Roles, and Obligations

The Health Care Provider's Role and Obligations

In 1986, the American Medical Association and Council on Ethical and Judicial Affairs stated the following:

> For humane reasons, with informed consent, a physician may do what is medically necessary to alleviate severe pain, or cease or omit treatment to permit a terminally ill patient whose death is imminent to die. However, he should not intentionally cause death. In deciding whether the administration of potentially life-prolonging medical treatment is in the best interest of the patient who is incompetent to act in his own behalf, the physician should determine what the possibility is for extending life under humane and comfortable conditions and what are the prior expressed wishes of the patient and attitudes of the family or those who have responsibility for the custody of the patient. *(51)*

Even if death is not imminent but a patient's coma is beyond doubt irreversible and there are adequate safeguards to confirm the accuracy of the diagnosis and with the concurrence of those who have responsibility for the care of the patient, it is not unethical to discontinue all means of life-prolonging medical treatment.

Life-prolonging medical treatment includes medication and artificially or technologically supplied respiration, nutrition or hydration. In treating a terminally ill or irreversibly comatose patient, the physician should determine whether the benefits of treatment outweigh its burdens. At all times, the dignity of the patient should be maintained.

Practical Aspects of Informed Consent

Each day, millions of medical procedures are administered to patients for the diagnosis or treatment of disease or for research purposes. Appropriate consent should be sought and obtained prior to each medical procedure. CPR and emergency interventions are exempt from this process *(52)*. CPR is undertaken under the doctrine of presumed consent; that in the absence of clear and convincing evidence to the contrary, it is presumed that the patient would choose life over death. With minors or incompetent adults, the power of consent is relinquished to the responsible relative or appointed surrogate under the doctrine of "substituted judgment" *(53)*.

Informed consent has three legs: full disclosure, patient competence to choose, and the assurance that the patient's decision is out of the exercise of free will *(54)*.

Full disclosure requires the treating physician to explain to his or her patient details of the proposed procedure including all possible foreseen (and unforeseen) complications; all alternate ways of treatment and the merits and risks of each of these alternatives; and the physician's own results with the proposed procedure, including success and complication rates vis-á-vis those of other physicians. Patient competence stipulates that the patient is able to comprehend and process all available information, that the patient is able to evaluate and choose between these options, and that the patient is allowed to ask any pertinent questions that enable him or her to make a choice. The exercise of free will, while allowing for the physician to express his or her own bias regarding the preferred course of treatment, requires that the patient's choice of a certain treatment to be made in a rational, deliberate, calculated, and objective manner. Importantly, the decision should not be subject to coercion, manipulation, emotional encumbrances, nor undue pleadings or threats.

The truthful reality in medical practice is that the satisfaction of all these theoretical requirements of the consent process is unimaginable in practice and implausible, even in theory.

In the first place, most patients are either totally or near totally ignorant about most complex medical technologies and the pathophysiology of disease and its outcomes, let alone the jargon of medical terminologies (the American Medical Association has an informative physician's tape on the subject). Patients' knowledge about medical issues often derives from a limited experience with a relative or a friend or from distorted information from the news media or the Internet. Even when such information is gleaned from authentic medical sources, it is interpreted out of context by the lay public and tainted by the patient's own limited personal experiences.

Second, full disclosure is unrealistic and may be cruel (55). A personal experience illustrates the peril of full disclosure. During the explanation of the cardiac catheterization procedure and the litany of all possible complications to the patient, the patient's 300 lb., 6- foot tall husband suffered neurocardiogenic syncope, fell unconscious to the floor, and sustained a deep laceration to the forehead. He later complained he did not desire to hear all the details provided. Physicians have recognized the flaws of "full disclosure" for centuries. Over the years, the imperative of informed consent has metamorphasized into a legal formality requiring the patient to sign a lengthy and printed form written in legal jargon and containing a litany of possible complications whose primary purpose is to protect the physician (and hospital) or to meet legal requirements, rather than to duly inform the patient (56).

But if the consent process is riddled with flaws and misconceptions, is there a better substitute? For example, what about the substituted judgment standard? This standard stipulates that the patient may relinquish medical decision-making to a trusted relative or friend. The doctrine assumes that the chosen surrogate's decisions are exact replicas of the patient's own when the patient is incapable or unable to make his or her own medical decisions. Unfortunately, such assumptions are more likely to prove to be wrong than right. Surrogates are often encumbered by feelings of guilt, fear of loss of a loved one, concern about the possibility of being accused of not doing enough for the patient, or may simply be driven by self interests and personal gain (57,58). Surrogates who are not fully informed about the patient's chances for recovery or have unrealistic expectations from a medical intervention; those who lack the will to make tough choices to forgo life-prolonging means; and those who have agendas of their own further undermine the validity of the substitute judgment standard.

Because patients cannot fully understand all the medical implications of health care decisions, it is desirable and possibly even imperative to have all medical decision making done as a shared exercise between the physician and his adult competent patient or the patient's chosen surrogate. In practice, such decision making is almost always *physician-guided*, and with few exceptions, the physician's recommendation carries the day. This fact is especially true the longer and the more trusting the relationship between a particular patient and his or her chosen doctor. There are precious few instances in which a patient declines a recommendation from a physician that the patient has known and trusted for many years. Under most situations of ill health or an imminent death, there is a one best medical course of treatment. Experienced physicians should recommend this one best course after weighing the probability, extent, and duration of benefit against possible risks, taking into account the extent of the patient's illness and physician's skill and experience.

The Wide Gulf Between What the Dying Patient Wants and What the Doctor Honors

Peter Singer et al. (59) interviewed 126 patients belonging to three groups: those maintained on dialysis, sufferers of AIDS, and residents of long-term care facilities. Patients identified five domains of quality end-of-life care in the following order of importance:

1. Receiving adequate pain and symptom treatment.
2. Avoiding inappropriate prolongation of dying.
3. Achieving a sense of control.

4. Relieving the burden on loved ones.
5. Strengthening relationships with loved ones.

These romantic, emotion-based concepts are foreign to physicians who are accustomed to dealing with probabilities and the results of laboratory testing and high-tech imaging. It is no wonder that the Study to Understand Prognoses and Preferences for Outcomes and Treatment (SUPPORT) showed that many Americans suffer needlessly before dying *(60)* and that a recent report showed that 80% of Americans rated their medical care as excellent or very good, whereas less than 30% of the respondents said the same thing about care for the dying *(2)*.

BARRIERS TO END-OF-LIFE CONVERSATIONS

The most common professional problem in end-of-life care is failure to make a deliberate, mutual (with patient, family, and other physicians) decision to make the transition from curative to palliative care, based on the timely recognition of medical futility. Treatment norms that contribute to this problem are difficult to change. Not uncommonly, individual physicians do not fully accept the mortality of themselves or their patients. Medical futility decisions are among the most emotionally and ethically difficult, involving issues such as advanced age, dementia, severe brain injury, disabling stroke, extremely low birth weight, and congenital defects with severe handicaps and limited life expectancy. At a time when decisions have become increasingly difficult, physicians have felt a sense of loss of control over patient care, not only from competing autonomy of patients and surrogates, but also from pressures of third-party payers, managed care, soaring hospital costs, and even practice guidelines imposed by peers.

Young physicians are trained to fight death and preserve life through diligent battle with each and every physiological problem. They are often not trained to recognize or deal with medical futility *(61,62)*. Training that emphasizes evidence-based thinking, reinforced by objective testing, does not lend itself to intellectual comfort with the uncertainty of predicting prognosis, much less time of death. Statistical models designed to help physicians predict prognosis in critically ill patients are not highly predictive for the individual patient *(60,63,64)*. For patient protection, "medical futility" must be declared very sparingly to avoid overzealous use in questionably curable patients, erring on the side of aggressive care.

Physicians often have limited knowledge and skill in palliative care and fail to recognize that discontinuation of futile, curative treatment is often necessary to allow the best possible palliative care. Instead, medical teams frequently inflict CPR, the ultimate invasive and traumatic treatment, on dying patients as their "last rite." Medical personnel grossly overestimate the success of CPR (>30%) and the public sees a 67% television survival rate, whereas actual results are much worse: 10%–20% survival for in-hospital arrest (3.5% if over 85 years old) and 5% for out-of-hospital arrest (1% in elderly nursing home patients) *(65–68)*. Institutional policies further discourage futility decisions, such as the requirement to resuscitate all patients unless a DNRO is written and the written or unwritten requirement to obtain acceptance of DNR status by all family members before orders can be written *(69–72)*. Vast educational, cultural, ethical, and religious differences exist among patients and physicians that impact attitudes about how to care for such individuals. The issue of "who should decide" whether to continue life support and curative efforts in a broad spectrum of medical conditions has led to legal battles and landmark decisions *(73)*. Major conflicts over end-of-life care, however, are unusual. Much more commonly, physicians and families choose to continue aggressive, curative treatment efforts until death rather than embark on the difficult and emotional journey of seeking and communicating the earliest possible recognition and acceptance of medical futility to allow the earliest, most merciful transition to palliative care.

CONFRONTING THE HISTORICAL
NEAR-IRRELEVANCE OF LIVING WILLS

Teno et al. *(74)* examined 688 living wills as a part of the SUPPORT study. The authors noted only a minority of Americans (generally less than 30%) have living wills. Of those, 50% do not have orders of *no* CPR when they asked not to be resuscitated. In 87% of the living wills, general statements were used. In only 1 in 30 living wills was there language specific enough as to apply to the patient's condition. The conclusion was that currently used living wills have little relevance to patient care.

Based on our human experience, people have survived almost every imaginable illness. We tend to reason that almost any illness is potentially reversible, be it a stroke, a fracture, a cardiac arrest or pneumonia. Living wills that speak about terminal illness, irreversible conditions, heroic measures, or artificial means must be interpreted by the treating physician and by the patient's appointed surrogate, who are likely to believe that any illness is reversible, and are prone to err on the side of continued aggressive treatment. Similarly, physicians find end-of-life decisions, which are often based on less than absolutely certain data, extremely difficult, both intellectually and emotionally. As physicians and families protect themselves from facing the grief and hopelessness of death, they often unknowingly transform a potentially peaceful death into a harsh one. Physicians must learn through the eyes and experiences of their own patients. They should recognize and communicate to the family when life has permanently lost all value and therefore allow a peaceful death.

A properly executed advance directive can be highly effective. Hammes et al. *(75)* demonstrated that, given the proper document, timing, education and support, almost 90% of individuals choose to execute advance care plans that become an integral section of the medical chart, and that in the vast majority of instances the dying patients receive their chosen treatment. No one can belittle the success achieved by Hammes et al. The fact that La Crosse, Wisconsin is an enclave of fairly homogeneous people of northern European descent served by one clinic (Gundersen Lutheran Medical Center) may provide insight into the unusual success Hammes documented. Such success offers a challenge to all organizations dealing with end-of-life care to provide a mechanism for ensuring a graceful exit and a good death.

Project GRACE is a 501(c)3 nonprofit organization located in Clearwater, Florida. Among other things, its board has developed and tested an advance care plan that has the following virtues:

1. It is endorsed by numerous medical societies, including the Florida Medical Association, and is one page, with an additional page that defines most end-of-life medical conditions and treatment options.
2. It is medical scenario-specific, listing the four most common conditions that lead to imminent death or permanent loss of what most individuals would consider quality of life.
3. It allows the potential future patient the option to choose "yes" or "no" to each of four most common life-prolonging treatment efforts for each of the four incurable illnesses.

The document is written in simple language, which has been tested for clarity of understanding among individuals at an eighth grade level. The Project GRACE Advance Care Plan Document has been adopted by the majority of hospitals in the Tampa Bay, Florida area *(76,77)*.

THE HIGH COST OF DYING IN AMERICA

Most of the recent innovations in medicine have been employed to extend the life of people past middle age. Dr. Daniel Callahan, director of the Hastings Center in New York and outspoken critic of wasteful medical care at the end of life, quotes Dr. Jerome Avorn, health economist of the Harvard Medical School, who writes, "With the exception of the birth control pill, most of medical technology interventions developed since the 1950s have their most widespread impact on people who are past their fifties—the further past their fifties, the greater the impact *(78)*.

Over the past three decades, health care costs in America have increased threefold as a percentage of the gross national product (GNP). Today, America devotes one-seventh of its GNP to health care; most of these expenditures are spent on the oldest segment of the population. One of the most widely quoted statistics in medical and economic circles derives from the 1986 publication from the Center for Health Statistics, which showed that 30% of Medicare expenditures are incurred during the last year of life. Furthermore, for the 6% of the elderly Medicare patients who die each year, 50% of all medical costs are spent during the last 2 months of life, and 40% goes toward care during the last month *(79)*. According to one of America's leading economists, Victor Fuchs, "One of the biggest challenges facing policy makers for the rest of this century will be how to strike an appropriate balance between care for the dying and health services for the rest of the population" *(80)*.

IS HEALTH IN THE UNITED STATES THE BEST IN THE WORLD?

In the United States, we spend more health dollars per citizen than any other nation on earth, yet we are not healthier and we do not live longer than people in most civilized nations. Dr. Barbara Starfield reminds us of the Institute of Medicine's report "To Err Is Human," documenting that 20% to 30% of US patients receive unnecessary surgery or other interventions and that 44,000 to 98,000 among them die each year as a result of medical errors *(81)*. Dr. Starfield compares the US health care system with 12 other distinguished nations: Japan, Sweden, Canada, France, Australia, Germany, Spain, Finland, the Netherlands, the United Kingdom, Denmark, and Belgium. The United States ranks 12th (second from the bottom on overall performance) among this select group of nations *(79)*.

The Year 2000 World Health Organization's (WHO) report using disability-adjusted life expectancy shows similar data. The report ranked the United States as 15th among 25 industrialized countries *(82)*. The WHO measured each nation's overall health system performance by its achievement of three goals: the provision of good health, responsiveness to the expectations of the population, and the fairness of the individuals' financial contribution toward their health care. Health was measured by life expectancy adjusted for the likelihood of a range of disabilities and produced the following ranking:

1. Japan: 74.5 years
2. Australia: 73.2 years
3. France: 73.1 years
4. Sweden: 73.0 years
5. Spain: 72.8 years
6. United States: 70 years

The United States ranked better when judged on attention to individual choice and care, ranking first when responsiveness was judged by a nation's respect for the dignity of individuals, the confidentiality of health records, prompt attention in emergencies, and choice of provider:

1. United States
2. Switzerland
3. Luxembourg
4. Denmark
5. Germany

However, when financial fairness was measured by the equal distribution of the health cost faced by each household, the United States ranked extremely low:

1. Columbia
2. Luxembourg
3. Belgium
4. Djibouti
5. Denmark
6. United States

The full report is available on the WHO website: http://www.who.int/.

High spending does not necessarily translate into a better health system, according to the WHO. Among the 15 top-rated nations, the amount spent on health care as a percentage of the overall economy and on a per-person basis varied widely. These differences are shown in Table 1.

Yes, America has the most technologically advanced and most responsive system in the world. It has the best doctors, the best hospitals, and the best-equipped intensive care units. Also, the relatively poor health care performance cannot be blamed on the fact that Americans "behave badly," (i.e., smoking, drinking and perpetrating violence). This accusation is not supported by the data. In fact, Americans tend to smoke less and consume less alcohol than most other Western countries. The reasons for the poor performance of our health care system are no doubt complex and multifaceted. However, contributing causes may be that Americans undergo more surgeries, consume more medications and are hospitalized more often than citizens of other, better-rated nations *(83)*.

Table 1
Health Care Spending Among Top-Rated Nations

Country	Health spending as percentage of GDP	Per capita spending	Population
1. France	9.8%	$2369	59 million
2. Italy	9.3	1855	57 million
3. San Marino	7.5	2257	26,000
4. Andorra	7.5	1368	75,000
5. Malta	6.3	551	386,000
6. Singapore	3.1	876	3.5 million
7. Spain	8.0	1071	39 million
8. Oman	3.9	370	2.4 million
9. Austria	9.0	2277	8.2 million
10. Japan	7.1	2373	126 million
11. Norway	6.5	2283	4.4 million
12. Portugal	8.2	845	9.8 million
13. Monaco	8.0	1264	33,000
14. Greece	8.0	905	10 million
15. Iceland	7.9	2149	279,000
16. United States	13.7	4187	276 million

GDP, gross domestic product. (From ref. *83*.)

THE FUTILITY DEBATE: FAR FROM FUTILE

More than 750 recent medical publications on medical futility have failed to bring medical and lay personnel to a consensus, to the point that the "futility movement" has "fallen" *(84)*. Inability to resolve the "debate" over ethical, philosophical, and definitional issues has been assumed to be the primary reason that the futility concept has failed. A review of the multiple complex forces contributing to futile care at end-of-life described earlier, however, suggests that resolution of the debate alone will not eliminate futile treatment. Searching for consensus on the meaning of medical futility remains worthwhile, however, and may be necessary before the other forces can be overcome.

The issues raised in the "futility debate" have centered around disagreements over the following:

1. an acceptable definition of medical futility or even whether it is possible to define futility;
2. whether or not physicians have the right or obligation to withhold treatments that they judge to be futile; and

3. whether or not patients have the right to demand any form of treatment if they feel it will be beneficial to them (i.e., the struggle between the autonomy of patients and the autonomy of physicians).

Numerous authors have offered definitions of medical futility, pointing to its recognition since antiquity by Hippocrates and Plato *(85,86)*. Futile treatments have generally been subdivided into two types:

1. physiological or quantitative futility (very low statistical probability of achieving the desired physiological response; and
2. qualitative futility (in which treatment may have a physiological effect, but fails to "benefit" the patient as a whole) *(87)*.

Much of the futility debate has centered around futile CPR *(88–91)*. A broader, more comprehensive definition of medical futility was proposed by Drane and Coulehan in 1993 *(92)* as treatment that does not alter a person's persistent vegetative state; does not alter diseases or defects that make a baby's survival beyond infancy impossible; leaves permanently unrestored a patient's neurocardiorespiratory capacity, capacity for relationship, or moral agency; or will not help free a patient from permanent dependency on total intensive care support.

We have proposed an operational definition of medical futility *(93)* that requires that the physician combine clinical experience and scientific data with the concepts of both qualitative and quantitative futility through three questions: (a) Is death imminent? (b) If treatment leads to full recovery, is the best quality of life that can be hoped for undesirable? (c) Is the statistical probability of recovery extremely low? *(See* Fig. 1.) A negative answer to any of these questions indicates that continued efforts toward curative care are futile. In borderline futile situations, the potential for continued life-prolonging treatment efforts to cause harm or prolong suffering must be carefully weighed against their (often minimal) potential for benefit. Examples of the practical application of this definition are offered through a published list of common futile medical conditions (Table 2).

Whether "futile" or other terminology is used, most physicians are fully aware that predictably ineffective "curative" medical care is prevalent, is expensive, and contributes immeasurably to the pain and suffering of many dying patients. Some physicians have attempted to use the concept of medical futility to justify unilateral decisions to withhold treatment options or withdraw treatment. Arguments have been based on the physician's ethical obligations of beneficence (benefit), nonmaleficence (avoid harming), and justice (wise use of resources) versus the patient's autonomy (which is the basis of informed consent, personal

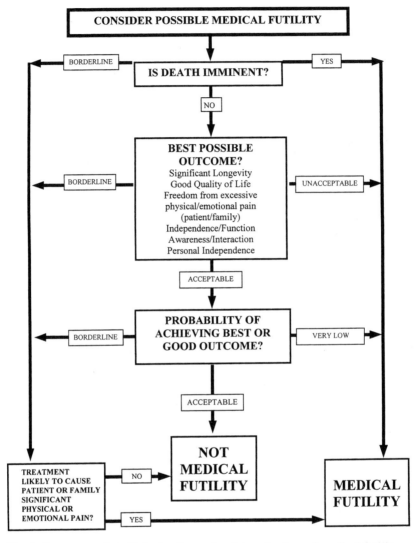

Fig. 1. Recommended clinical pathway for determination of medical futility.

right to accept or reject treatment, and advance care planning) *(94)*. The patient's or surrogate's belief that patient autonomy to refuse treatment extends equally to the right to demand treatment sometimes results in inappropriate demands for futile treatment. A counterargument is that the treating physician's ethical obligations logically limit the patient's autonomous choices to those options the physician can ethically offer *(93)*. Despite ethical considerations, it is unusual for a physician to withdraw or withhold treatment over the objections of the patient or family.

Table 2
Medical Futility

Rationale for futility:
I = death is imminent
II = best possible outcome is unacceptable
III = probability of achieving good outcome is very low

Definite futilty	Frequent futility	Not futile
Metastatic cancer, untreatable or multiple treatment failures (I, II, III)	Widespread cancer, incurable (II)	Treatable cancer, with potential cure or significant probability of remission
End-stage CHF, unable to wean off ventilator or keep out of hospital (nontransplant candidate) (I,II)	Severe, class IV CHF, despite maximal medical therapy (nontransplant candidate) (II)	CHF amenable to medical therapy and/or with reversible or treatable underlying cause
End-stage chronic lung disease, on ventilator, unable to wean (not heart-lung transplant candidate) (II)	End-stage chronic lung disease, post respiratory failure, requiring continuous oxygen (nontransplant candidate) (II, III)	Moderately severe to severe chronic lung disease amenable to medical therapy and oxygen; acute, reversible respiratory failure
ESRD with severe, irreversible dysfunction of other organ systems (heart, lung, liver, CNS, or bone marrow); not dialysis or transplant candidate (I,II)	ESRD with multiorgan system failure, low probability of recovery (III)	Acute, reversible renal failure and chronic renal failure, transplant and/or dialysis candidate
End-stage liver disease, hepatic encaphalopathy or coma (nontransplant candidate) (I,II)	Severe chronic or acute liver dysfunction plus multiorgan system failure (CHF, renal failure, or respiratory failure) (III)	Non-end-stage chronic liver disease and acute, potentially reversible hepatic dysfunction

(continued)

Table 2 (Continued)

Rationale for futility:
I = death is imminent
II = best possible outcome is unacceptable
III = probability of achieving good outcome is very low

Definite futilty	Frequent futility	Not futile
Severe myelodysplasia with severe pancytopenia and bleeding and/or infection (I, II, III)	Myelodysplasia with severe reduction in at least two of three types of blood cells with infection or bleeding (III)	Reversible bone marrow failure and chronic anemia amenable to transfusion therapy
Severe, irreversible dementia, totally dependent for activities of daily living, bedfast, disoriented (II)	Severe or moderately severe and progressive Ddementia, bedfast or severely dependent or with severe behavioral dysfunction (agitation, hostility) (II)	Mild or moderate dementia with intact communication and some activities of daily living independence
Severe immune compromise (HIV, organ transplantation, active chemotherapy for incurable cancer) plus incurable, life-threatening infection (I, II)	Sepsis plus multiple organ system failure (III)	Severe infection with potential for recovery
Irreversible coma/persistent vegetative state, 1 year after head injury or 3 months after CVA or anoxic brain injury (II, III)	Severe brain dysfunction (CVA, trauma, infection, anoxia), persistent for 2 weeks with no improvement; Severe brain stem or high spinal stroke or injury, irreversible (locked in syndrome) (II, III)	Acute coma or dementia, without severe, irreversible brain injury

386

Extreme (>90% third degree) burn injury (II, III)	Extensive burns (third degree over much of body); sepsis (II,III)	Limited but severe burns, skin graft candidate, absent sepsis
Prolonged cardiac asystole or electrical-mechanical dissociation (>10 minutes), unresponsive to ACLS (I, III)	Electrical-mechanical dissociation in setting of severe cardiac disease and cardiac arrest with critical aortic stenosis (I, III)	Witnessed cardiac arrest post CPR, successful defibrillation and adequate blood pressure, absent end-stage heart or other organ disease (acute setting)
Advanced age in ICU with extremely poor prognosis predictive model scores (SUPPORT, APACHE, SAPS, MMP) (III)	Advanced age in hospital with poor prognosis predictive model scores (SUPPORT, APACHE, SAPS, MMP) (III)	Advanced age alone (functionally, medically and mentally intact; some independence and interaction)
Absence of neonatal potential for higher brain development (anencephaly) (I, II)	Congenital defects associated with extreme mental retardation and inability to achieve independence or survive beyond infancy (II)	Congenital defects with potential for longevity and development (Trisomy 21)
Congenital organ defects incompatible with survival and development (nontransplant candidate) (I, II)	Congenital defects associated with moderately severe to severe mental retardation plus organ defects	Congenital defects associated with nonfatal organ dysfunction or transplant candidate

CHF, congestive heart failure; ESRD, end-stage renal disease; CNS, central nervous system; CVA, cerebrovascular accident; ACLS, advanced cardiac life support; CPR, cardiopulmonary resuscitation; ICU, intensive care unit; SUPPORT, Study to Understand Prognoses and Preferences for Outcomes and Treatment; APACHE, Acute Physiology and Chronuc Health Evaluation; SAPS, Assessment of Positive Symptoms; MMP, matrix metalloproteinase.

Such disputes are typically settled by "giving in" to futile treatment or recommending that another physician take over (who will usually provide the requested treatment).

Actually, unresolved disagreements among patients, surrogates and physicians are relatively infrequent. The much more common error, however, is that medical futility is simply never acknowledged by anyone. In reality, physicians dismiss treatments as "futile," or simply unlikely to provide benefit to patients, routinely during medical care. Doctors unilaterally make these decisions based upon their unique medical skills and knowledge. This reality makes the "futility debate" over whether physicians can unilaterally decide to offer specific treatments irrelevant— doctors simply do and must make these decisions all the time.

The critical issue in the physician's role in dealing with medical futility arises when that physician suspects that all curative or life-prolonging treatment options can no longer benefit the patient. The choice must then be made between concluding that all further curative care attempts are futile or continuing with attempts at curative or life-prolonging treatment. No matter how grave, the physician is typically less than 100% certain of the prognosis and is personally reluctant to "give up" on the patient. After acknowledging "medical futility," the physician must choose to deliver extremely bad news to the family, then launch into the difficult, time-consuming process of helping the family deal with anger, grief, and acceptance. It is no surprise that the physician often continues aggressive, curative care, despite personal recognition of medical futility.

The "futility debate," thus, ultimately centers around the question of whether physicians are willing to embrace their unique responsibility as the professional advocates for patients in recognizing when patients are "there," when all reasonable hope of mastery of disease has vanished. Like all other medical decisions, it is not necessary or possible for all physicians to agree upon exactly what circumstances must exist in all patient conditions. In fact, the decision should and must be unique to each patient. What is needed is for all physicians to recognize the compelling obligation to apply all available data and skill to making the decision that medical futility exists at a specific point in the patient's life that is neither before hope for cure has gone, nor after futile treatment has deprived the patient of the best possible death.

The physician should not feel alone, nor generally attempt to communicate medical futility alone. Communication with and support from physician colleagues, nurses and, when available, a dedicated palliative care team is critical to effective communication and acceptance. Though commonly overlooked, clergy and other spiritual support can serve as an invaluable resource for the patient and family. When possible, the patient's priest, minister, or rabbi should be routinely informed and brought into discussions and decisions by the health care team. Physicians should also recognize their own spirituality in making agonizing futility decisions and their own "priesthood" role in the spiritual care of the patient and family *(95)*.

The question of patient vs physician autonomy or "who should decide?" remains a critical issue. The answer lies in the question, "who should decide what?" and must logically and ethically depend on the capabilities and vested interests of the individuals involved. The physician's role should always be to delineate the reasonable spectrum of treatment choices, from most aggressive to most conservative (including the recognition of medical futility), while the patient or surrogate must choose among medically plausible and reasonable treatment options, based upon personal goals and values. In the vast majority of medically futile situations, lack of benefit of curative treatment efforts is clear to the physician. Given a choice, the well-informed patient or surrogate will almost always choose good palliative care over futile, sometimes punishing, "curative" care.

When treatment is not clearly futile, but may offer little benefit with significant risk or morbidity, the informed patient or surrogate must make the decision to accept or reject treatment based upon personal values. The critical ingredient is communication. Communication often breaks down when physicians, patients and families choose to continue to pursue false "hopes" of improbable or impossible cure, rather than going through the painful, sometimes lengthy grieving process of recognizing and dealing with futility. However, it is only through the timely recognition and communication that futility exists (by physicians) and the acceptance (by patients and families) that curative or life-prolonging treatment is no longer beneficial that patients and physicians can be freed to redefine "hope" as a comfortable death with dignity, through unrestricted palliative care.

COMMUNICATION IN THE FACE OF MEDICAL FUTILITY: PHYSICIANS' "DOS AND DON'TS"

Communication skills are a vital component of healing, especially when the physician is the bearer of bad news during the last stages of disease *(96)*. The temptation to offer a dying patient the option of one more intervention, even if such an intervention has a low probability of benefiting the patient, is all too great. Physicians fighting death and disease can sometimes unknowingly inflict great harm. Exaggerated promises

Table 3
Physician's Guide to Effective
Patient/Family Communication on End-of-Life Care

Dos

- Clearly lay out medical facts, options and consequences.
- Give an accurate and realistic expectation of prognosis to patient and family as soon into the illness as possible.
- Provide a time frame for probable expectation of improvement and propose plans for a finite duration of continued aggressive, curative care.
- Openly show compassion, empathy, personal grief, respect, and love for the patient and family.
- Assure patient and family you will be with them; ensure relief of suffering; and inform them constantly of ongoing reassessment of the appropriateness of treatment.
- Regularly communicate your thinking about prognosis and goals of care to other physicians and nurses through progress notes and direct communication; encourage/expect the same from colleagues.
- As a consultant, provide information about the impact of severity of illness in your area of expertise on the overall prognosis.

(continued)

lead to unfulfilled hopes and unreasonable demands from patients and families, followed by great disappointments. The medical profession can never be more greatly impoverished than when the physician's self-interests are made to masquerade as altruism; or when unbeneficial, high-technology intervention is offered to a dying patient in the name of compassion; or when the physician's love of technology exceeds his or her love for fellow man. No wonder many citizens, not groundlessly, accuse the medical profession of being driven by self-interest, even avarice. Truthfulness and self-restraint dictate prudence in always giving patients and families realistic expectations. Upholding the primacy of patients' self-interest should reign supreme in all medical decisions, whether the aim is to restore health or ensure a peaceful dying. Table 3 should guide the treating physicians as they talk to their patients and relevant family members about end-of-life medical treatment issues.

EVIDENCE-BASED AVOIDANCE
OR WITHDRAWAL OF INTERVENTIONS

Realistic knowledge of prognosis in cardiac patients is critical in making treatment choices. Unfortunately, most prospective studies are supported by drug or device companies who cherry-pick among patients.

Table 3 (Continued)

Dos

- Advise against procedures you are requested to perform, if futile.
- Hope for the best, prepare for the worst; communicate that approach to patient and family.
- Constantly strive to identify new, appropriate, achievable goals.
- Ask "How do you think your loved one would feel about this situation?"
- Ask "What kind of life did he/she live? Was it important to be active/ healthy?"
- Reassure families that "Whatever decision is thoughtfully made in his/her best interest is the best one, no matter what the (unpredictable) outcome."
- Clearly communicate that "No Resuscitation" does not mean "No Care" and make sure it doesn't!
- Listen, ask, seek to understand, and feedback what you are hearing from patients and families for confirmation of their fears and wishes.
- Prepare the family for the expected breathing pattern and other characteristics of dying; assure them the patient is not suffering; and sedate enough to eliminate even the *appearance* of suffering.
- Involve and utilize other physicians, clergy, palliative care nurses, social services, pain management, Hospice, psychology, psychiatry, bioethics committee.

Don'ts

- Don't impose your own values or culture on the patient or family.
- Don't show impatience, condescension, anger, or defensiveness.
- Don't avoid contact with the patient/family.
- Don't perform surgery or other procedures on the patient that will not alter the outcome of the illness or provide comfort care, even if requested by family or a colleague.
- Don't avoid recognizing futility by reasoning that you can never be absolutely sure of the outcome.
- Don't provide "good news" about improvements in physiologic parameters when they do not change the overall (poor) prognosis.
- Don't say "We need this critical care unit bed for another patient."
- Don't say "We can't justify the cost."
- Don't say "There's nothing we can do."
- Don't use words such as "futile" when describing the situation or treatment to patient or family.
- Don't ask "Do you want us to stop this or do everything?"
- Don't say "I don't know about that, you'll have to ask the other doctor."
- Don't criticize others involved in the patient's care.
- Don't withhold needed analgesia or sedation in dying patients.
- Don't give mixed messages from different doctors and nurses.
- Don't exhibit or lay guilt or blame.
- Don't allow a significant time of false hope to elapse, then suddenly deliver bad news when there is no apparent change in condition.

They often comprise of mostly younger men with a limited number of chronic diseases *(97)*. The results are then often applied to treating older patients, most of whom are women who have multiple health problems. For example, at least half of heart failure patients have impaired renal function, yet the vast majority of studies exclude such patients *(98)*. Lower body compression treatments, regular infusion of inotropes, brain peptide infusion, biventricular pacing, automatic implantable cardioverter defibrillator implantation, and left ventricular-assist devices are routinely chosen for frail, elderly patients, based on evidence obtained from younger, healthier patients. There is overwhelming evidence from heart failure studies that patients with markedly reduced oxygen consumption and left ventricular ejection fraction, particularly those who have elevated serum uric acid levels, tend to die during the first year of follow-up, unless heart transplantation is indicated and undertaken promptly *(99–101)*. Retrospective analysis of Medicare patients with six or more chronic conditions have a similar, prohibitively high mortality during the first year of follow-up *(102)*. Kenneth Rockwood has shown that demented, frail, elderly, patients who depend on others to carry out the majority of their daily activities also behave similarly when confronted with an acute complication such as a fracture, pneumonia, or a stroke *(103)*.

Physicians must also have knowledge of the expected impact of treatment on the individual. In another retrospective study, a 95% increase in complications occurred from interventions in Medicare patients having four or more chronic conditions *(104)*.

Yes, people senesce at different rates; persons from rich neighborhoods tend to live longer. They tend to take care of themselves and to seek medical care sooner *(105)*. However, all end up dying. Interventions that are attended by a high mortality or morbidity should be generally advised against. Only procedures that improve life's quality should be undertaken in dying patients, such as the removal of a gangrenous limb or treatment of a painful cystitis, an intractable constipation, or urinary retention. It is the physician's sacred duty to fight premature or unexpected dying, but not to delay expected, imminent death.

THE RULE OF DOUBLE EFFECT

The rule of double effect differentiates between the intent and foreseeable result of an action *(106)*. The rule comes into play when large doses of opiates or more drastic measures, such as unconscious sedation, are needed to ease the passing of a dying patient. Heavy sedation is especially needed in patients dying of respiratory failure or when removing ventilator support from terminally ill patients. Dying patients deserve as much medication as necessary to relieve pain; they never "get addicted." Sedation to unconsciousness must be resorted to rarely, when the suffering is intolerable or convulsions can't be otherwise controlled. The American Medical Association has recommended that every practicing physician use large enough doses of analgesics and sedatives to alleviate the suffering of their dying patient, even if that hastens the moment of death. When physicians are inexperienced or uncertain about sedation of the dying patient, proper consultation from a specialist should always be sought.

Allowing nature to take its course is simply not interfering in nature's will to end life, once it has lost all meaning. It is ethically, morally, and legally right to discontinue mechanical ventilation for a patient who will either never wake up or who cannot be weaned from a ventilator and does not desire to continue such an existence; in other words, it is right to "let die," but not to "make die." Although the result is the same in both instances, the intent is totally different, thus, the "rule of double effect" *(107)*. To subject a dying person to needless and punishing suffering is contrary to the core values of medicine. An injection of potassium chloride to end a life, on the other hand, is illegal and immoral. To kill your patient in order to put him or her out of his or her misery is not permissable by law or ethics *(108)*.

PHYSICIAN-ASSISTED SUICIDE AND EUTHANASIA

Euthanasia is illegal in the United States. Among the US states, physician-assisted suicide is legal only in Oregon *(109)*. Euthanasia and physician-assisted suicide are legal in the Netherlands, and more recently, in Switzerland *(110,111)*. Physician-assisted suicide is always voluntary. An example is that the doctor prescribes a lethal dose of barbiturates at the patient's request, which the patient has the option of taking at the time it is needed. The patient controls the time of dying. Euthanasia may be voluntary or involuntary. Voluntary active euthanasia means that the physician ends the life (and suffering) of the patient by an intravenous injection (usually of potassium chloride) when asked to do so. Involuntary active euthanasia refers to a situation in which the physician in charge ends the life of the patient at the time and with the method of his choosing without being asked to do so by the patient; such patients may be very old, demented, or wheelchair bound. In other words, the doctor views the patient as a burden to self and society.

In Oregon the "Death with Dignity Act" received a majority vote in 1995 and again in November 1997, allowing for physician-assisted suicide with the following safeguards:

- The patient's request must be in writing and must be witnessed.
- A consulting physician must certify that the patient's condition is terminal.
- A 15-day waiting period must elapse between the patient's request and obtaining the suicide prescription.

The physician must ensure that the patient's decision is voluntary by providing information about diagnosis, prognosis and other options, such as hospice care and referral to a state-licensed psychologist or psychiatrist if there is any suspicion that the patient may be asking for assisted suicide as a result of depression and not because of suffering caused by the underlying disease.

The populations of both Oregon and the Netherlands are characterized as being relatively stable, of northern European extraction, well educated, and influenced by religion to a limited degree. A comparison between the experiences of Oregon and the Netherlands has been undertaken by Willems et al. *(112)*. In Oregon, less than one-third of those who ask for lethal prescriptions receive it and some of these do not use it; less than 1 in 1000 of those who die do so assisted by physicians; and none receive physician-assisted suicide primarily because they perceive themselves to be a burden on others. By contrast, in the Netherlands almost 3% of those who die, die through euthanasia or physician-assisted suicide, with euthanasia being the preferred method. Furthermore, being perceived as a burden on others or society is a common reason for euthanasia in the Netherlands.

The actual prevalence of euthanasia by health care workers and families is unknown, but it is not surprising that a significant number of people contemplate or actually perform euthanasia or physician-assisted suicide when faced with the alternative of helplessly watching an agonal death. A recent survey of 3299 US oncologists indicated that 6.5% "supported" and 3.7% had performed euthanasia; 22.7% supported physician-assisted suicide for terminally ill patients with unremitting pain despite optimal analgesia, and 10.8% had performed or assisted in the death of their patients *(113)*. This surprising data may be attributed to the unavailability of adequate palliative care, even to oncologists, who should have the most experience and access to resources.

An unforeseen benefit of the passage of the Death with Dignity Act in Oregon is that terminally ill patients talk to their doctors about medical care at the end of life. Additionally, fewer Oregonians die in hospitals or undergo life-prolonging interventions and CPR. Many have an advance care plan, opt for palliative care and use hospice care *(114)*. The rare frequency of physician-assisted suicide in Oregon suggests that when communication and access to adequate control of pain and suffering is readily available, extremely few turn to euthanasia or suicide at the end of life.

COMMUNITY EFFORTS IN END-OF-LIFE CARE

Many communities in America are realizing that end-of-life care should be a community-wide effort that has many components and one head. The function of a controlling agency is more important than whether it is affiliated with a medical school. Components should include the following:

- Education of medical students, physicians (whether in primary care or specialty practice), professional and paraprofessional healthcare workers, ethics councils, and the public-at-large.
- Development and implementation of specific community services, such as hospital-based primary and secondary palliative care facilities and hospice care.
- Revised legislation regarding management of pain and suffering, CPR policies in and outside of the hospital, revision/standardization of advance care plan documentation, and remuneration and indemnity issues.
- Inclusion of end-of-life care initiatives in other, nonmedical organizations dealing with the elderly, including religious organizations, funeral homes, financial planners, estate lawyers, and secular community service, nonprofit organizations.
- Promotion of research in the most effective process of delivering excellent palliative care, the impact of advance care planning, the limits of medical interventions, and the discovery of more accurate predictors of medical prognosis.

HOW TO MEASURE DYING WELL IN AMERICA

In its 2002 report, Last Acts, the largest nonprofit organization dealing with end-of-life issues in the United States, identified the following goals *(2)*:

- More state policies should support good advance care planning.
- A higher proportion of deaths should occur at home.
- Hospice care must be more widely used.
- Hospitals should offer more pain and palliative care services.
- Fewer elderly people should spend a week or more in an intensive care unit during the last 6 months of life.
- More nursing homes should better manage their resident's pain.
- States should enact laws for better pain control.
- More physicians and nurses should be trained and certified in palliative care.

We would like to fully support these goals, ultimately striving to assure that more families will feel that their dying loved ones receive the best possible care; care given with honesty and compassion, with due regard to the individual's expressed wishes. As physicians, we must rise above the time-driven pressures and technological temptations of our era and to rejoin the priesthood of medicine, serving our patients as their compassionate, loving friends.

After all, "To die well is the height of wisdom of life" (Sören Kierkegaard, 1813-1855).

REFERENCES

1. U.S. Census Bureau. Population Projections. www.census.gov.
2. Last Acts: Means to a Better End: A Report on Dying in America Today. 2002, p. 2.
3. Basta L. Life and Death on Your Own Terms. Prometheus Books, Amherst, NY, 2001, p. 172.
4. Basta L. Is medical intervention wasted on the old? Am J Geriatr Cardiol 2000;9(5): 86–93.
5. Lunney JR, Lynn J, Foley DJ, Lipson S, Guralnik JM. JAMA 2003;289(18):2387–2392.
6. Gallup Poll. 1996: Nationwide Gallup survey conducted for NHO, Fall 1996.
7. *Union Pacific Railway Co. v. Botsford*, 141 U.S. 250, 251 (1891).
8. See *Schloendorff v. Society of New York Hospital*, 211 N.Y. 125, 105 N.E. 92 (1914) (Cardozo, J.).
9. Throughout this section, Florida statutes are cited for illustration purposes. State laws very in some respects. Local and state laws should always be consulted in specific situations.
10. *Sistruck v. Hoshall*, 530 So.2d 935 (Fla. 1st DCA 1988), review dismissed 534 So.2d 398, 401.
11. *Schloendorf v. Society of New York Hospital*, 211 N.Y. 125, 129–130, 105 N.E. 92, 93 (1914), quoted in *Cruzan v. Director, Missouri Department of Health*, 110 S.Ct 2841, 2847 (1990).
12. *Valcin v. Public Health Trust of Dade County*, 473 So.2d 1297, 1300 n.2 (Fla. 3d DCA 1984). *See also* Florida Standard Jury Instructions for Civil Cases, 3.5m, 4.2, and 5.3.
13. *Fl. Stat* § 381.004; *Fl. Stat.* § 381.0041.
14. *Fl. Stat.* § 390.001(4).
15. *Fl. Stat.* § 400.002(j).
16. *Fl. Stat.* § 400.6095(2).
17. *See* for example *Fl. Stat.* § 768.13 and 766.103(3).
18. *Fl. Stat.* § 401.45(3)(a) F.A.C. 10D–66.325.
19. *Fl. Stat.* § 401.445.
20. *Fl. Stat.* § 766.103(3).
21. *Fl. Stat.* Chapter 394.
22. *Fl. Stat.* Chapter 397.
23. *Fl. Stat.* § 392.51 – 392.655 (1994).
24. *Fl. Stat.* § 384.287.
25. *In Re: Matter of Dubreuil*, 629 So2d 819, 822 (1993); *Public Health Trust of Dade County v. Wons*, 541 So.2d 96 (Fla. 1989); *Saltz v. Perlmutter*, 379 So.2d 359 (Fla. 1980); *Fl. Const.* Art. I § 23.
26. *In Re: Matter of Dubreuil*, 629 So.2d 819 (Fla. 1994).
27. *Guardianship of Browning v. Herbert*, 568 So.2d 4,12 (Fla. 1990).
28. *Fl. Stat.* § 765.203 *et. seq.*
29. *Fl. Stat.* § 765.401.

30. *Fl. Stat.* § 765.205.
31. *In Re: Guardianship of Browning v. Herbert,* 568 So.2d 4,13 (Fla. 1990).
32. *Matter of Jobes,* 108 N.J. 394, 415, 529 A.2d 434, 444 (1987), aff'd 438 Pa. Super 610, 652 A.2d 1350 (1996).
33. *Fl. Stat.* § 765.105.
34. *Fl. Stat.* § 765.104.
35. *Fl. Stat.* § 765.302.
36. *Fl. Stat.* § 765.302(1).
37. *Fl. Stat.* § 765.302(3).
38. *Fl. Stat.* § 765.304(2)(a).
39. *Fl. Stat.* § 765.304(2)(b).
40. *Fl. Stat.* § 765.304(2)(c).
41. Pub. L. 101–508, §§ 4206, 4751, amending 42 USC §§ 1395cc and 1396a.
42. *Fl. Stat.* § 765.101(11).
43. *Guardianship of Browning,* 568 So.2d 4,11 (Fla. 1990).
44. *Fiori v. Commonwealth,* n.2, 543 Pa. 592, 598, 673 A.2d 905, 908 (1996) citing *In re Conroy,* 98 N.J 321, 372–73, 486 A.2d 1209, 1239 (1985); *In re Grant,* 109 Wash.2d 545, 559–62, 747 P.2d 445, 452–54 (1987).
45. *Fl. Stat.* 765.101(17) (1993).
46. *Fl. Stat.* 765.306 (1993).
47. *Fl. Stat.* § 765.306 (1993) *See also In Re: Guardianship of Browning,* 568 So.2d 4,16 (Fla. 1990).
48. *Fl. Stat.* § 765.305(1) (1993).
49. *Fl. Stat.* § 765.305(2) (1993).
50. *Fl. Stat.* § 401.45(1)(a).
51. AMA Council on Ethical and Judicial Affairs, March 15, 1986.
52. Rabkin MT, Dillerman, Rice NR. Orders not to resuscitate. N Engl J Med 1976; 7:364–366.
53. Cohen-Mansfield J, Droge JA, Billing N. The utilization of durable power of attorney for health care among hospitalized elderly patients. J Am Geriatr Soc 1991;39: 1174–1178.
54. Campbell A, Charlesworth M, Gillett G, Jones G. Medical Ethics. Oxford University Press, Melbourne, Oxford, NY, 1997, pp. 20–22.
55. Tobias JS, Soulami RL. Fully informed consent can be needlessly cruel. Br M J 1993;307:1435–1439.
56. Weinberg SL. Reflections on advocacy: ethics and benefits. The golden age of medical science and the dark age of health care delivery. ACC 2000;184–188.
57. Hardwig J. The problem of proxies with interests of their own: toward a better theory of proxy decisions. Ethics 1991;4:41–46.
58. Buchanan AE, Brock DW. Deciding for Others: The Ethics of Surrogate Decision-Making. Cambridge University Press, New York, NY, 1990.
59. Singer PA, Martin DK, Kelner M. Quality end-of-life care, patients' perspectives. JAMA 1999;281:163–168.
60. Knaus WA, Harrell FE Jr, Lynn J, et al. The SUPPORT prognostic model: objective estimates of survival for seriously ill hospitalized adults. Ann Int Med 1995;22: 191–203.
61. Brenner MJ. The curative paradigm in medical education: striking a balance between caring and curing. The Pharos 1999;62(3):4–9.
62. Ramsetty AN. Walking through the valley of the shadow of death: a student's perspective on death and the medical profession. The Pharos 1999;62(3):11–15.

63. Lemeshow S, Teres D, Klar J, et al. Mortality Probability Models (MPM II) based on an international cohort of intensive care unit patients. JAMA. 1993;270:2478–2486.

64. Rowan KM, Kerr JH, Major E, et al. Intensive Care Society's APACHE II study in Britain and Ireland—I: Variations in case mix of adult admissions to general intensive care units and impact on outcome. BMJ 1993;307:972–977.

65. Wagg A, Kinirons M, Stewart K. Cardiopulmonary resuscitation: doctors and nurses expect too much. J R Coll Physicians of London 1995;29:20–24.

66. Diem SJ, Lantos JD, Tulsky JA. Cardiopulmonary resuscitation on television. Miracles and misinformation. N Engl J Med 1996;334:1578–1582.

67. Basta L., Plunkitt K., Shassy R., Gamouras G. Cardiopulmonary resuscitation in the elderly: defining the limits of appropriateness. Am J Geriatr Cardiol 1998;7:46–55.

68. Schonwetter RS, Walker RM, Kramer DR, Robinson BE. Resuscitation decision making in the elderly: the value of outcome data. J Gen Intern Med 1993;8:295–300.

69. Marsh FH, Staver A. Physician authority for unilateral DNR orders. J Leg Med 1991;12:115–165.

70. Blackhall LJ. Must we always use CPR?. N Engl J Med 1987;317:1281–1285.

71. Layson RT, McConnell T. Must consent always be obtained for a do-not-resuscitate order? Arch Intern Med 1996;156:2617–2620.

72. Plunkitt K, Matar F, Basta L. Therapeutic CPR or consent DNR—A dilemma looking for an answer. J Am Coll Cardiol 1998;32:2095–2097.

73. Paola FA, Anderson JA. The process of dying. In: Sanbar SS, Gibofsky A, Firestone MR, LeBlang TR eds. Legal Medicine (4th ed.), Mosby, St. Louis, MO,1988, pp. 352–364.

74. Teno JM, Licks s, Lynn J, et al. Do advance directives provide instructions that direct care? J Amer Geriatr Soc 1997;45:508–512.

75. Hammes BJ, Rooney BL. Death and end-of-life planning in one midwestern community. Arch Intern Med 1998;158(4):383–390.

76. Brooks RG. Project GRACE: Florida's panel to study end-of-life care: an interim appraisal. Clin Cardiol 2000;23(Suppl.II):II–1–2.

77. Basta LL, McIntosh HD. Project GRACE (Guidelines for Resuscitation And Care at End-of-Life). Clin Cardiol 2000;23(Suppl.II):II–3–5.

78. Callahan D. Limiting health care for the old. In: Jecker N ed. Aging and Ethics: Philosophical Problems in Gerontology. Humana Press, Totowa, NJ, 1991, pp. 219–226.

79. National Center for Health Statistics. National Hospital Discharge Survey. Advance Data from Vital and Health Statistics. 1986 Summary. Hyattsville, MD, Public Health Service, DHHS Publication No. 145 [PHS] 87–1250, 1987:1–16.

80. Fuchs VR. The Future of Health Policy. Harvard University Press, Cambridge, MA, 1993.

81. Kohn L, Corrigan J, Donaldson M. To Err Is Human: Building a Safe Health System. National Academy Press, Washington DC, 1999.

82. World Health Report 2000. Available at http://www.who.int/whr/2000/en/report.htm; Accessed June 28, 2000.

83. Dalen JE. Health care in America: the good, the bad, and the ugly. Arch Intern Med 2000;160:2573–2576.

84. Helft P, Seigler M, Lantos J. The rise and fall of the futility movement. N Engl J Med 2000;343:293–295.

85. Hippocrates. Selections from the Hippocratic corpus: the art. In: Jones WHS, trans., Reiser SJ, Dyck AJ, Curran WJ eds. Ethics in Medicine. Historical Perspectives and Contemporary Concerns. MIT Press, Cambridge, MA, 1977, pp. 6–7.

86. Plato (Grube GM, trans.). The Republic Hackett Publishing, Indianapolis, IN, 1981, pp. 76–77.
87. Schneiderman LJ, Jecker NS, Jonsen AR. Medical futility: Its meaning and ethical implications. Ann Intern Med 1990;112:949–954.
88. Marsh FH, Staver A. Physician authority over unilateral DNR orders. J Legal Med 1991;12:115–165.
89. Blackhall LJ. Must we always use CPR? N Engl J Med 1987;317:1281–1285.
90. Layson RT, McConnell T. Must consent always be obtained for a do-not-resuscitate order? Arch Intern Med 1996;156:2617–2620.
91. Plunkitt K, Matar F, Basta L. Therapeutic CPR or consent DNR—a dilemma looking for an answer. J Am Coll Cardiol 1998;32:2095–2097.
92. Drane JF, Coulehan JL. The concept of futility: patients do not have a right to demand medically useless treatment. Health Prog 1993;74:28–32.
93. Doty WD, Walker RM. Medical futility. Clin Cardiol 2000;23(Suppl.II):II–6–16.
94. Beauchamp TL, Childers JF. Principles of Biomedical Ethics (5th ed.). Oxford University Press, New York, NY, 2001.
95. Gregory SR. Growth at the edges of medical education: Spirituality in American Medical Education. The Pharos 2003:66(2)14–19.
96. Larson DG, Tobin DR. End-of-life conversations: evolving practice and theory. JAMA 2000;284:1573–1578.
97. Basta L. Routine implantation of cardioverter/defibrillator devices in patients aged 75 years and older with prior myocardial infarction and left ventricular ejection fraction <30: antagonist viewpoint. Am J Geriatr Cardiol 2003;12(6):363–365.
98. Aronow WS. Treatment of heart failure in older persons. Congest Heart Fail 2003; 9(3):142–147.
99. Anker SD, Doehner W, Rauchhaus M, et al. Uric acid and survival in chronic heart failure: validation and application in metabolic, functional, and hemodynamic staging. Circulation 2003;107:1991–1997.
100. Aaronson KD, Schwartz JS, Chen TM, et al. Development and prospective validation of a clinical index to predict survival in ambulatory patients referred for cardiac transplant evaluation. Circulation. 1997;95:2660–2667.
101. Mancini D, LeJemtel T, Aaronson K. Peak Vo$_2$: a simple yet enduring standard. Circulation. 2000;101:1080–1082.
102. Walter LC, Brand RJ, Counsell SR, et al. Develoment and validation of a prognostic index for 1-year mortality in older adults after hospitalization. JAMA 2001;285 (23):2987–2994.
103. Rockwood, K. What do we treat patients for? Am J Med 2001;110(2):151–152.
104. Wolff JL, Starfield B, Anderson G. Prevalence, expenditures and complications of multiple chronic conditions in the elderly. Arch Intern Med 2002;162(20): 2269–2276.
105. Hadler NM. A ripe old age. Arch Intern Med 2003;163:1261–1262.
106. Quill TE, Dresser R, Brock DW. The rule of double effect—a critique of its role in end-of-life decision making. N Engl J Med 1997 337(24):1768–1771.
107. Council on Ethical and Judicial Affairs, American Medical Association. Decisions near the end of life. JAMA 1992;276:2229–2233.
108. Dyer C. Rheumatologist convicted of attempted murder. Br Med J 1992;325:731.
109. Oregon Death with Dignity Act, Oregon Revised Statutes § 127:800–897, 1997.
110. Williams CJ. Netherlands OKs assisted suicide. Los Angeles Times, April 11, 2001, sec. A.
111. Dutch Parliament Passes Bill Legalizing Euthanasia. Associated Press Release, November 28, 2000.

112. Willems DL, Daniels CR, van der Wal G, van der Maas PJ, Emanuel EJ. Attitudes and practices concerning the end of life: a comparison between physicians from the United States and from the Netherlands. Arch Intern Med 2000;160:63–68.
113. Emanuel EJ, Fairclough D, Clarridge BC, et al. Attitudes and practices of U.S. oncologists regarding euthanasia and physician-assisted suicide. Ann Intern Med 2000;133:527–532.
114. Sullivan AD, Hedberg K, Fleming D. Legalized physician-assisted suicide in Oregon—the second year. N Engl J Med 2000;342:598–604.

INDEX

National Cholesterol Education
Program ATPIII, 309
NCN, *see* National Cardiovascular
Network
Neuroendocrine dysregulation, 60,
62, 64, 74
Neurotransmitters, 4
New York Heart Association
(NYHA), 214, 216, 218, 219,
221, 280
Nitrates, 112–113, 146, 214, 216,
355, 357
Nitroglycerin, 113, 145, 146, 169, 286
Nonautonomic vascular responses,
355
Nonsteroidal anti-inflammatory
agents (NSAIDs), 357
Norepinephrine (NE), 4, 13
North American Society of Pacing
and Electrophysiology
(NASPE), 290
NSAIDs, *see* Nonsteroidal anti-
inflammatory agents
NYHA, *see* New York Heart Asso-
ciation

O

Obesity, 82, 87–88, 114
Off-pump coronary artery bypass
graft, 184–185
OSA, *see* Sleep apnea, obstructive
Oxygen, peak consumption of, 6

P

Pacemakers, 218
PAD, *see* Peripheral arterial disease
PAD Awareness, Risk and Treatment:
New Resources for Survival
(PARTNERS), 301–302
Palliative care, 365–366, 377–378,
388–389, 394–395
Parasympathetic system, 354–355
Paroxysmal supraventricular tachy-
cardia (PSVT), 265–266

PARTNERS, *see* PAD Awareness,
Risk and Treatment: New
Resources for Survival
Patient Self Determination Act, 372
PCI, *see* Percutaneous coronary
intervention
PDGF-B, *see* Platelet-derived
growth factor-B
Percutaneous coronary intervention
(PCI), 164, 166, 169
for angina, 165–168
antiplatelet therapy, 172–174
anti-thrombotic therapy, 172–
173
vs CABG, 160–164
CURE and, 147
outcomes of, 168–172
treatment goals, 160
trials of, in elderly, 164–165
Perioperative stroke, 187–188
Peripheral arterial disease (PAD),
antiplatelet drug therapy, 310–
312
claudication treatment, 312–313
clinical history, 302
diabetes and, 302, 308
invasive therapeutic approaches,
313–314
physical examination, 302–305
risk-factor modification, 307–
310
vascular laboratory testing, 305–
307
Permeability, 34
PET, *see* Positron emission tomography scanning
Pharmacodynamics,
age-related changes,
in adrenergic system, 353–
354
in central nervous system
responses, 355
in coagulation, 356